Springer Texts in Statistics

Springer Texts in Statistics (STS) includes advanced textbooks from 3rd- to 4th-year undergraduate courses to 1st- to 2nd-year graduate courses. Exercise sets should be included. The series editors are currently Genevera I. Allen, Richard D. De Veaux, and Rebecca Nugent. Stephen Fienberg, George Casella, and Ingram Olkin were editors of the series for many years.

More information about this series at http://www.springer.com/series/417

Johannes Lederer

Fundamentals of High-Dimensional Statistics

With Exercises and R Labs

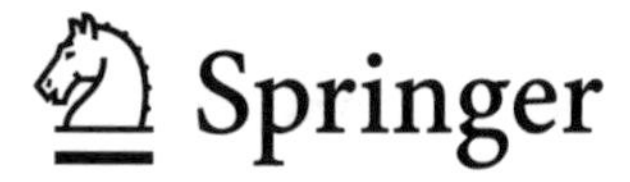

Johannes Lederer
Statistics, Machine Learning
& Data Science
Ruhr-University Bochum
Bochum, Germany

ISSN 1431-875X ISSN 2197-4136 (electronic)
Springer Texts in Statistics
ISBN 978-3-030-73794-8 ISBN 978-3-030-73792-4 (eBook)
https://doi.org/10.1007/978-3-030-73792-4

This Springer imprint is published by the registered company Springer Nature Switzerland AG.
The registered company address is: Gewerbestrasse 11, 6330 Cham, Switzerland

To my family

Preface

This textbook is designed for beginning graduate and advanced undergraduate students in statistics, biostatistics, and bioinformatics, but it may also be useful to a broader audience. Particular emphasis is put on

- Step-by-step introductions to the mathematical tools and principles
- Exercises that complement the main text, many of them with detailed solutions
- Computer labs that convey practical insights and experience
- Suggestions for further reading

This approach should give the reader a smooth start in the field.

I am grateful to Dr. Marco Rossini for the inspiring discussions about drafts of this book and about statistics in general. I also thank Yannick Düren, Shih-Ting Huang, Dr. Tobias Kaufmann, Janosch Kellermann, Mike Laszkiewicz, Mahsa Taheri, and Dr. Fang Xie for their valuable suggestions and corrections.

Johannes Lederer
Bochum, Germany
January 2020

Exercises, Labs, and Literature

In addition to the main text, the book contains exercises, labs, and literature notes. The diamond ratings ◊/♦, ◊◊/♦♦, ◊◊◊/♦♦♦ next to an exercise number indicate the difficulty of the problem and if solutions are provided: the more diamonds, the harder or longer the solution of an exercise, and filled diamonds mean that there are solutions at the back of the book (however, I still recommend strongly to attempt all exercises seriously without looking up the solutions first).

The labs are written in `R`. We propose the use of the `Rstudio` IDE, which is available for free on the Web. Make sure to have downloaded the packages that are included with the `library()` command; this can be done conveniently within `Rstudio` via the `Packages` panel. To access the manuals of the various functions, you can use the `Help` panel. ◘ Fig. 1 shows how the lab exercises look like (top panel) and how to solve them (bottom panel). The labs are interpreted with `R` version 3.5.2; your outputs might slightly differ if you use a different version of `R` (especially the `set.seed()` function changed with version 3.6.0).

Further notes and references are indicated by numbered superscripts (such as "[...] copy-number variation (CNV).[2]") in the main text and stated in the Notes and References sections toward the end of each chapter.

Finally, we denote sections that can be skipped at first reading with an asterisk (such as "2.4 Hölder Inequality*").

Plot the sine() function from 0 to 2π.

```
t <- seq(0, 2 * pi, 0.01)
y <- REPLACE
plot(t, y, type="l", las=1, xlab="angle", ylab="sine")
```

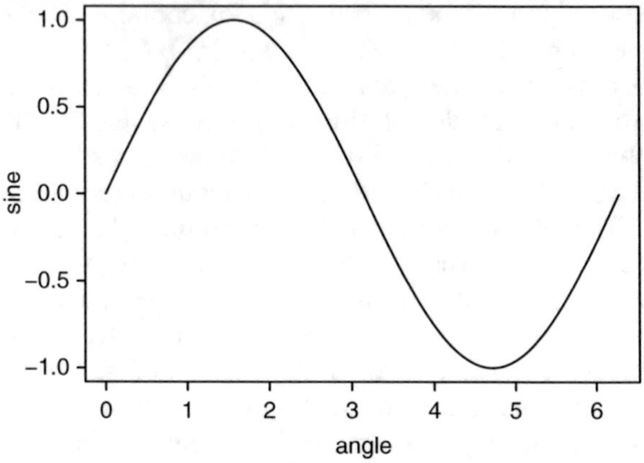

Plot the sine() function from 0 to 2π.

```
t <- seq(0, 2 * pi, 0.01)
y <- sin(t)
plot(t, y, type="l", las=1, xlab="angle", ylab="sine")
```

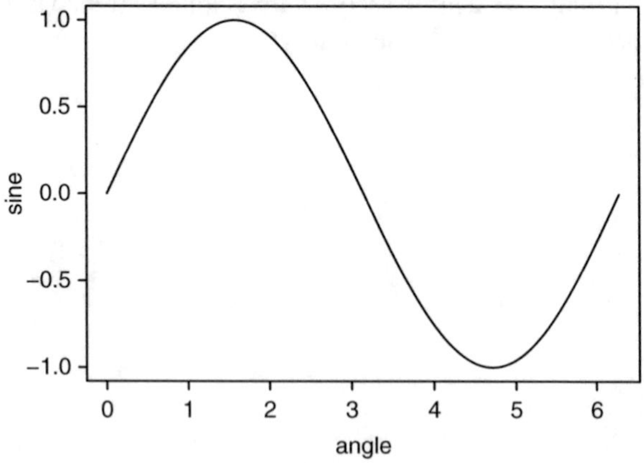

Fig. 1 Example R lab (top panel) and corresponding solution (bottom panel). The reader is supposed to replace the keyword REPLACE by the correct code

Notation

Here, we introduce some notation that we will use throughout the book.

Basic Quantities Lowercase letters a denote numbers; calligraphic lowercase letters $\mathscr{f}$ real-valued functions; boldface lowercase letters $\boldsymbol{a}$ (column) vectors; boldface, calligraphic lowercase letters $\boldsymbol{\mathscr{f}}$ vector-valued functions; capital letters A matrices; calligraphic capital letters $\mathscr{A}$ sets; Greek letters λ real-valued parameters; boldface Greek letters $\boldsymbol{\lambda}$ vector-valued parameters; capital Greek letters Λ matrix-valued parameters; and additional hats $\widehat{\lambda}$, $\widehat{\boldsymbol{\lambda}}$, $\widehat{\Lambda}$ parameter estimates.

Basic Functions The logarithm is taken with respect to the basis e, that is, $\log e = 1$. The smallest integer larger or equal to a given $a \in \mathbb{R}$ is denoted by $\lceil a \rceil$. The *support of a vector* $\boldsymbol{a} \in \mathbb{R}^p$ is denoted by $\operatorname{supp}[\boldsymbol{a}] := \{j \in \{1, \ldots, p\} : a_j \neq 0\}$. Minima over the empty set are set to infinity: $\min_{\boldsymbol{a} \in \varnothing} \mathscr{f}[\boldsymbol{a}] := \infty$ for every function $\mathscr{f}$. The *signum function* $\operatorname{sign} : \mathbb{R} \to \mathbb{R}$ is defined via $\operatorname{sign}[a] := \mathbb{1}\{a \geq 0\} - \mathbb{1}\{a \leq 0\}$. The *cardinality of a set* $\mathscr{A}$, that is, the number of elements in $\mathscr{A}$, is denoted by $|\mathscr{A}| \in \{0, 1, \ldots, \infty\}$. The sum of two sets $\mathscr{A}$, $\mathscr{B}$ that are defined over the same vector space is $\mathscr{A} + \mathscr{B} := \{\boldsymbol{a} + \boldsymbol{b} : \boldsymbol{a} \in \mathscr{A},\ \boldsymbol{b} \in \mathscr{B}\}$, and $a\mathscr{B} := \{a\boldsymbol{b} : \boldsymbol{b} \in \mathscr{B}\}$.

Norms and the Standard Inner Product A function $\|\cdot\| : \mathbb{R}^p \to \mathbb{R}$ is called a *norm* on $\mathbb{R}^p$ if it 1. satisfies the *triangle inequality* ($\|\boldsymbol{a} + \boldsymbol{b}\| \leq \|\boldsymbol{a}\| + \|\boldsymbol{b}\|$ for all $\boldsymbol{a}, \boldsymbol{b} \in \mathbb{R}^p$), 2. is *absolutely homogenenous* ($\|a\boldsymbol{b}\| = |a|\|\boldsymbol{b}\|$ for all $a \in \mathbb{R}$, $\boldsymbol{b} \in \mathbb{R}^p$), and 3. is *positive definite* ($\|\boldsymbol{a}\| = 0$ if and only if $\boldsymbol{a} = \boldsymbol{0}_p$).

Assumptions 1–3 imply that norms are non-negative: $0 = \|\boldsymbol{0}_p\| = \|\boldsymbol{a} - \boldsymbol{a}\| \leq \|\boldsymbol{a}\| + \|-\boldsymbol{a}\| = \|\boldsymbol{a}\| + |-1|\|\boldsymbol{a}\| = 2\|\boldsymbol{a}\|$, that is, $\|\boldsymbol{a}\| \geq 0$ for all $\boldsymbol{a} \in \mathbb{R}^p$; Assumption 2 implies that norms are symmetric: $\|-\boldsymbol{a}\| = \|(-1) \cdot \boldsymbol{a}\| = |-1|\|\boldsymbol{a}\| = \|\boldsymbol{a}\|$; Assumption 2 also implies that norms are scalable: $\|\boldsymbol{b}/\|\boldsymbol{b}\|\| = \|\boldsymbol{b}\|/\|\boldsymbol{b}\| = 1$ for all $\boldsymbol{b} \neq \boldsymbol{0}_p$. The ℓ_q-functions on $\mathbb{R}^p$, where $q \in [0, \infty]$ and $p \in \{1, 2, \ldots\}$, are defined for $q \in (0, \infty)$ as

$$\begin{aligned} \ell_q \ &: \mathbb{R}^p \to \big[0, \infty\big)\,; \\ &\boldsymbol{a} \mapsto \|\boldsymbol{a}\|_q := \left(\sum_{j=1}^{p} |a_j|^q\right)^{1/q}, \end{aligned}$$

for $q = 0$ as

$$\begin{aligned} \ell_0 \ &: \mathbb{R}^p \to \{0, 1, \ldots\}\,; \\ &\boldsymbol{a} \mapsto \|\boldsymbol{a}\|_0 := \big|\big\{j \in \{1, \ldots, p\} \,:\, a_j \neq 0\big\}\big|\,, \end{aligned}$$

and for $q = \infty$ as

$$\begin{aligned} \ell_\infty \ &: \mathbb{R}^p \to \big[0, \infty\big)\,; \\ &\boldsymbol{a} \mapsto \|\boldsymbol{a}\|_\infty := \max_{j \in \{1, \ldots, p\}} |a_j|\,. \end{aligned}$$

The ℓ_q-functions are norms if and only if $q \geq 1$ (see 1. in Exercise 2.2); accordingly, we often refer to those functions as ℓ_q-norms. The ℓ_2-norm is also called *Euclidean norm*; the ℓ_∞-norm is also called *sup-norm* or *max-norm*.

The (standard) *inner product* on $\mathbb{R}^p$ is the function $\langle\cdot,\ \cdot\rangle : \mathbb{R}^p \times \mathbb{R}^p \to \mathbb{R}$ defined through $\langle \boldsymbol{a},\ \boldsymbol{b}\rangle := \boldsymbol{a}^\top \boldsymbol{b} = \sum_{j=1}^{p} a_j b_j$ for $\boldsymbol{a}, \boldsymbol{b} \in \mathbb{R}^p$. The inner product is 1. *symmetric* ($\langle \boldsymbol{a},\ \boldsymbol{b}\rangle = \langle \boldsymbol{b},\ \boldsymbol{a}\rangle$ for all $\boldsymbol{a}, \boldsymbol{b} \in \mathbb{R}^p$), 2. *linear* ($\langle a\boldsymbol{b},\ \boldsymbol{c}\rangle = a\langle \boldsymbol{b},\ \boldsymbol{c}\rangle$ and $\langle \boldsymbol{a}+\boldsymbol{b},\ \boldsymbol{c}\rangle = \langle \boldsymbol{a},\ \boldsymbol{c}\rangle + \langle \boldsymbol{b},\ \boldsymbol{c}\rangle$ for all $a \in \mathbb{R}$, $\boldsymbol{a}, \boldsymbol{b}, \boldsymbol{c} \in \mathbb{R}^p$), and 3. *positive definite* ($\langle \boldsymbol{a},\ \boldsymbol{a}\rangle \geq 0$ for all $\boldsymbol{a} \in \mathbb{R}^p$ and $\langle \boldsymbol{a},\ \boldsymbol{a}\rangle = 0$ if and only if $\boldsymbol{a} = \boldsymbol{0}_p$). Two vectors $\boldsymbol{a}, \boldsymbol{b} \in \mathbb{R}^p$ are *orthogonal* if $\langle \boldsymbol{a},\ \boldsymbol{b}\rangle = 0$.

Intervals and the Extended Real Line We denote by $[a, b]$ the interval between $a \in \mathbb{R}$ and $b \in \mathbb{R}$ that contains the endpoints ($a, b \in [a, b]$), by $[a, b)$ and $(a, b]$ the intervals between a and b that contain the left end right endpoint, respectively ($a \in [a, b)$, $b \notin [a, b)$, $a \notin (a, b]$, $b \in (a, b]$), and by (a, b) the interval between a and b that does not contain the endpoints ($a, b \notin (a, b)$).

The real line extended by $\{-\infty, +\infty\}$ is denoted by $[-\infty, \infty] := \mathbb{R} \cup \{-\infty, +\infty\}$. Similarly, $[0, \infty] := [0, \infty) \cup \{\infty\}$, $(0, \infty] := (0, \infty) \cup \{\infty\}$, and so forth. We use the conventions $0 \cdot (\pm\infty) := (\pm\infty) \cdot 0 := 0$, $a/(\pm\infty) := 0$ for $a \in \mathbb{R}$, $a \cdot (\pm\infty) := (\pm\infty) \cdot a := \pm\infty$ for $a \in (0, \infty]$, and $a \cdot (\pm\infty) := (\pm\infty) \cdot a := \mp\infty$ for $a \in [-\infty, 0)$, which are all continuous extentions of the rules on $\mathbb{R}$, and the convention $0/0 := 0$, which renders our expressions most concise (note that $0/0$ cannot be obtained by extending the rules on $\mathbb{R}$ continuously: if it were, then $0/0 = \lim_{a \to 0}(a/a) = 1$ and at the same time $0/0 = (2 \cdot 0)/0 = 2 \cdot (0/0) = 2$, which is a contradiction). The ordering of the values in $[-\infty, \infty]$ is as expected: for example, $a < \infty$ for all $a \in [-\infty, \infty)$.

Index Sets and Matrices The complement of a set $\mathcal{A}$ with respect to an ambient set $\mathcal{B}$ is denoted by $\mathcal{A}^{\complement} := \mathcal{B} \setminus \mathcal{A}$. For example, the complement of $\{1, 2\}$ with respect to $\{1, \ldots, p\}$, where $p \in \{3, 4, \ldots\}$, is $\{3, \ldots, p\}$. Typically, it is clear what the ambient set is, so that there is no further mention of it.

Consider a vector $\boldsymbol{c} \in \mathbb{R}^l$ and a corresponding index set $\mathcal{A} \subset \{1, \ldots, l\}$ with size $a := |\mathcal{A}|$. We denote $\boldsymbol{c}_{\mathcal{A}} \in \mathbb{R}^a$ as the vector that consists of the coordinates of $\boldsymbol{c}$ with indexes in $\mathcal{A}$. For example, for $\boldsymbol{c} = (3, 4, 5)^\top$ and $\mathcal{A} = \{1, 3\}$, it holds that $\boldsymbol{c}_{\mathcal{A}} = (3, 5)^\top$. The special case $\mathcal{A} = \varnothing$ is taken into account by setting $\boldsymbol{c}_\varnothing := 0$.

Consider a matrix $C \in \mathbb{R}^{l \times m}$ and corresponding index sets $\mathcal{A} \subset \{1, \ldots, l\}$ and $\mathcal{B} \subset \{1, \ldots, m\}$ with sizes $a := |\mathcal{A}|$ and $b := |\mathcal{B}|$, respectively. We denote $C_{\mathcal{A}} \in \mathbb{R}^{l \times a}$ as the matrix that consists of the columns of C with indexes in $\mathcal{A}$, and we denote $C_{\mathcal{B}\mathcal{A}} \in \mathbb{R}^{l \times m}$ as the matrix that consists of the rows and columns of C with indexes in $\mathcal{B}$ and $\mathcal{A}$, respectively. For example,

$$C = \begin{pmatrix} 1\,2\,3 \\ 4\,5\,6 \end{pmatrix}, \ \mathcal{A} = \{2, 3\}, \ \mathcal{B} = \{1\} \Rightarrow C_{\mathcal{A}} = \begin{pmatrix} 2\,3 \\ 5\,6 \end{pmatrix}, \ C_{\mathcal{B}\mathcal{A}} = \begin{pmatrix} 2\,3 \end{pmatrix}.$$

However, we typically assume that the coordinates of the vectors/the rows and columns of the matrices are shuffled such that $\mathscr{A} = \{1, \ldots, a\}$ and $\mathscr{B} = \{1, \ldots, b\}$. This allows us to write, for example, $\boldsymbol{c} = (\boldsymbol{c}_{\mathscr{A}}^\top, \boldsymbol{c}_{\mathscr{A}^\complement}^\top)^\top$ and

$$C = \begin{pmatrix} C_{\mathscr{B}\mathscr{A}} & C_{\mathscr{B}\mathscr{A}^\complement} \\ C_{\mathscr{B}^\complement\mathscr{A}} & C_{\mathscr{B}^\complement\mathscr{A}^\complement} \end{pmatrix}.$$

We finally use the convention $C_{\mathscr{A}}^\top := (C_{\mathscr{A}})^\top$.

A brief review of matrix algebra can be found in ▶ Sect. B.2.

Miscellaneous The expression $\boldsymbol{z} \sim \mathscr{N}_p[\boldsymbol{\mu}, \Sigma]$, $\boldsymbol{\mu} \in \mathbb{R}^p$, $\Sigma \in \mathbb{R}^{p \times p}$, states that $\boldsymbol{x}$ is a random vector that follows a Gauss distribution in p dimensions with mean vector $\boldsymbol{\mu}$ and covariance matrix Σ. In $p = 1$ dimensions, we write $z \sim \mathscr{N}[\mu, \sigma^2]$, where $\mu \in \mathbb{R}$ is the mean and $\sigma^2 \in (0, \infty)$ the variance.

Given a positive integer $p \in \{1, 2, \ldots\}$, we define $\mathbf{0}_p := (0, \ldots, 0)^\top \in \mathbb{R}^p$.

Contents

Introduction

Contents

J. Lederer, *Fundamentals of High-Dimensional Statistics*, Springer Texts in Statistics,
https://doi.org/10.1007/978-3-030-73792-4_1

high-dimensional statistics

High-dimensional statistics specializes in models that have many parameters. Its basic concept is to complement classical estimators with terms that formalize prior information. This inclusion of prior information allows us to use data much more efficiently.

1.1 Embracing High-Dimensionality

The genomics revolution of the 1990s enabled researchers to fully sequence the genomes of a variety of species, including simple bacteria as well as complex eukaryotes such as conifers, gilled mushrooms, and primates including humans, whose genome consists of about 3 billion base pairs.[1] Genomes vary across different species and within species. The genomic diversity among individuals of a species is called *genetic variation.*

One source of genetic variation is copy number variation (CNV).[2] Genomes often contain repeats of long nucleotide sequences; CNV describes differences in the multiplicity of such repeats across individuals. CNVs can encompass entire *genes*, which are functional units of up to several million base pairs. The human genome contains about 20 000 protein-coding genes, and there is strong evidence that CNVs of these protein-coding genes (or of parts of these genes) influence traits such as the predisposition to certain diseases.[3]

A statistical framework for assessing the influence of CNVs is linear regression. Say, $y \in \mathbb{R}$ is a subject's C4 blood level, a biomarker for hereditary angioedema (a disease that causes severe swellings), and $x_1, \ldots, x_p \in \{0, 1, 2, \ldots\}$ the numbers of copies in the genome of each of the p genes under consideration, where $p \approx 20\,000$ if all protein-coding genes are considered. The linear regression model

$$y = \beta_0 + \beta_1 x_1 + \cdots + \beta_p x_p + u \qquad (1.1)$$

connects the *outcome variable* y with the *predictor variables* $x_1, \ldots, x_p$. The *intercept* β_0 quantifies the base level of the biomarker; the *model parameters* $\beta_1, \ldots, \beta_p \in \mathbb{R}$ quantify the influence of the corresponding genes on the level of the biomarker: the larger $|\beta_i|$, the more important is the role of gene i. Measurement errors, non-genomic influences, and so forth are summarized in the *noise vari-*

able $u \in \mathbb{R}$. The goal of a statistical analysis is to estimate the unknown quantities of interest $\beta_1, \ldots, \beta_p$ from the observations of y and $x_1, \ldots, x_p$ in n subjects.

The classical approach to estimating model parameters in linear regression models is least-squares. Why is least-squares problematic here? The first suspect are the *data*: the number of genes for which the copy numbers are available can be of the same order or even larger than the number of study subjects. To see if this causes problems, we first focus on a single gene, that is, $y = \beta_0 + \beta_1 x_1$ and $p = 1$. Estimating the parameter β_1 by using the toy data set A on the left-hand side in ◘ Table 1.1, which consist of $n = 7$ observations of the biomarker y and of the gene's copy number x_1, is straightforward: a standard least-squares (see 1. in Exercise 1.1) yields $\widehat{\beta_1} = 1.61$, and the corresponding model fits the data reasonably well in terms of the (adjusted) coefficient of determination[4]—see the bottom of ◘ Table 1.1. Estimating β_1 by using the data set B on the right-hand side in ◘ Table 1.1, which contains the copy numbers of 7 additional genes, seems more difficult. However, we can just neglect the measurements of $x_2, \ldots, x_8$ and proceed as before:[5] we can run a

◘ Table 1.1 Two regression-type data sets (top panel) and estimated models for y in terms of the x's (bottom panel). Although the data set on the right is more comprehensive than the data set on the left, both data sets are equally suited for regressing y on x_1: one can just ignore the values for $x_2, \ldots, x_8$. But having the values for $x_2, \ldots, x_8$ allows for estimating more refined models that are based not only on x_1. For example, the lasso model that is based on all of $x_1, \ldots, x_8$ has a better fit that the simple model (the larger the adjusted coefficient of determination denoted by R_a^2, the better the fit; $R_a^2 = 1$ means that the model predictions and the observations match perfectly); refer to Exercise 1.1 for the calculations

A			*B*								
y	x_1		y	x_1	x_2	x_3	x_4	x_5	x_6	x_7	x_8
0.0	0		0.0	0	2	0	0	1	0	1	0
2.1	1		2.1	1	0	2	3	2	0	0	3
2.7	0		2.7	0	0	0	2	2	1	1	1
5.9	3		5.9	3	0	1	0	0	0	2	0
7.3	3		7.3	3	4	0	1	1	1	0	0
0.0	0		0.0	0	2	0	0	3	0	0	0
2.0	1		2.0	1	0	2	1	0	0	0	1

Estimated model	Fit measured in R_a^2
$y = 0.66 + 1.92x_1 + u$	0.83
$y = 0.22 + 1.78x_1 + 0x_2 + 0x_3 + 0x_4 + 0x_5$ $+2.11x_6 + 0x_7 + 0x_8 + u$	0.98

least-squares that uses only the realizations of y and x_1, which yields again $\widehat{\beta}_1 = 1.61$. Hence, data per se is not the problem.

What causes new challenges is instead how such data is *used*. So far, we fit a model with a small number of parameters as compared to the number of samples: $p = 1$ and $n = 7$, that is, $p \gg n$. We call such models *low-dimensional*. But the data set B can also be used to fit a model of the form $y = \beta_0 + \beta_1 x_1 + \cdots + \beta_8 x_8 + u$ to account for all eight genes simultaneously. The number of model parameters is now $p = 8$, while the number of samples is still $n = 7$. We call models where $p \approx n$ or even $p \gg n$ *high-dimensional*. In such models, the classical least-squares estimator is unreliable, even ambiguous (see ▶ Sect. 1.2): for estimating this many parameters, the data just do not contain a sufficient amount of information.

high-dimensional model

However, information can come in many shapes and forms, not only as observations of y's and x's. For example, biological research indicates that hereditary diseases are often associated with only a small number of genes. Statistically speaking, we can expect that most of the parameters $\beta_1, \ldots, \beta_8$ in our model are equal to zero. We call such models *sparse*. High-dimensional estimators, such as the lasso estimator (see ▶ Sect. 2.2), include such prior information. Using the lasso estimator yields the model $\widehat{y} = 0.17 + 1.43x_1 + 0x_2 + 0x_3 + 0x_4 + 0x_5 + 1.97x_6 + 0x_7 + 0x_8$ (see 2. in Exercise 1.1), which improves the fit of the one-gene-model substantially—see the bottom of ◘ Table 1.1. The model accounts for *all* eight genes, but it focuses the attention on two of them. This is the general idea of high-dimensional statistics: exploiting information beyond the bare data to find meaningful patterns (here, an accurate model based on only two genes) in complex data (here, the copy numbers of eight genes).[6]

sparse model

High-dimensional statistics comes into play whenever one fits complex models (p large) and is even indispensable in high-dimensional models (p large and $p \approx n$ or even $p \gg n$)—see ◘ Table 1.2. Complex models arise naturally in *Big Data*, where the total number of measurements is large (both n and p large). Applications include predicting shopping habits based on extensive customer profiles, finding weaknesses in opposing soccer teams by tracking every action of their players, and optimizing the fertilization of crops by using fine-grained geospatial data. Nevertheless,

Table 1.2 Typical scopes of classical statistics (such as least-squares estimation) and high-dimensional statistics (such as lasso estimation). The larger the number of parameters p as compared to the number of samples n, the more essential is high-dimensional statistics

	Classical statistics	High-dimensional statistics
$n \not\gg 1$	–	–
$n \gg 1, p \not\gg 1$	✓	–
$n, p \gg 1, p \ll n$	✓	✓
$n, p \gg 1, p \approx n$ or $p \gg n$	–	✓

high-dimensional statistics is not limited to large data sets: in our toy example, the total number of measurements across y and $x_1, \ldots, x_8$ is only $n \times (1+p) = 7 \times (1+8) = 63$. Also, high-dimensionality can be an issue in basically any model class. Our workhorse in this book is linear regression, but the insights can be transferred readily to other types of models such as logistic regression, tensor regression, and graphical modeling (see ▶ Chap. 3 for the latter). Altogether, high-dimensional statistics is useful in a very wide variety of applications.

1.2 Statistical Limitations of Classical Estimators

Here, we illustrate that classical estimators often fail in high-dimensional models. Consider n data points $(y_1, (x_1)_1, \ldots, (x_p)_1), \ldots, (y_n, (x_1)_n, \ldots, (x_p)_n)$ from a linear regression model of the form (1.1). We summarize the observations of y in the *outcome* $\boldsymbol{y} := (y_1, \ldots, y_n)^\top \in \mathbb{R}^n$, the observations of $x_1, \ldots, x_p$ in the *design matrix* $X \in \mathbb{R}^{n \times p}$ defined through $X_{ij} := (x_j)_i$, the model parameters (which remain the same across all data points) in the *regression vector* $\boldsymbol{\beta} := (\beta_1, \ldots, \beta_p)^\top \in \mathbb{R}^p$ (we drop the intercept without loss of generality[7]), and the instantiations of u in the *noise* $\boldsymbol{u} := (u_1, \ldots, u_n)^\top \in \mathbb{R}^n$. These definitions allow us to coalesce the relationships specified by (1.1) into a single vector-valued equation:

$$\boldsymbol{y} = X\boldsymbol{\beta} + \boldsymbol{u}. \tag{1.2}$$

least-squares estimator

The goal of linear regression is to estimate the unknown regression vector $\boldsymbol{\beta}$ from the data $(\boldsymbol{y}, X)$. The classical approach to this is the *least-squares estimator*

$$\widehat{\boldsymbol{\beta}}_{\mathrm{ls}} \in \underset{\boldsymbol{\alpha}\in\mathbb{R}^p}{\arg\min}\, \|\boldsymbol{y} - X\boldsymbol{\alpha}\|_2^2\,, \tag{1.3}$$

which minimizes the data-fitting function $\boldsymbol{a} \mapsto \|\boldsymbol{y} - X\boldsymbol{a}\|_2^2 = \sum_{i=1}^n (y_i - (X\boldsymbol{a})_i)^2$. In other words, the least-squares approach selects model parameters such that the corresponding linear model approximates the data best. However, a good fit to the data is not the same as a good estimation of $\boldsymbol{\beta}$. In the following, we study the least-squares' performance at this latter task in terms of the *prediction error* $\|X\boldsymbol{\beta} - X\widehat{\boldsymbol{\beta}}_{\mathrm{ls}}\|_2^2$ and *prediction risk* $\mathbb{E}[\|X\boldsymbol{\beta} - X\widehat{\boldsymbol{\beta}}_{\mathrm{ls}}\|_2^2]$. The prediction error measures how well the estimator disentangles the data-generating part $X\boldsymbol{\beta}$ from the noise $\boldsymbol{u}$.

Since the least-squares function $\boldsymbol{a} \mapsto \|\boldsymbol{y} - X\boldsymbol{a}\|_2^2$ is convex (see 1. in Exercise 1.4) and differentiable, we can characterize $\widehat{\boldsymbol{\beta}}_{\mathrm{ls}}$ through derivatives of that function:

$$\begin{aligned}\widehat{\boldsymbol{\beta}}_{\mathrm{ls}} \in \underset{\boldsymbol{\alpha}\in\mathbb{R}^p}{\arg\min}\, \|\boldsymbol{y} - X\boldsymbol{\alpha}\|_2^2 \quad &\Leftrightarrow \\ &\frac{\partial}{\partial \alpha_k}\|\boldsymbol{y} - X\boldsymbol{\alpha}\|_2^2\Big|_{\boldsymbol{\alpha}=\widehat{\boldsymbol{\beta}}_{\mathrm{ls}}} = 0 \quad \forall k \in \{1, \ldots, p\}.\end{aligned}$$

The derivatives on the right-hand side can be computed explicitly:

$$\begin{aligned}&\frac{\partial}{\partial \alpha_k}\|\boldsymbol{y} - X\boldsymbol{\alpha}\|_2^2 \\ &= \frac{\partial}{\partial \alpha_k}\sum_{i=1}^n \Big(y_i - \Big(\sum_{j=1}^p X_{ij}\alpha_j\Big)\Big)^2 \quad \text{definition of the } \ell_2\text{-norm} \\ &= \sum_{i=1}^n 2\Big(y_i - \Big(\sum_{j=1}^p X_{ij}\alpha_j\Big)\Big)\cdot(-X_{ik}) \quad \text{sum and chain rules}\end{aligned}$$

$$= -2\sum_{i=1}^{n}\Bigl(X_{ki}^{\top}y_i - \Bigl(\sum_{j=1}^{p}X_{ki}^{\top}X_{ij}\alpha_j\Bigr)\Bigr)$$

rearranging factors; $X_{ik} = X_{ki}^{\top}$

$$= -2\bigl(X^{\top}\boldsymbol{y} - X^{\top}X\boldsymbol{\alpha}\bigr)_k\,.$$

evaluating the sums

Hence, setting $\boldsymbol{\alpha} = \widehat{\boldsymbol{\beta}}_{\text{ls}}$ and using the right-hand side of the least-squares' characterization in the foregoing display, we find that a vector $\widehat{\boldsymbol{\beta}}_{\text{ls}}$ is a solution of the least-squares estimator if and only if

$$-2\bigl(X^{\top}\boldsymbol{y} - X^{\top}X\widehat{\boldsymbol{\beta}}_{\text{ls}}\bigr)_k = 0 \quad \forall k \in \{1, \ldots, p\}\,,$$

which is equivalent to the vector equality

$$X^{\top}X\widehat{\boldsymbol{\beta}}_{\text{ls}} = X^{\top}\boldsymbol{y}\,.$$

The matrix $X^{\top}X$ will appear throughout the book; we call it the *Gram matrix*. For simplicity, we assume that $X^{\top}X$ is invertible (see Exercise 1.2 for a generalization). We can then multiply both sides of the display by $(X^{\top}X)^{-1}$, which identifies

Gram matrix

$$\widehat{\boldsymbol{\beta}}_{\text{ls}} = (X^{\top}X)^{-1}X^{\top}\boldsymbol{y} \tag{1.4}$$

as the unique least-squares estimator. The prediction error is then

$$\|X\boldsymbol{\beta} - X\widehat{\boldsymbol{\beta}}_{\text{ls}}\|_2^2$$

$$= \|X\boldsymbol{\beta} - X(X^{\top}X)^{-1}X^{\top}\boldsymbol{y}\|_2^2$$

mentioned form of $\widehat{\boldsymbol{\beta}}_{\text{ls}}$

$$= \|X\boldsymbol{\beta} - X(X^{\top}X)^{-1}X^{\top}(X\boldsymbol{\beta} + \boldsymbol{u})\|_2^2$$

linear regression model introduced at the beginning of the section

$$= \|X(X^{\top}X)^{-1}X^{\top}\boldsymbol{u}\|_2^2\,.$$

simplifying the terms

We now replace the design matrix X by a singular value decomposition of it (see Lemma B.2.11). For this, consider orthogonal (and therefore, invertible—see Definition B.2.8) square matrices $U \in \mathbb{R}^{n\times n}$, $V \in \mathbb{R}^{p\times p}$ and a diagonal matrix $D \in \mathbb{R}^{n\times p}$ (that is, $D_{ij} = 0$ if $i \neq j$) such that

$$X = UDV^\top .$$

With these definitions, the previous display gives

$$\begin{aligned}
&\|X\boldsymbol{\beta} - X\widehat{\boldsymbol{\beta}}_{\text{ls}}\|_2^2 \\
&= \|UDV^\top\big((UDV^\top)^\top UDV^\top\big)^{-1}(UDV^\top)^\top \boldsymbol{u}\|_2^2 \\
&\qquad\qquad\text{combining the two previous displays} \\
&= \|UDV^\top\big(VD^\top U^\top UDV^\top\big)^{-1} VD^\top U^\top \boldsymbol{u}\|_2^2 \\
&\qquad\qquad (AB)^\top = B^\top A^\top \text{ for all } A, B \\
&= \|UDV^\top\big(V^\top\big)^{-1}\big(D^\top U^\top UD\big)^{-1} V^{-1} VD^\top U^\top \boldsymbol{u}\|_2^2 \\
&\qquad\qquad (AB)^{-1} = B^{-1}A^{-1} \text{ for all invertible matrices } A, B \\
&= \|UD(D^\top D)^{-1}D^\top U^\top \boldsymbol{u}\|_2^2 \\
&\qquad\qquad U^\top U = \mathrm{I}_{n\times n} \text{ since } U \text{ orthogonal by assumption;} \\
&\qquad\qquad V^\top(V^\top)^{-1} = V^{-1}V = \mathrm{I}_{p\times p} \text{ invertible} \\
&= \big(UD(D^\top D)^{-1}D^\top U^\top \boldsymbol{u}\big)^\top UD(D^\top D)^{-1}D^\top U^\top \boldsymbol{u} \\
&\qquad\qquad \text{definition of the } \ell_2\text{-norm} \\
&= \big(D(D^\top D)^{-1}D^\top U^\top \boldsymbol{u}\big)^\top U^\top UD(D^\top D)^{-1}D^\top U^\top \boldsymbol{u} \\
&\qquad\qquad (AB)^\top = B^\top A^\top \text{ for all } A, B \\
&= \|D(D^\top D)^{-1}D^\top U^\top \boldsymbol{u}\|_2^2 . \\
&\qquad\qquad U^\top U = \mathrm{I}_{n\times n}\text{; again definition of the } \ell_2\text{-norm}
\end{aligned}$$

Next, since D is diagonal, we get for all $k, l \in \{1, \ldots, p\}$

$$(D^\top D)_{kl} = \sum_{m=1}^{n} D_{mk}D_{ml} = \begin{cases} D_{kk}^2 & \text{if } k = l; \\ 0 & \text{otherwise}. \end{cases}$$

Since $X^\top X$ is invertible by assumption, it holds that $D_{kk} \neq 0$. Together with the result above, this implies that $(D^\top D)^{-1}$ exists and is diagonal with diagonal elements $1/D_{11}^2, \ldots, 1/D_{pp}^2$. Using this, and also $p \leq n$ since $X^\top X$

is invertible by assumption (see 1. of Exercise 1.2), we find for all $i, j \in \{1, \ldots, n\}$

$$
\begin{aligned}
&(D(D^\top D)^{-1}D^\top)_{ij} \\
&= \sum_{k,l=1}^{p} D_{ik}(D^\top D)^{-1}_{kl} D_{lj} && \text{matrix algebra} \\
&= \sum_{k=1}^{p} D_{ik}(1/D^2_{kk}) D_{kj} && \text{previous observation} \\
&= \begin{cases} D_{ii}(1/D^2_{ii})D_{ii} = 1 & \text{if } i = j \text{ and } i \le p\,; \\ 0 & \text{otherwise}\,, \end{cases} && D \text{ diagonal; } p \le n
\end{aligned}
$$

so that

$$D(D^\top D)^{-1}D^\top = \begin{pmatrix} \mathrm{I}_{p\times p} & \\ & \mathbf{0}_{(n-p)\times(n-p)} \end{pmatrix}.$$

We can plug this back into the earlier display to find

$$\|X\boldsymbol{\beta} - X\widehat{\boldsymbol{\beta}}_{\mathrm{ls}}\|_2^2 = \|(U^\top \boldsymbol{u})_{\{1,\ldots,p\}}\|_2^2\,.$$

The term $\|(U^\top \boldsymbol{u})_{\{1,\ldots,p\}}\|_2$ is the *effective noise* of the least-squares estimator: the larger this term, the larger the prediction error of the least-squares estimator.

effective noise of the least-squares estimator

As a concrete example, consider X fixed and $\boldsymbol{u} \sim \mathcal{N}_n[\mathbf{0}_n, \sigma^2 \mathrm{I}_{n\times n}]$ for a $\sigma \in (0, \infty)$. Then, $(U^\top \boldsymbol{u})_{\{1,\ldots,p\}} \sim \mathcal{N}_p[\mathbf{0}_p, \sigma^2 \mathrm{I}_{p\times p}]$, and the effective noise has a Chi-squared distribution with p degrees of freedom and a scaling of σ^2; in particular, taking expectations over the noise, we get the average prediction risk (see 1. in Exercise 5.4)

$$\mathbb{E}\left[\frac{\|X\boldsymbol{\beta} - X\widehat{\boldsymbol{\beta}}_{\mathrm{ls}}\|_2^2}{n}\right] = \frac{\sigma^2 p}{n}\,. \tag{1.5}$$

This result demonstrates that least-squares provides accurate prediction only in traditional settings where $p/n \ll 1$, that is, $p \ll n$—or if the variance of the noise σ^2 is very small. (This observation is related to the overfitting phenomenon, which we discuss in ► Sect. 2.2.) Thus, for the high-dimensional settings that are the focus of this book, we need to introduce different approaches.

1.3 Incorporating Prior Information

In genome studies, the number of genes p under consideration can be much larger than the number of subjects n, and we have seen in the previous section that the classical least-squares estimator is then uninformative. But biological research also indicates that phenotypical traits are often determined by only a small number of genes. High-dimensional estimators incorporate such biological information into the data analysis.

Statistical estimators in general ensure that the selected model parameters agree with data. This agreement is measured by *data-fitting functions*. For example, $\boldsymbol{a} \mapsto \|\boldsymbol{y} - X\boldsymbol{a}\|_2^2$ measures how well the parameters agree with regression data $(\boldsymbol{y}, X)$. Many classical estimators minimize such functions over a set of candidate parameters $\mathscr{B}$ for given data Z.

data-fitting function

High-dimensional estimators ensure in addition that the selected model parameters agree with prior information. This agreement is measured by *prior functions*; for example, $\boldsymbol{a} \mapsto \|\boldsymbol{a}\|_0 := |\{j : a_j \neq 0\}|$ measures how well the parameters agree with sparsity. Typical high-dimensional estimators then simply combine data-fitting functions and prior functions:

prior function

high-dimensional estimator

$$\widehat{\boldsymbol{\beta}} \in \underset{\boldsymbol{\alpha} \in \mathscr{B}}{\arg\min}\left\{\text{DataFitting}[Z, \boldsymbol{\alpha}] + r\,\text{Prior}[\boldsymbol{\alpha}]\right\}. \qquad (1.6)$$

We call the combined function $\boldsymbol{a} \mapsto \text{DataFitting}[Z, \boldsymbol{\alpha}] + r\,\text{Prior}[\boldsymbol{\alpha}]$ the estimator's *objective function*. The *tuning parameters* $r \in [0, \infty]$ weigh the prior information: setting $r = 0$ gives classical estimators, which include no prior information, while increasing r moves the estimates in the direction specified by the prior function.

objective function

Traditional names for the prior function are *penalty* and *regularizer;* the first name speaks to the idea of penalizing unrealistic or unfavorable models, the second name originates in nonparametric statistics, where one is interested in functions that are sufficiently regular (which typically means smooth). By introducing the word "prior," we want to circumvent the negative connotations that penalty and regularizer might have (do we impose a penalty on unruly model parameters?) and establish a connection to Bayes statistics: similarly as the prior distribution in the Bayes literature, our prior term does not incorporate any data, and it formulates our knowledge or beliefs about the parameter space. Still, we will use the different names interchangeably in the following.

The most important feature of high-dimensional estimators is that they can provide accurate estimates even if the model is high-dimensional. High-dimensional estimators achieve this essentially by using the prior information to trade a small bias against a large gain in variance. In linear regression with fixed design X, the prediction risk, bias, and variance of an estimator $\widehat{\boldsymbol{\beta}}$ are related through

$$\underbrace{\mathbb{E}\Big[\|X\boldsymbol{\beta} - X\widehat{\boldsymbol{\beta}}\|_2^2\Big]}_{\text{risk}} = \underbrace{\big(\|\mathbb{E}[X\widehat{\boldsymbol{\beta}}] - X\boldsymbol{\beta}\|_2\big)^2}_{\text{bias}} + \underbrace{\mathbb{E}\Big[\|X\widehat{\boldsymbol{\beta}} - \mathbb{E}[X\widehat{\boldsymbol{\beta}}]\|_2^2\Big]}_{\text{variance}}.$$

This decomposition follows from

$$\begin{aligned}
&\mathbb{E}\Big[\|X\boldsymbol{\beta} - X\widehat{\boldsymbol{\beta}}\|_2^2\Big]\\
&= \mathbb{E}\Big[\|X\boldsymbol{\beta} - \mathbb{E}[X\widehat{\boldsymbol{\beta}}] + \mathbb{E}[X\widehat{\boldsymbol{\beta}}] - X\widehat{\boldsymbol{\beta}}\|_2^2\Big]\\
&\hspace{6cm}\text{adding a zero-valued term}\\
&= \mathbb{E}\Big[\|\mathbb{E}[X\widehat{\boldsymbol{\beta}}] - X\boldsymbol{\beta}\|_2^2 + 2\langle X\boldsymbol{\beta} - \mathbb{E}[X\widehat{\boldsymbol{\beta}}],\ \mathbb{E}[X\widehat{\boldsymbol{\beta}}] - X\widehat{\boldsymbol{\beta}}\rangle\\
&\quad + \|X\widehat{\boldsymbol{\beta}} - \mathbb{E}[X\widehat{\boldsymbol{\beta}}]\|_2^2\Big] \qquad \text{expanding the squared term}\\
&= \mathbb{E}\Big[\|\mathbb{E}[X\widehat{\boldsymbol{\beta}}] - X\boldsymbol{\beta}\|_2^2\Big] + 2\mathbb{E}\Big[\langle X\boldsymbol{\beta} - \mathbb{E}[X\widehat{\boldsymbol{\beta}}],\ \mathbb{E}[X\widehat{\boldsymbol{\beta}}] - X\widehat{\boldsymbol{\beta}}\rangle\Big]\\
&\quad + \mathbb{E}\Big[\|X\widehat{\boldsymbol{\beta}} - \mathbb{E}[X\widehat{\boldsymbol{\beta}}]\|_2^2\Big]\\
&\hspace{3cm}\text{linearity of expectations and inner products}\\
&= \|\mathbb{E}[X\widehat{\boldsymbol{\beta}}] - X\boldsymbol{\beta}\|_2^2 + 2\langle X\boldsymbol{\beta} - \mathbb{E}[X\widehat{\boldsymbol{\beta}}],\ \mathbb{E}\big[\mathbb{E}[X\widehat{\boldsymbol{\beta}}] - X\widehat{\boldsymbol{\beta}}\big]\rangle\\
&\quad + \mathbb{E}\Big[\|X\widehat{\boldsymbol{\beta}} - \mathbb{E}[X\widehat{\boldsymbol{\beta}}]\|_2^2\Big]\\
&\hspace{2cm}X \text{ is fixed and, therefore, } \mathbb{E}[X\widehat{\boldsymbol{\beta}}] \text{ and } X\boldsymbol{\beta} \text{ are fixed;}\\
&\hspace{6cm}\text{linearity of expectations}\\
&= \|\mathbb{E}[X\widehat{\boldsymbol{\beta}}] - X\boldsymbol{\beta}\|_2^2 + \mathbb{E}\Big[\|X\widehat{\boldsymbol{\beta}} - \mathbb{E}[X\widehat{\boldsymbol{\beta}}]\|_2^2\Big].\\
&\hspace{1cm}\text{second term is equal to zero due to } \mathbb{E}[\mathbb{E}[X\widehat{\boldsymbol{\beta}}]] = \mathbb{E}[X\widehat{\boldsymbol{\beta}}]\\
&\hspace{4cm}\text{and the linearity of expectations}
\end{aligned}$$

If the noise is Gauss-distributed according to $\boldsymbol{u} \sim \mathcal{N}_n[\mathbf{0}_n, \sigma^2 \mathrm{I}_{n\times n}]$ and $X^\top X$ invertible, the bias of the least-squares estimator (1.3) is zero:

$$\begin{aligned}
&\mathbb{E}\big[X\widehat{\boldsymbol{\beta}}_{\mathrm{ls}}\big] - X\boldsymbol{\beta}\\
&= \mathbb{E}\big[X(X^\top X)^{-1}X^\top \boldsymbol{y}\big] - X\boldsymbol{\beta} && \text{explicit form of the least-squares estimator (1.4)}\\
&= \mathbb{E}\big[X(X^\top X)^{-1}X^\top (X\boldsymbol{\beta} + \boldsymbol{u})\big] - X\boldsymbol{\beta} && \text{linear regresson model (1.2)}\\
&= X\boldsymbol{\beta} + X(X^\top X)^{-1}X^\top \mathbb{E}[\boldsymbol{u}] - X\boldsymbol{\beta} && (X^\top X)^{-1}X^\top X = \mathrm{I}_{n\times n};\ \text{linearity of expectations}\\
&= X\boldsymbol{\beta} - X\boldsymbol{\beta} = \mathbf{0}_n\,. && \mathbb{E}[\boldsymbol{u}] = \mathbf{0}_n \text{ by assumption}
\end{aligned}$$

The variance of the least-squares estimator is, however,

$$\begin{aligned}
&\mathbb{E}\Big[\|X\widehat{\boldsymbol{\beta}}_{\mathrm{ls}} - \mathbb{E}[X\widehat{\boldsymbol{\beta}}_{\mathrm{ls}}]\|_2^2\Big]\\
&= \mathbb{E}\Big[\|X\boldsymbol{\beta} - X\widehat{\boldsymbol{\beta}}_{\mathrm{ls}}\|_2^2\Big] && \mathbb{E}[X\widehat{\boldsymbol{\beta}}_{\mathrm{ls}}] = X\boldsymbol{\beta} \text{ according to the preceding result}\\
&= \sigma^2 p\,. && \text{Eq. (1.5)}
\end{aligned}$$

In other words, the average prediction risk $\mathbb{E}[\|X\boldsymbol{\beta} - X\widehat{\boldsymbol{\beta}}_{\mathrm{ls}}\|_2^2/n] = \sigma^2 p/n$ only consists of variance. In contrast, the prior terms "push" high-dimensional estimators toward the prior knowledge and, thereby, generate a bias: $\mathbb{E}[X\widehat{\boldsymbol{\beta}}] \neq X\boldsymbol{\beta}$—cf. ▶ Chap. 5, especially Exercise (5.3). But this bias is typically small, and there can be a substantial gain in variance. In consequence, high-dimensional estimators can have much lower risks than the least-squares estimator: for example, we will show in ▶ Chap. 6 that the lasso estimator allows us to replace the least-squares estimator's effective noise $\|(U^\top \boldsymbol{u})_{\{1,\dots,p\}}\|_2$, which determines the least-squares' variance, by the lasso estimator's effective noise $2\|X^\top \boldsymbol{u}\|_\infty$. This then leads to the risk bound[8,9]

$$\mathbb{E}\left[\frac{\|X\boldsymbol{\beta} - X\widehat{\boldsymbol{\beta}}_{\mathrm{lasso}}\|_2^2}{n}\right] \leq \frac{as\sigma^2 \log p}{n}$$

for $s := \|\boldsymbol{\beta}\|_0 = |\{\beta_j \neq 0\}|$ the number of actually influential predictors and $a \in (0, \infty)$ a reasonably small constant if again $\boldsymbol{u} \sim \mathcal{N}_n[\mathbf{0}_n, \sigma^2 \mathrm{I}_{n\times n}]$, and the predictors are not too much correlated. The important difference to the earlier risk bound for the least-squares is that this one is linear in the number of *relevant* predictors s and only logarithmic in the *total* number of predictors p, which can allow us to accurately estimate complex models (p large) if these models are sparse (s small): instead of $n \gg \sigma^2 p$, we now only require $n \gg \sigma^2 s \log p$.

1.4 Regularization for Increasing the Numerical Stability*

The idea of prior functions predates high-dimensional statistics considerably. For example, it was understood already in the middle of the last century that prior functions can increase the numerical stability in inverse problems. We connect this early research with the modern statistical topics of this book by comparing least-squares to the ridge estimator, an estimator that has its roots in the classical literature on inverse problems but is also used in contemporary high-dimension statistics. We will find that least-squares estimation is like a dog that calmly walks next to its keeper at most times but immediately goes on a wild chase all around the park when a rabbit comes into sight. The additional prior function in the ridge estimator is the leash for keeping the dog under control, and the corresponding tuning parameter balances between the safety of the wildlife and the dog's freedom: the larger the tuning parameter, the tighter the leash.

To illustrate the stabilizing effect of prior functions, we study least-squares and ridge estimation on the data family in ◘ Table 1.3. These data specify the outcome $y = (1,2)^\top \in \mathbb{R}^2$ and the design matrix $X = ((1,2)^\top, (d,2)^\top) \in \mathbb{R}^{2\times 2}$, where d takes values in $\mathbb{R}$. We will vary d to evaluate the estimators' robustness against small changes in the data.

◘ Table 1.3 Regression-type data indexed by $d \in \mathbb{R}$. The least-squares estimator on these data is not unique when $d = 1$ and not continuous in d at $d = 1$, while the ridge estimator is always unique and continuous in d. This illustrates that regularization can have numerical benefits even for seemingly simple data

y	x_1	x_2
1	1	d
2	2	2

We first consider least-squares estimation. For $d \neq 1$, the least-squares estimator has the unique solution $\widehat{\boldsymbol{\beta}}_{\text{ls}} = (1,0)^\top$. To see this, note first that $\|\boldsymbol{y} - X\boldsymbol{a}\|_2^2 \geq 0$ for all $\boldsymbol{a} \in \mathbb{R}^2$. Since the $\|\boldsymbol{y} - X\boldsymbol{a}\|_2^2 = 0$ for $\boldsymbol{a} = (1,0)^\top$, the vector $\widehat{\boldsymbol{\beta}}_{\text{ls}} = (1,0)^\top$ must indeed be a solution of the least-squares estimator. Now, one can also check that $X^\top X$ is invertible if $d \neq 1$. Since the least-squares objective function $\boldsymbol{a} \mapsto \|\boldsymbol{y} - X\boldsymbol{a}\|_2^2$ is strictly convex for $X^\top X$ invertible (see 2. in Exercise 1.4), and since strictly convex functions have unique minima (see 4. in Exercise 1.4), it follows that $\widehat{\boldsymbol{\beta}}_{\text{ls}}$ is the unique least-squares solution.

We can also calculate the least-squares estimator for $d \neq 1$ by using our previously established formula:

$$\widehat{\boldsymbol{\beta}}_{\text{ls}} = \left(X^\top X\right)^{-1} X^\top \boldsymbol{y}$$

▶ Sect. 1.2

$$= \left(\begin{pmatrix} 1 & 2 \\ d & 2 \end{pmatrix}\begin{pmatrix} 1 & d \\ 2 & 2 \end{pmatrix}\right)^{-1}\begin{pmatrix} 1 & 2 \\ d & 2 \end{pmatrix}\begin{pmatrix} 1 \\ 2 \end{pmatrix}$$

plugging in the data from ◘ Table 1.3

$$= \begin{pmatrix} 5 & 4+d \\ 4+d & 4+d^2 \end{pmatrix}^{-1}\begin{pmatrix} 1 & 2 \\ d & 2 \end{pmatrix}\begin{pmatrix} 1 \\ 2 \end{pmatrix}$$

matrix multiplication

$$= \frac{1}{4-8d+4d^2}\begin{pmatrix} 4+d^2 & -4-d \\ -4-d & 5 \end{pmatrix}\begin{pmatrix} 1 & 2 \\ d & 2 \end{pmatrix}\begin{pmatrix} 1 \\ 2 \end{pmatrix}$$

$$\begin{pmatrix} a_{11} & a_{12} \\ a_{21} & a_{22} \end{pmatrix}^{-1} = \begin{pmatrix} a_{22} & -a_{12} \\ -a_{21} & a_{11} \end{pmatrix} / (a_{11}a_{22} - a_{12}a_{21})$$

$$= \frac{1}{4-8d+4d^2}\begin{pmatrix} 4-4d & -2d+2d^2 \\ -4+4d & 2-2d \end{pmatrix}\begin{pmatrix} 1 \\ 2 \end{pmatrix}$$

matrix multiplication

$$= \frac{1}{4-8d+4d^2}\begin{pmatrix} 4-8d+4d^2 \\ 0 \end{pmatrix}$$

matrix–vector multiplication

$$= \begin{pmatrix} 1 \\ 0 \end{pmatrix}.$$

vector–constant multiplication

One can verify readily that $\widehat{\boldsymbol{\beta}}_{\text{ls}}$ is a solution also for $d = 1$, but it is then no longer the only solution. For $d = 1$, it holds that $X(-a,a)^\top = \mathbf{0}_2$ for all $a \in \mathbb{R}$. Therefore, all vectors of the form $\widehat{\boldsymbol{\beta}}^a_{\text{ls}} := \widehat{\boldsymbol{\beta}}_{\text{ls}} + (-a,a)^\top = (1-a,a)^\top$ satisfy $X\widehat{\boldsymbol{\beta}}^a_{\text{ls}} = X\widehat{\boldsymbol{\beta}}_{\text{ls}}$, and consequently, $\|\boldsymbol{y} - X\widehat{\boldsymbol{\beta}}^a_{\text{ls}}\|_2^2 =$

$\|\boldsymbol{y} - X\widehat{\boldsymbol{\beta}}_{\mathrm{ls}}\|_2^2$. Hence, in the case $d = 1$, *all* vectors $\widehat{\boldsymbol{\beta}}_{\mathrm{ls}}^a$, $a \in \mathbb{R}$, are least-squares solutions.

This ambiguity of the least-squares estimator leads to a numerical instability. The ℓ_2-difference between a response for $d = 1$ (which can be any vector of the form $\widehat{\boldsymbol{\beta}}_{\mathrm{ls}}^a$) and the response for $d \neq 1$ (which must be $\widehat{\boldsymbol{\beta}}_{\mathrm{ls}} = \widehat{\boldsymbol{\beta}}_{\mathrm{ls}}^a$ with $a = 0$) is

$$\|\widehat{\boldsymbol{\beta}}_{\mathrm{ls}}^a - \widehat{\boldsymbol{\beta}}_{\mathrm{ls}}\|_2 = \|(1-a, a)^\top - (1,0)^\top\|_2 = \sqrt{2}|a|\,.$$

Since a can be arbitrarily large, the response for $d = 1$ can differ arbitrarily much from the response for $d \neq 1$—however close d is to 1. Hence, the least-squares procedure is discontinuous in the data: an ever so small change in the observations can lead to a dramatically different least-squares response.

We now aim at removing this numerical instability. For this, we replace the least-squares estimator by the *ridge estimator*[10]

ridge

$$\widehat{\boldsymbol{\beta}}_{\mathrm{ridge}}[r] \in \operatorname*{arg\,min}_{\boldsymbol{\alpha} \in \mathbb{R}^p} \bigl\{ \|\boldsymbol{y} - X\boldsymbol{\alpha}\|_2^2 + r\|\boldsymbol{\alpha}\|_2^2 \bigr\}\,, \tag{1.7}$$

where $r \in (0, \infty)$ is a tuning parameter and $\|\boldsymbol{\alpha}\|_2^2 = \sum_{j=1}^p (\alpha_j)^2$. Since the ridge estimator's objective function is still differentiable, we can proceed as in ▶ Sect. 1.2 to find that $\widehat{\boldsymbol{\beta}}_{\mathrm{ridge}}[r]$ is a solution of the ridge estimator if and only if

$$\bigl(X^\top X + r\mathrm{I}_{p\times p}\bigr)\widehat{\boldsymbol{\beta}}_{\mathrm{ridge}}[r] = X^\top \boldsymbol{y}\,.$$

The crux is that the matrix $X^\top X + r\mathrm{I}_{p\times p}$ is *always* invertible. Indeed, for every $\boldsymbol{a} \in \mathbb{R}^p \setminus \{\boldsymbol{0}_p\}$,

$$\begin{aligned}
&\boldsymbol{a}^\top\bigl(X^\top X + r\mathrm{I}_{p\times p}\bigr)\boldsymbol{a} \\
&= \boldsymbol{a}^\top X^\top X\boldsymbol{a} + r\boldsymbol{a}^\top \mathrm{I}_{p\times p}\boldsymbol{a} && \text{linearity of matrices} \\
&= (X\boldsymbol{a})^\top X\boldsymbol{a} + r\boldsymbol{a}^\top\boldsymbol{a} && \text{3. in Lemma B.2.1 (reversion of transposition) and definition of the identity matrix} \\
&= \|X\boldsymbol{a}\|_2^2 + r\|\boldsymbol{a}\|_2^2 && \text{definition of the } \ell_2\text{-norm} \\
&> 0\,, && \text{norms are positive definite; } r > 0,\ \boldsymbol{a} \neq \boldsymbol{0}_2
\end{aligned}$$

which implies that $X^\top X + r\mathrm{I}_{p\times p}$ is invertible. Hence, we can write

$$\widehat{\boldsymbol{\beta}}_{\text{ridge}} = \left(X^\top X + r\mathrm{I}_{p\times p}\right)^{-1} X^\top \boldsymbol{y}, \tag{1.8}$$

irrespective of whether $X^\top X$ itself is invertible or not. This shows in particular that the ridge estimator is always unique.

We now use the formula to calculate the ridge estimator on the data in ◘ Table 1.3:

$$\begin{aligned}
\widehat{\boldsymbol{\beta}}_{\text{ridge}}[r] &= \left(X^\top X + r\mathrm{I}_{p\times p}\right)^{-1} X^\top \boldsymbol{y} \\
&= \left(\begin{pmatrix} 1 & 2 \\ d & 2 \end{pmatrix}\begin{pmatrix} 1 & d \\ 2 & 2 \end{pmatrix} + \begin{pmatrix} r & 0 \\ 0 & r \end{pmatrix}\right)^{-1} \begin{pmatrix} 1 & 2 \\ d & 2 \end{pmatrix}\begin{pmatrix} 1 \\ 2 \end{pmatrix} \\
&= \begin{pmatrix} 5+r & 4+d \\ 4+d & 4+d^2+r \end{pmatrix}^{-1} \begin{pmatrix} 1 & 2 \\ d & 2 \end{pmatrix}\begin{pmatrix} 1 \\ 2 \end{pmatrix} \\
&= \frac{1}{4-8d+4d^2+(9+d^2)r+r^2} \\
&\quad \times \begin{pmatrix} 4+d^2+r & -4-d \\ -4-d & 5+r \end{pmatrix}\begin{pmatrix} 1 & 2 \\ d & 2 \end{pmatrix}\begin{pmatrix} 1 \\ 2 \end{pmatrix} \\
&= \frac{1}{4-8d+4d^2+(9+d^2)r+r^2} \\
&\quad \times \begin{pmatrix} 4-4d+r & -2d+2d^2+2r \\ -4+4d+dr & 2-2d+2r \end{pmatrix}\begin{pmatrix} 1 \\ 2 \end{pmatrix} \\
&= \frac{1}{4-8d+4d^2+(9+d^2)r+r^2} \\
&\quad \times \begin{pmatrix} 4-8d+4d^2+5r \\ (4+d)r \end{pmatrix} \\
&= \frac{1}{4(1-d)^2+(9+d^2)r+r^2} \begin{pmatrix} 4(1-d)^2+5r \\ (4+d)r \end{pmatrix}.
\end{aligned}$$

The individual steps mirror those for the least-squares estimator for $d \neq 0$. Since the denominator of the factor is strictly positive for every $r > 0$, this result shows in particular that the ridge estimator is continuous in d (see also Exercise 1.5). Thus, the ridge estimator is stable with respect to small changes in the observations.

The continuity is due to the additional regularization term in the ridge estimator's objective function. We would thus expect that the stronger the regularization, that is, the larger the tuning parameter, the more stable the estimates are with respect to changes in the data. To support this, we derive two limits from the preceding result: First, we find that the limit of $\widehat{\boldsymbol{\beta}}_{\text{ridge}}[r]$ for $r \to \infty$ exists for all $d \in \mathbb{R}$ and is equal to the zero-vector:

$$\lim_{r\to\infty} \widehat{\boldsymbol{\beta}}_{\text{ridge}}[r] = \lim_{r\to\infty} \frac{1}{r^2} \begin{pmatrix} 5r \\ (4+d)r \end{pmatrix} = \begin{pmatrix} 0 \\ 0 \end{pmatrix} \qquad \text{for all } d \in \mathbb{R}\,.$$

In this sense, the ridge estimator is perfectly stable when $r \to \infty$. Second, we find that the limit of $\widehat{\boldsymbol{\beta}}_{\text{ridge}}[r]$ for $r \to 0^+$ also exists for all d and equals a least-squares solution:

$$\lim_{r\to 0^+} \widehat{\boldsymbol{\beta}}_{\text{ridge}}[r] =$$

$$\begin{cases} \lim\limits_{r\to 0^+} \frac{1}{10r+r^2} \begin{pmatrix} 5r \\ 5r \end{pmatrix} = \lim\limits_{r\to 0^+} \frac{1}{1+r/10} \begin{pmatrix} 1/2 \\ 1/2 \end{pmatrix} = \begin{pmatrix} 1/2 \\ 1/2 \end{pmatrix} & \text{for } d = 1\,; \\ \frac{1}{4(1-d)^2} \begin{pmatrix} 4(1-d)^2 \\ 0 \end{pmatrix} = \begin{pmatrix} 1 \\ 0 \end{pmatrix} & \text{for } d \neq 1\,, \end{cases}$$

which are the least-squares estimators $\widehat{\boldsymbol{\beta}}_{\text{ls}}^{1/2}$ and $\widehat{\boldsymbol{\beta}}_{\text{ls}} = \widehat{\boldsymbol{\beta}}_{\text{ls}}^{0}$, respectively. That the two limits for $d = 1$ and $d \neq 1$ differ is another display of the instability of the least-squares estimator; a graphical explanation of where the two different solutions come from is given in ◘ Fig. 1.1. More generally, one can derive that the smaller the regularization, the better the approximation of least-squares solutions (see Exercise 1.6 for such a calculation).

In summary, the prior function stabilizes the least-squares estimator and removes potential ambiguity. The corresponding tuning parameter allows one to balance stability and closeness to the standard least-squares estimator. The dimensionality of the data ($n = p = 2$) shows that these effects are not tied to high dimensions, but the numerical stability is an extra benefit when using high-dimensional estimators in high-dimensional statistics.

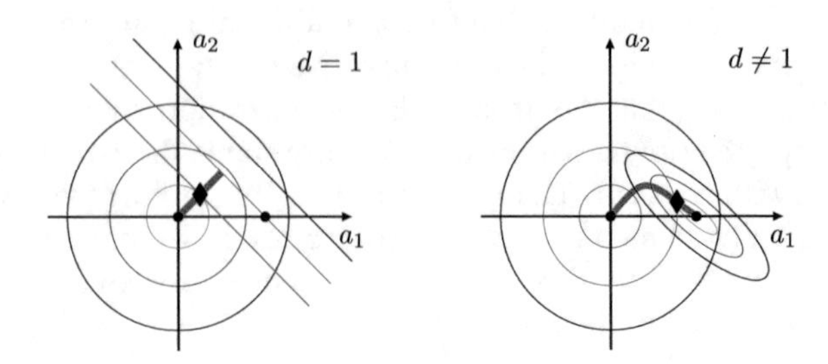

Fig. 1.1 An illustration of why the limiting solutions of the ridge estimator on the data of Table 1.3 differ for $d = 1$ and $d \neq 1$. The round black dots denote $(1, 0)^\top$, which is a minimum of $\boldsymbol{a} \mapsto \|\boldsymbol{y} - X\boldsymbol{a}\|_2^2$ for every $d \in \mathbb{R}$, and $(0, 0)^\top$, which is the minimum of $\boldsymbol{a} \mapsto r\|\boldsymbol{a}\|_2^2$ for every $r \in (0, \infty)$. The lines (left plot) and ellipses (right plot) indicate points that have the same values in $\boldsymbol{a} \mapsto \|\boldsymbol{y} - X\boldsymbol{a}\|_2^2$. The three concentric circles indicate points that have the same values in $\boldsymbol{a} \mapsto r\|\boldsymbol{a}\|_2^2$. The thick brown lines indicate coordinates of the ridge estimators; each point on the brown lines corresponds to an estimator with a given value of the tuning parameter r: the larger r, the closer the corresponding ridge estimator is to the origin. Since the ridge estimators are minimizers of functions of the form $\boldsymbol{a} \mapsto \|\boldsymbol{y} - X\boldsymbol{a}\|_2^2 + r\|\boldsymbol{a}\|_2^2$, they correspond to points (indicated by black diamonds) where a line/ellipse (in blue) generated by the least-squares function "touch" a circle (in red) generated by the prior function. See also Exercise 1.7 for details

1.5 Outlook

In the remainder of this book, we study the principles of high-dimensional statistics in further detail. In ▸ Chap. 2, we deepen our discussion of sparse, high-dimensional regression models to highlight different schemes of regularization. These models are also the basis for illustrating tuning-parameter calibration, inference, and theory later in the book. In ▸ Chap. 3, however, we also introduce graphical models to describe networks. In ▸ Chap. 4, we then calibrate tuning parameters to balance data and prior information. In ▸ Chap. 5, we construct confidence intervals for the coordinates of estimators to quantify uncertainty. In ▸ Chaps. 6 and 7, we finally develop theories to establish mathematical evidence for the features and limitations of high-dimensional estimators.

1.6 Exercises

1.6.1 Exercises for ▸ Sect. 1.1

Exercise 1.1 ♦♦ In this exercise, we confirm the models of ◘ Table 1.1. If you are not sufficiently familiar with the lasso estimator yet, come back to this exercise after reading ▸ Chap. 2.

1. Use `R` to build the least-squares model based on data set A and to check the model's adjusted R^2 value. You can use the `lm()` function.
2. Use `R` to build the lasso model based on data set B and to check the model's adjusted R^2 value. For this, load the `glmnet` package for the lasso estimator and run `coef(glmnet(y=y, x=x, lambda=1))` with the appropriate `y` and `x`, which, in our case, provides the first two model parameters that enter the lasso path (as a bonus exercise, you can confirm this). Then, run the `lm()` function on the two selected model parameters to obtain the corresponding least-squares model.

   Hint: Details on the lasso estimator will follow in the next section.

1.6.2 Exercises for ▸ Sect. 1.2

Exercise 1.2 ♦♦♦ In this exercise, we generalize the results of ▸ Sect. 1.2 to cases where the Gram matrix $X^\top X$ is not necessarily invertible. We show in particular that least-squares prediction is expected to be accurate only if $\text{rank}[X] \ll n$.

Our derivations use the Moore–Penrose matrix inverse.[11] A matrix $A^+ \in \mathbb{R}^{p\times n}$ is called a *Moore–Penrose matrix inverse* of $A \in \mathbb{R}^{n\times p}$ if the following four conditions are met: 1. $AA^+A = A$; 2. $A^+AA^+ = A^+$; 3. $(AA^+)^\top = AA^+$; and 4. $(A^+A)^\top = A^+A$. Moore–Penrose matrix inverses always exist and are unique. One can also check readily that for an invertible square matrix A, the regular matrix inverse A^{-1} satisfies the mentioned four conditions; hence, Moore–Penrose matrix inverses generalize regular matrix inverses.

Moore-Penrose inverse

1. Show that the Gram matrix $X^\top X$ is always positive *semi*-definite: $(X^\top X)^\top = X^\top X$ and $\boldsymbol{\alpha}^\top X^\top X\boldsymbol{\alpha} \geq 0$ for all $\boldsymbol{\alpha} \in \mathbb{R}^p$.

2. Invertibility then requires positive definiteness: $\alpha^\top X^\top X\alpha > 0$ for all $\alpha \in \mathbb{R}^p$ (see 4. in Lemma B.2.5). Show that if the Gram matrix $X^\top X$ is invertible, then $p \leq n$. Conclude that the treatment in ▶ Sect. 1.2 applies only to settings where the number of model parameters is at most as large as the number of samples.
3. Show that $\arg\min_{\alpha\in\mathbb{R}^p} \|y - X\alpha\|_2^2$ contains only one point if and only if $X\gamma \neq \mathbf{0}_n$ for all $\gamma \in \mathbb{R}^p \setminus \{\mathbf{0}_p\}$. Conclude that the least-squares estimator is not unique if $X^\top X$ is not invertible.
4. Show that all $\widehat{\gamma}_{\text{ls}}, \widehat{\beta}_{\text{ls}} \in \arg\min_{\alpha\in\mathbb{R}^p} \|y - X\alpha\|_2^2$ provide the same prediction: $X\widehat{\gamma}_{\text{ls}} = X\widehat{\beta}_{\text{ls}}$.
5. Show that $\widehat{\beta}_{\text{ls}} = X^+y$ is always a solution of the least-squares estimator, where X^+ is a Moore–Penrose inverse of X.
6. Consider the singular value decomposition $X = UDV^\top$ used in the main text.
   (i) Show that D^+ defined as diagonal matrix with diagonal elements $D^+_{ii} := 1/D_{ii}$ if $D_{ii} \neq 0$ and $D^+_{ii} := 0$ otherwise is a Moore–Penrose inverse of D.
   (ii) Show that DD^+ is diagonal with rank$[X]$ ones on its diagonal and zeros everywhere else.
   (iii) Show that $X^+ = VD^+U^\top$ is a Moore–Penrose inverse of X.

7. Show that for every least-squares solution $\widehat{\beta}_{\text{ls}}$, it holds that

$$\|X\beta - X\widehat{\beta}_{\text{ls}}\|_2^2 = \|UDD^+U^\top u\|_2^2 .$$

8. Conclude that if $u \sim \mathcal{N}_n[\mathbf{0}_n, \sigma^2 \mathrm{I}_{n\times n}]$ for a $\sigma \in (0,\infty)$, we have the risk bound

$$\mathbb{E}\left[\frac{\|X\beta - X\widehat{\beta}_{\text{ls}}\|_2^2}{n}\right] = \frac{\sigma^2\,\text{rank}[X]}{n} . \tag{1.9}$$

   Here, the expectation is taken over the noise u, while the design is assumed to be fixed.
9. Bonus: Show that $(X^\top X)^+X^\top$ is a Moore–Penrose inverse of X, where $(X^\top X)^+$ is a Moore–Penrose inverse of $X^\top X$. Conclude that $\widehat{\beta}_{\text{ls}} = (X^\top X)^+X^\top y$ is always a least-squares estimator.

1.6.3 Exercises for ▶ Sect. 1.3

Exercise 1.3 ♦♦ In this exercise, we motivate the ridge and lasso estimators from a Bayes perspective. For this, we consider a linear regression model

$$y = X\boldsymbol{\beta} + \boldsymbol{u}$$

with outcome $\boldsymbol{y} \in \mathbb{R}^n$, design matrix $X \in \mathbb{R}^{n\times p}$, regression vector $\boldsymbol{\beta} \in \mathbb{R}^p$, and noise $\boldsymbol{u} \sim \mathcal{N}_n[\mathbf{0}_n, \sigma^2 \mathrm{I}_{n\times n}]$. We assume the design X to be fixed. In a frequentist framework, $\boldsymbol{\beta}$ is also fixed, which means in particular that the outcome is distributed according to $\boldsymbol{y} \sim \mathcal{N}_n[X\boldsymbol{\beta}, \sigma^2\mathrm{I}_{n\times n}]$. In a hierarchical Bayes framework, on the other hand, $\boldsymbol{\beta}$ follows some prior distribution, and, instead of the outcome itself, the outcome *given* the regression vector is distributed according to $\boldsymbol{y} \mid \boldsymbol{\beta} \sim \mathcal{N}_n[X\boldsymbol{\beta}, \sigma^2\mathrm{I}_{n\times n}]$. Adopting the Bayes viewpoint, we study the *maximum a posteriori estimator*

$$\widehat{\boldsymbol{\beta}}_{\text{map}} \in \underset{\boldsymbol{\alpha}\in\mathbb{R}^p}{\arg\max}\, \ell[\boldsymbol{\alpha} \mid \boldsymbol{y}]\,,$$

where the posterior likelihood $\ell[\boldsymbol{\alpha} \mid \boldsymbol{y}]$ is the logarithm of the density of $\boldsymbol{\alpha} \mid \boldsymbol{y}$ as a function of $\boldsymbol{\alpha}$.

Assume that the regression vector is distributed independently of the noise and has strictly positive density[12] g, which implies that $\ell[\boldsymbol{\alpha} \mid \boldsymbol{y}]$ is proportional to $f_{\boldsymbol{\alpha}}[\boldsymbol{y}]g[\boldsymbol{\alpha}]$, where $f_{\boldsymbol{\alpha}}$ is the density of $\mathcal{N}_n[X\boldsymbol{\alpha}, \sigma^2\mathrm{I}_{n\times n}]$. Establish the following two relationships between the map estimator and the frequentist estimators lasso and ridge.

1. Show that in case of a multivariate normal prior distribution $\boldsymbol{\beta} \sim \mathcal{N}_p[\mathbf{0}_p, \tau^2\mathrm{I}_{p\times p}]$, the map estimator coincides with the ridge estimator

$$\widehat{\boldsymbol{\beta}}_{\text{ridge}} \in \underset{\boldsymbol{\alpha}\in\mathbb{R}^p}{\arg\min}\big\{ \|\boldsymbol{y} - X\boldsymbol{\alpha}\|_2^2 + r\|\boldsymbol{\alpha}\|_2^2 \big\}$$

   with tuning parameter $r = \sigma^2/\tau^2$. Hint: Use the identity $\max_{\boldsymbol{\alpha}\in\mathbb{R}^p} \ell[\boldsymbol{\alpha} \mid \boldsymbol{y}] = \min_{\boldsymbol{\alpha}\in\mathbb{R}^p} -\log[f_{\boldsymbol{\alpha}}[\boldsymbol{y}]g[\boldsymbol{\alpha}]]$.
2. Show that in case of a multivariate Laplace (double-exponential) prior distribution with density $e^{-\|\boldsymbol{\beta}\|_1/\tau}/(2\tau)^p$, the map estimator coincides with the lasso

$$\widehat{\boldsymbol{\beta}}_{\text{lasso}} \in \underset{\boldsymbol{\alpha}\in\mathbb{R}^p}{\arg\min}\big\{ \|\boldsymbol{y} - X\boldsymbol{\alpha}\|_2^2 + r\|\boldsymbol{\alpha}\|_1 \big\}$$

   with tuning parameter $r = 2\sigma^2/\tau$.

We conclude that the ridge and lasso estimators can be formulated as map estimators of hierarchical Bayes frameworks.

3. Show that in general,

$$\widehat{\boldsymbol{\beta}}_{\text{map}} \in \underset{\boldsymbol{\alpha}\in\mathbb{R}^p}{\arg\min}\{\,\|\boldsymbol{y}-X\boldsymbol{\alpha}\|_2^2 - 2\sigma^2 \log g[\boldsymbol{\alpha}]\,\}\,.$$

We conclude that there is a general correspondence between map estimators and regularized least-squares estimators.[13]

1.6.4 Exercises for ► Sect. 1.4

Exercise 1.4 ♦ In this exercise, we verify and extend the claims about convexity in ► Sects. 1.2 and 1.4. According to Definition 2.5.1 in the following section, a function $f : \mathbb{R}^p \to \mathbb{R}$ is *convex* if and only if

$$f[w\boldsymbol{a}+(1-w)\boldsymbol{b}] \le wf[\boldsymbol{a}]+(1-w)f[\boldsymbol{b}] \quad \text{for all } w \in [0,1];\ \boldsymbol{a},\boldsymbol{b} \in \mathbb{R}^p\,.$$

The function f is *strictly convex* if

$$f[w\boldsymbol{a} + (1-w)\boldsymbol{b}] < wf[\boldsymbol{a}] + (1-w)f[\boldsymbol{b}] \quad \text{for all } w \in (0,1);\ \boldsymbol{a},\boldsymbol{b} \in \mathbb{R}^p,\ \boldsymbol{a} \neq \boldsymbol{b}\,.$$

Refer also to ► Sect. 2.5.

1. Show that the least-squares objective function $\boldsymbol{a} \mapsto \|\boldsymbol{y} - X\boldsymbol{a}\|_2^2$ is convex.
2. Show that the least-squares objective function $\boldsymbol{a} \mapsto \|\boldsymbol{y} - X\boldsymbol{a}\|_2^2$ is strictly convex if and only $X^\top X$ invertible.
3. Give an example of a convex but not strictly convex function that has multiple minima and one that has only one minimum. Bonus: Is the function $\boldsymbol{a} = (a_1, a_2)^\top \mapsto a_1^2 a_2^2$ convex?
4. Show that in contrast, the minima of *strictly* convex functions, say $f : \mathbb{R}^p \to \mathbb{R}$, are always unique.

Exercise 1.5 ◊◊ In this exercise, we study the continuity of the ridge estimator, which is related to its numerical stability. Specifically, use the data discussed in ► Sect. 1.4 to show that the ridge estimator with any fixed tuning parameter is a continuous function of the parameter d of the data in that section, that is: for all $r, u > 0$, there is a

$v > 0$ such that for all $d, d' \in \mathbb{R}$, $|d - d'| < v$, it holds that

$$\|\widehat{\boldsymbol{\beta}}_{\text{ridge}}[r, \boldsymbol{y}, X^d] - \widehat{\boldsymbol{\beta}}_{\text{ridge}}[r, \boldsymbol{y}, X^{d'}]\|_1 < u\,,$$

where $X^d = ((1,2)^\top, (d,2)^\top)$ (and analogously $X^{d'}$) is the design from ◘ Table 1.3 for given d, and $\widehat{\boldsymbol{\beta}}_{\text{ridge}}[r, \boldsymbol{y}, X^d]$ (and analogously $\widehat{\boldsymbol{\beta}}_{\text{ridge}}[r, \boldsymbol{y}, X^{d'}]$) is the ridge estimator with tuning parameter r on the data $(\boldsymbol{y}, X^d)$.

Exercise 1.6 ♦ In this exercise, we corroborate our statement that the smaller the tuning parameter, the better the ridge estimator approximates a least-squares solution. For this, consider the data discussed in ► Sect. 1.4 with $d = 1$. Show that

$$\|\widehat{\boldsymbol{\beta}}_{\text{ridge}}[r] - (1/2, 1/2)^\top\|_2 = \frac{r}{\sqrt{2}(10 + r)}$$

and conclude that the smaller the tuning parameter, the closer is the corresponding ridge estimator to a least-squares solution of the form $(1 - a, a)^\top$.

Exercise 1.7 ♦♦ In this exercise, we provide mathematical details on the plots of ◘ Fig. 1.1.

Consider again the data in ◘ Table 1.3.

1. Show that for all $d \in \mathbb{R}$ and $\boldsymbol{\alpha} = (\alpha_1, \alpha_2)^\top$, it holds that

$$\|\boldsymbol{y} - X\boldsymbol{\alpha}\|_2^2 = 5(\alpha_1 - 1)^2 + (4 + d^2)\alpha_2^2 + 2(4 + d)(\alpha_1 - 1)\alpha_2\,.$$

2. Verify that for $d = 1$, the equation simplifies to

$$\|\boldsymbol{y} - X\boldsymbol{\alpha}\|_2^2 = 5(\alpha_1 - 1 + \alpha_2)^2\,.$$

3. Conclude that for $d = 1$ and every $c \in [0, \infty)$, it holds that

$$\left\{\boldsymbol{\alpha} \in \mathbb{R}^2 \,:\, \|\boldsymbol{y} - X\boldsymbol{\alpha}\|_2^2 = c\right\} = \left\{\boldsymbol{\alpha} \in \mathbb{R}^2 \,:\, \alpha_2 = 1 - \alpha_1 \pm \sqrt{\frac{c}{5}}\right\}.$$

   This means that the function $\boldsymbol{\alpha} \mapsto \|\boldsymbol{y} - X\boldsymbol{\alpha}\|_2^2$ has level sets (a level set is a complete set of function arguments that have the same function value) specified by linear relationships between the coordinates. These level sets are indicated by the straight lines in the left panel of ◘ Fig. 1.1.

4. We consider now the level sets of ellipses centered at $(1, 0)^\top$ and parameterized by $\omega \in [0, 180°)$ and $a, b \in (0, \infty)$:

$$\left\{ \boldsymbol{\alpha} \in \mathbb{R}^2 \,:\, \frac{\left((\cos\omega)(\alpha_1 - 1) + (\sin\omega)\alpha_2\right)^2}{a^2} + \frac{\left(-(\sin\omega)(\alpha_1 - 1) + (\cos\omega)\alpha_2\right)^2}{b^2} = c \right\}.$$

The parameter c indexes the different level sets. Show that for $\omega \to 45°$, $a \to 1/\sqrt{10}$, and $b \to \infty$, these level sets converge to

$$\left\{ \boldsymbol{\alpha} \in \mathbb{R}^2 \,:\, 5(\alpha_1 - 1 + \alpha_2)^2 = c \right\}.$$

For this, recall that a sequence of sets $\mathscr{A}_1, \mathscr{A}_2, \ldots$ converges to $\mathscr{A}$ if for every point $a \in ((\cup_j \mathscr{A}_j) \cup \mathscr{A})$, there is an $n \in \{1, 2, \ldots\}$ such that either $a \in (\mathscr{A}_m \cap \mathscr{A})$ for all $m \geq n$ or $a \notin \mathscr{A}_m, a \notin \mathscr{A}$ for all $m \geq n$.In the case here, it suffices to show that $((\cos\omega)(\alpha_1 - 1) + (\sin\omega)\alpha_2)^2/a^2 + (-(\sin\omega)(\alpha_1 - 1) + (\cos\omega)\alpha_2)^2/b^2 \to 5(\alpha_1 - 1 + \alpha_2)^2$.

Conclude with 2. that for $d = 1$, we can think of the least-squares' level sets as 45°-rotated ellipses that are stretched infinitely in one direction.

5. We switch to $d \neq 1$ and write

$$\|\boldsymbol{y} - X\boldsymbol{\alpha}\|_2^2 = \frac{\left((\cos\omega)(\alpha_1 - 1) + (\sin\omega)\alpha_2\right)^2}{a^2} + \frac{\left(-(\sin\omega)(\alpha_1 - 1) + (\cos\omega)\alpha_2\right)^2}{b^2}$$

for $\omega \in [0°, 180°)$, $a, b \in (0, \infty)$. In the following, we compute the parameters ω, a, and b as functions of d and show that the least-squares function $\boldsymbol{\alpha} \mapsto \|\boldsymbol{y} - X\boldsymbol{\alpha}\|_2^2$ can indeed be written in that elliptic form. For this, verify first that

$$\begin{aligned}&\frac{\left((\cos\omega)(\alpha_1 - 1) + (\sin\omega)\alpha_2\right)^2}{a^2} + \frac{\left(-(\sin\omega)(\alpha_1 - 1) + (\cos\omega)\alpha_2\right)^2}{b^2}\\ &= \left(\frac{(\cos\omega)^2}{a^2} + \frac{(\sin\omega)^2}{b^2}\right)(\alpha_1 - 1)^2 + \left(\frac{(\sin\omega)^2}{a^2} + \frac{(\cos\omega)^2}{b^2}\right)\alpha_2^2\\ &\quad + 2\left(\frac{1}{a^2} - \frac{1}{b^2}\right)(\cos\omega)(\sin\omega)(\alpha_1 - 1)\alpha_2 .\end{aligned}$$

6. Compare the $(\alpha_1 - 1)$-terms of the formulations in 5. and 1. to show that if $a \neq b$, it holds that

$$(\cos\omega)^2 = \frac{5 - \frac{1}{b^2}}{\frac{1}{a^2} - \frac{1}{b^2}}\,.$$

7. Compare the α_2-terms of the formulations in 5. and 1. to show that if $a \neq b$, it holds that

$$\frac{1}{a^2} + \frac{1}{b^2} = 9 + d^2\,.$$

8. Use the previous two steps to show that if $a \neq b$, it holds that

$$(\cos\omega)^2(\sin\omega)^2 = \frac{5(4+d^2)b^4 - (9+d^2)b^2 + 1}{(9+d^2)^2 b^4 - 4(9+d^2)b^2 + 4}\,.$$

9. Show similarly as in the previous steps that $a \neq b$ for every $d \neq 1$. Conclude from 5.–7. that if $d \neq 1$, the least-squares function can indeed be written in the mentioned elliptic form with the parameters derived in 6.–7.
10. Compare the $(\alpha_1 - 1)\alpha_2$-terms of the formulations in 1. and 5. to show that

$$\frac{5(4+d^2) - \frac{9+d^2}{b^2} + \frac{1}{b^4}}{(9+d^2)^2 - \frac{4(9+d^2)}{b^2} + \frac{4}{b^2}} - \frac{(4+d)^2}{(9+d^2-\frac{2}{b^2})^2} = 0\,.$$

11. Use the above insights to draw level sets of the least-squares objective function $\boldsymbol{a} \mapsto \|\boldsymbol{y} - X\boldsymbol{a}\|_2^2$ for $d = 1$ and $d \neq 1$.

1.7 R Lab: Least-Squares vs. Ridge Estimation

In this lab, we compare the least-squares estimator with the ridge estimator.

Your task is to replace the keyword `REPLACE` by suitable code and to answer the questions posed in the text.

1.7.1 Generating Toy Data

Generate data according to $\boldsymbol{y} = X\boldsymbol{\beta} + \boldsymbol{u}$ with $X \in \mathbb{R}^{2\times 2}$ as in ◘ Table 1.3 with $d = 2$, $\boldsymbol{\beta} = (1, 1/2)^\top$, and $\boldsymbol{u} \sim \mathcal{N}_2[\mathbf{0}_2, (0.1)^2 \mathrm{I}_{2\times 2}]$. You might want to use the `rnorm()` function.

```
set.seed(11)
DesignFamily <- function(d)
{
  return(matrix(c(1, 2, d, 2), nrow=2, ncol=2))
}
design <- DesignFamily(2)
regression.vector <- c(1, 1/2)
outcome <- REPLACE
```

1.7.2 Implementing the Estimators

Implement the least-squares estimator (for $d \neq 1$). You might want to use the `solve()` function.

```
LsEstimator <- function(y, X)
{
  REPLACE
}
LsEstimator(outcome, design)
```

```
##              [,1]
## [1,] 1.0617625
## [2,] 0.4395672
```

Similarly, implement the ridge estimator.

```
RidgeEstimator <- function(y, X, r)
{
  REPLACE
}
RidgeEstimator(outcome, design, 1)
```

```
##              [,1]
## [1,] 0.6774037
## [2,] 0.6469656
```

1.7.3 Showing that the Ridge Estimator Approximates a Least-Squares Solution

Show that the ridge estimator approaches in ℓ_2-norm the least-squares solution when r goes to zero. For this, establish a function that compares the ℓ_2-differences between the ridge estimator and the least-squares: $\|\widehat{\beta}_{\text{ridge}} - \widehat{\beta}_{\text{ls}}\|_2$.

```
RidgeLsDifference <- function(r, y, X)
{
  REPLACE
}
tuning.parameter <- 0.001 * c(1:10000)
difference <- apply(as.matrix(tuning.parameter), 1, RidgeLsDifference,
                    y=outcome, design)
plot(x    = tuning.parameter,
     y    = difference,
     type = "l",
     lty  = 1,
     ylim = c(0, 1),
     yaxp = c(0, 1, 2),
     las  = 1,
     xlab = "tuning parameter",
     ylab = "differences")
```

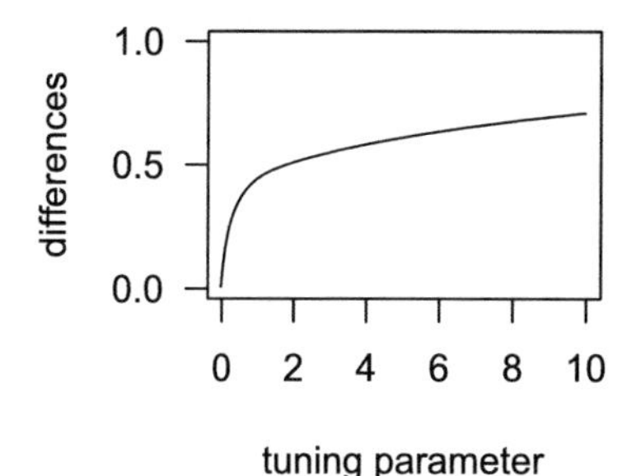

We find that the smaller the tuning parameter, the closer the ridge estimator is to the least-squares estimator. Eventually, for $r \to 0$, they coincide.

1.7.4 Comparing Estimation Errors

Compare the ℓ_2-estimator errors of the ridge estimator and the LS estimator: $\|\widehat{\boldsymbol{\beta}}^r_{\text{ridge}} - \boldsymbol{\beta}\|_2$ vs. $\|\widehat{\boldsymbol{\beta}}_{\text{ls}} - \boldsymbol{\beta}\|_2$.

```
RidgeError <- function(r, y, X)
{
  REPLACE
}
LsError <- function(y, X)
{
  REPLACE
}
tuning.parameter <- 0.001 * c(1:10000)
estimation.error <- apply(as.matrix(tuning.parameter), 1, RidgeError,
                          outcome, design)
```

```
plot(x     = tuning.parameter,
     y     = estimation.error,
     type = "l",
     lty  = 1,
     ylim = c(0, 0.8),
     yaxp = c(0, 0.8, 2),
     las  = 1,
     xlab = "tuning parameter",
     ylab = "estimation error")
abline(h=LsError(outcome, design), lty=4)
```

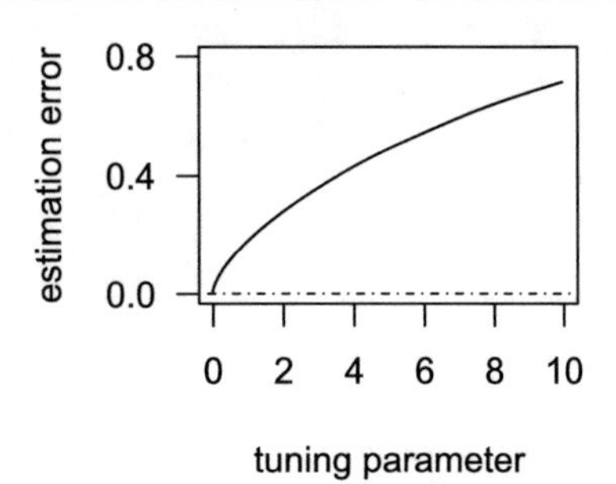

We observe in particular that the ℓ_2-error of the ridge estimator becomes large if the tuning parameter is large. What happens for $r \to \infty$?

1.7.5 Showing That the Ridge Estimator Is Continuous in the Data

Show that the ridge estimator is continuous in the variation of the design parameter d around the critical point $d_{\text{critical}} = 1$. For this, compute the ℓ_2-distances of ridge estimators on data with different design parameters d to the ridge estimator on data with fixed design parameter $d_{\text{critical}} = 1$. Set the tuning parameter to $r = 0.5$ throughout.

```
RidgeDifference <- function(d, r, y, d.critical)
{
  REPLACE
}
tuning_parameter_fixed <- 0.5
d.critical <- 1
d <- 0.01 * c(0:200)
differences <- apply(as.matrix(d), 1,  RidgeDifference,tuning_parameter_fixed, outcome,
                     d.critical)
plot(d, differences, type="l", lty=1, yaxp=c(0, 0.8, 2), las=1)
```

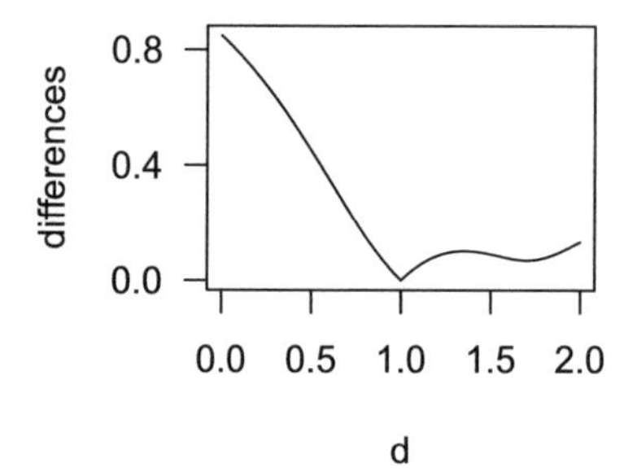

Since the curve is continuous at $d = 1$, we conclude that $\|\widehat{\beta}_{\text{ridge}}[d] - \widehat{\beta}_{\text{ridge}}[d_{\text{critical}}]\|_2 \to 0$ for $d \to d_{\text{critical}} = 1$, where $\widehat{\beta}_{\text{ridge}}[d]$ and $\widehat{\beta}_{\text{ridge}}[d_{\text{critical}}]$ denote the ridge estimators (with tuning parameter $r = 0.5$) on data indexed by d and d_{critical}, respectively. This means that the ridge estimator is continuous in the data as d varies around the critical point $d_{\text{critical}} = 1$.

Is the ridge estimator continuous as a function of d more generally?

1.7.6 Showing That the Coordinates of the Ridge Estimator Are Not Necessarily Monotone in the Tuning Parameter

Use the toy data to show that the individual coordinates of the ridge estimator are not necessarily monotone in the tuning parameter.

```
RidgeCoordinate <- function(r, y, d, coordinate)
{
  REPLACE
}
d <- 2
tuning.parameter <- 0.001 * c(1:10000)
coordinate_1 <- apply(as.matrix(tuning.parameter), 1, RidgeCoordinate, outcome, d, 1)
coordinate_2 <- apply(as.matrix(tuning.parameter), 1, RidgeCoordinate, outcome, d, 2)
plot(x     = tuning.parameter,
     y     = coordinate_1,
     type  = "l",
     col   = "black",
     las   = 1,
     yaxp  = c(0.4, 1, 3),
     xlab  = "tuning parameter",
     ylab  = "coordinate")
lines(tuning.parameter, coordinate_2, col="blue")
```

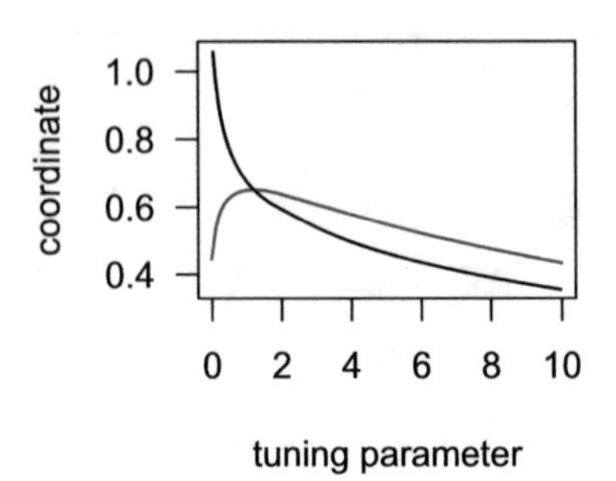

The curve of the second coordinate increases until about $r = 1.5$ and then decreases, which shows that the coordinates are not necessarily monotone in the tuning parameter. Nevertheless, both curves decrease monotonously approximately as c/r for r large, where $c \in (0, \infty)$ is a constant that can depend on the coordinate (and the data, of course), which corroborates our theoretical findings in the main text.

1.7.7 Comparing Ridge and Least-Squares on Economic Data

We apply the ridge estimator and the least-squares on the `longley` data that contains seven economic variables and is included in the standard `R` distributions. Take as outcome variable the `Employed` variable, and as predictor variables `GNP.deflator`, `GNP`, `Unemployed`, `Armed.Forces`, and `Population`. Also add a column of ones to design matrix to account for the intercept. (We regularize the intercept as any other variable.) Bonus: Write a version of the ridge estimator that does not regularize the intercept.) Hint: For easier manipulations later, use the `as.matrix()` function to convert all quantities to matrices.

```
outcome <- as.matrix(longley["Employed"])
design <- REPLACE
cbind(outcome, design)[1:5, ]
```

```
##      Employed Intercept GNP.deflator     GNP Unemployed Armed.Forces Population
## 1947   60.323         1         83.0 234.289      235.6        159.0    107.608
## 1948   61.122         1         88.5 259.426      232.5        145.6    108.632
## 1949   60.171         1         88.2 258.054      368.2        161.6    109.773
## 1950   61.187         1         89.5 284.599      335.1        165.0    110.929
## 1951   63.221         1         96.2 328.975      209.9        309.9    112.075
```

```
LsEstimator(outcome, design)
```

```
##                 Employed
## Intercept     92.461307827
## GNP.deflator  -0.048462828
## GNP            0.072003849
## Unemployed    -0.004038711
## Armed.Forces  -0.005604956
## Population    -0.403508682
```

```
RidgeEstimator(outcome, design, 1)
```

```
##                Employed
## Intercept     0.02227192
## GNP.deflator  0.21920075
## GNP          -0.01035088
## Unemployed   -0.01394317
## Armed.Forces -0.00579588
## Population    0.45119435
```

```
RidgeEstimator(outcome, design, 100)
```

```
##                 Employed
## Intercept     0.004790496
## GNP.deflator  0.252814814
## GNP          -0.012145722
## Unemployed   -0.012151700
## Armed.Forces -0.003817691
## Population    0.418655390
```

```
RidgeEstimator(outcome, design, 10000)
```

```
##                Employed
## Intercept    0.001724652
## GNP.deflator 0.101214227
## GNP          0.012424157
## Unemployed   0.043045876
## Armed.Forces 0.065315837
## Population   0.156333129
```

Are the ridge estimator's coordinates monotone in the tuning parameter here? Is the ridge estimator's magnitude in ℓ_2 monotone in the tuning parameter here?

1.7.8 Bonus: Checking the Theoretical Formulae of ▸ Sect. 1.4

We show that the formulae in ▸ Sect. 1.4 are correct. We first compare the least-squares estimator to the version in the script for three values of d:

```
LsEstimatorTheory <- c(1, 0)
outcome <- c(1, 2)
LsEstimator(outcome, DesignFamily(0)) - LsEstimatorTheory
```

```
##                [,1]
## [1,]  2.220446e-16
## [2,] -2.220446e-16
```

```
LsEstimator(outcome, DesignFamily(2)) - LsEstimatorTheory
```

```
##                [,1]
## [1,]  2.220446e-15
## [2,] -1.332268e-15
```

```
LsEstimator(outcome, DesignFamily(1.1)) - LsEstimatorTheory
```

```
##                [,1]
## [1,] -3.375078e-14
## [2,]  6.217249e-14
```

These results confirm the theoretical formulae within the bounds of numerical precision.

We now compare the ridge estimator to the version in the script for three values of d and r:

```
RidgeEstimatorTheory <- function(d, r)
{
  return(1 / (4 - 8 * d + 4 * d^2 + (9 + d^2) * r + r^2) *
         c(4 - 8 * d + 4 * d^2 + 5 * r, (4 + d) * r))
}
RidgeEstimator(outcome, DesignFamily(0), 1) - RidgeEstimatorTheory(0, 1)
```

```
##                [,1]
## [1,] -1.110223e-16
## [2,]  0.000000e+00
```

```
RidgeEstimator(outcome,DesignFamily(2), 0.1) - RidgeEstimatorTheory(2, 0.1)
```

```
##                    [,1]
## [1,]   1.665335e-15
## [2,]  -6.245005e-16
```

```
RidgeEstimator(outcome, DesignFamily(1.1), 0.5) - RidgeEstimatorTheory(1.1, 0.5)
```

```
##                  [,1]
## [1,] 2.775558e-16
## [2,] 1.110223e-16
```

We find again equivalence within numerical precision.

1.7.9 Bonus: A Technical Note

Consider the following two functions:

```
Function_1 <- function(y, X)
{
  return(solve(t(X) %*% X) %*% t(X) %*% y)
}
Function_2 <- function(y, X)
{
  return(solve(t(X) %*% X, t(X) %*% y))
}
y <- c(1, 2)
X <- matrix(c(1, 2, 0, 2), nrow=2, ncol=2)
Function_1(y, X)
```

```
##                    [,1]
## [1,]   1.000000e+00
## [2,]  -2.220446e-16
```

```
Function_2(y, X)
```

```
##        [,1]
## [1,]      1
## [2,]      0
```

What is the difference between the two functions?

To keep the code as close as possible to the script, we have generated all labs' results by using the solve function as in `Function_1`. However, the faster and numerically more stable version is `Function_2`, which solves a system of equations instead of inverting a matrix and subsequently multiplying that inverse with a vector.

Implement the least-squares and the ridge as suggested by both `Function_1` and `Function_2` and compare the results for this lab. Are there any differences?

1.8 Notes and References

1. References for the sequencing of the human genome are Kidd et al. (2008) and citations therein. An example for early research on regression-type relationships in this context is Dettling and Bühlmann (2004), for gene–gene regulatory networks Dobra et al. (2004).
2. Other types of genomic variations include single-nucleotide polymorphisms (SNPs) (Judson et al., 2002), which are substitutions of single nucleotides, and insertion–deletions (INDELs) (Mills et al., 2006), which are insertions or deletions of small nucleotide sequences. In general, the abundant ways in which genomes can vary make genomics a prototypical field of application for high-dimensional statistics.
3. Associations between diseases and CNVs of different ranges are described in Almal and Padh (2012).
4. Actually, dropping data is common: for example, data sets usually come with "meta"-data such as the name of the lab the measurements were taken in, the machines used in the experiments, and so on—still, such information is rarely included in statistical analyses.
5. High-dimensional statistics is often associated with the phrase "curse of dimensionality," insinuating that high-dimensionality is an unwanted but inevitable side effect of modern data. This view probably roots in the wealth of mathematical and algorithmic challenges high-dimensional spaces are known to bring about. An archetypical example for those challenges is that volumes are very difficult to estimate in $\mathbb{R}^p$ with p large, because the number of intersection points needed to form lattices with fixed distances between adjacent points increases exponentially in the number of dimensions of the ambient space (see ◘ Fig. 1.2). But from a statistical perspective, we should follow ▶ Sect. 1.1 in viewing high-dimensionality as an *opportunity* generated by modern data: Only rich enough data can bear the large parameter spaces of models that unravel phenomena in fine detail. Accordingly, we could associate high-dimensional statistics with the phrase *blessing of dimensionality*.
6. We just assume that one of the predictors is reserved for modeling the intercept: for example, if $x_1 = 1$ for all observations, then $\beta_1 x_1 = \beta_1$ is the intercept.
7. Some of the earliest theoretical results for the lasso estimator have been derived in Greenshtein and Ritov (2004).
8. Such risk bounds can be derived by combining our power-two bounds of ▶ Chap. 6 with ideas from Bellec and Tsybakov (2017).
9. The field of *inverse problems* studies the reconstruction of the factors that have produced given observations from the observations

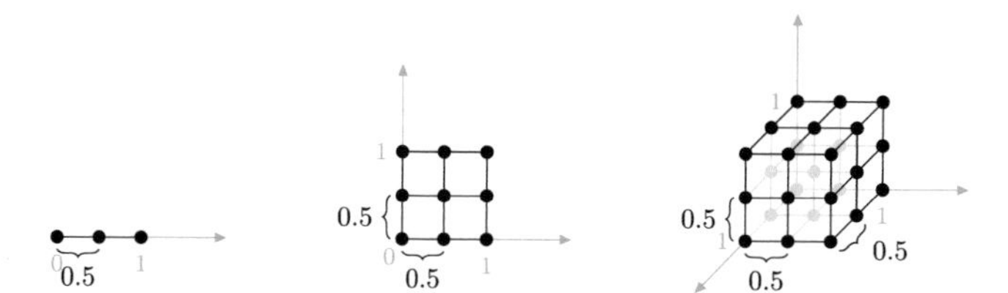

Fig. 1.2 One can pick $\lfloor 1/d+1 \rfloor$ points from the unit interval such that these points have mutual Euclidean distance $d \in (0, \infty)$ (the left panel depicts the case $d = 0.5$), at least $\lfloor 1/d + 1 \rfloor^2$ of such points from the unit square (middle panel), and at least $\lfloor 1/d + 1 \rfloor^3$ such points from the unit cube (right panel). In general, one can pick at least $\lfloor 1/d+1 \rfloor^p$ points from the p-dimensional unit cube such that the points have distance d between each other, which is an exponential increase in p

themselves. For example, the calculation of the mass distribution of the earth from the earth's gravity field is an inverse problem (because the earth's gravity field is the effect of the earth's mass distribution and not the other way around); the calculation of the earth's gravity field from the earth's mass distribution would be the corresponding *forward problem*. A general reference for inverse problems is Engl et al. (1996); an early paper that establishes a connection between inverse problems and numerical stability is Tikhonov (1943).

10 An early paper on the Ridge estimator in regression is Hoerl and Kennard (1970).

11 There are several equivalent definitions of the Moore–Penrose matrix inverse; the stated one is due to Penrose (1955, p. 406), see Albert (1972, Theorem 3.9 on p. 28) for a textbook reference. Existence and uniqueness of Moore–Penrose matrix inverses follow, for example, from Penrose (1955, Theorem 1 on p. 406) and Albert (1972, Theorem 3.4 on p. 19).

12 We consider densities with respect to the appropriate Lebesgue measures unless stated otherwise.

13 This connection has been highlighted through the introduction of the Bayes lasso estimator (Park and Casella, 2008) and discussed further in the context of tuning-parameter calibration (Bu and Lederer, 2017, Section 2.3).

Linear Regression

Contents

J. Lederer, *Fundamentals of High-Dimensional Statistics*, Springer Texts in Statistics,
https://doi.org/10.1007/978-3-030-73792-4_2

Linear regression relates predictor variables and outcome variables, such as gene copy numbers and the level of a biomarker. The assumed linearity of the relationships makes the models convenient both mathematically and computationally. And since the data can be arbitrarily transformed beforehand, such as by including polynomials of the copy numbers as predictor variables or by replacing the level of the biomarker in the outcome variable by its logarithm, linear regression can also effectively model non-linear relationships. This simplicity and flexibility have made linear regression the most popular statistical framework across the sciences and standard textbook material. But the standard methods for linear regression, such as the least-squares estimator, premise that the number of parameters is small as compared to the number of samples, which limits their usefulness in modern, data-intensive research, where the increasing granularity of data has prompted interest in increasingly complex models. More recent high-dimensional methods, in contrast, allow for models with many more parameters. These methods are the topic of this chapter.

2.1 Overview

We first formalize the framework of linear regression. We assume that there are n real-valued observations $y_1, \ldots, y_n \in \mathbb{R}$ and corresponding vector-valued observations $\boldsymbol{x}_1, \ldots, \boldsymbol{x}_n \in \mathbb{R}^p$; each pair $(y_i, \boldsymbol{x}_i)$ is called a *sample*. The samples are modeled according to

$$y_i = \boldsymbol{x}_i^\top \boldsymbol{\beta} + u_i \qquad \text{for all } i \in \{1, \ldots, n\},$$

where the vector $\boldsymbol{\beta} \in \mathbb{R}^p$ that summarizes the *model parameters* $\beta_1, \ldots, \beta_p \in \mathbb{R}$ is called the *regression vector* (which is the same across the samples) and $u_1, \ldots, u_n \in \mathbb{R}$ the *noise* (which can be different from one sample to another). The regression vector captures the linear relationship between y_i and $\boldsymbol{x}_i$; the noise comprises everything else, such as measurement errors, non-linear relationships, and so forth. We call these models *linear regression models*.

The most common examples of such models are Gaussian linear regression models with fixed design, where $u_1, \ldots, u_n$ are i.i.d. distributed according to $\mathcal{N}_1[0, \sigma^2]$ for a $\sigma \in (0, \infty)$, and where $\boldsymbol{x}_1, \ldots, \boldsymbol{x}_n$ are fixed vectors. We will use Gaussian models throughout the book to illustrate ideas, but we keep otherwise our derivations universal, that is, we allow for arbitrary noise distributions and random designs.

We summarize the above equations in

$$y = X\boldsymbol{\beta} + \boldsymbol{u}, \tag{2.1}$$

where $\boldsymbol{y} = (y_1, \ldots, y_n)^\top \in \mathbb{R}^n$ is called *outcome vector* or just *outcome*, $X = (\boldsymbol{x}_1^\top, \ldots, \boldsymbol{x}_n^\top)^\top \in \mathbb{R}^{n \times p}$ *design matrix*, and $\boldsymbol{u} = (u_1, \ldots, u_n)^\top \in \mathbb{R}^n$ *noise vector* or just *noise*. Moreover, the columns $\widetilde{\boldsymbol{x}}_j$ of the design matrix X (that is, $X = (\widetilde{\boldsymbol{x}}_1, \ldots, \widetilde{\boldsymbol{x}}_p)$) are called *predictors*.[1]

The pair $(\boldsymbol{y}, X)$ is the *data*. The data is known to the statistician, while the regression vector and the noise are not. Our goal is to draw inferences from the data about the regression vector, that is, to unravel the relationships between outcome and design. We call this process *linear regression*.

How difficult linear regression is mainly depends on four model specifications. First, linear regression becomes easier with increasing sample size n (more information available) and more challenging with increasing model size p (more parameters to estimate). Most challenging are models with $p \approx n$ or even $p \gg n$. We call such models *high-dimensional*.

Second, linear regression becomes easier with increasing amounts of prior information (more specific regularization possible). Estimators that complement least-squares with functions to leverage this prior information are called *regularized least-squares estimators*.

Third, linear regression becomes more challenging with increasing magnitudes of the noise u_i (data less informative). For prediction and estimation, where we are interested in $X\boldsymbol{\beta}$ and $\boldsymbol{\beta}$, respectively, the decisive factor is the absolute strength of the noise; for support recovery, where we are interested in $\text{supp}[\boldsymbol{\beta}]$, the decisive factor is the strength of the noise relative to the magnitudes of the parameters β_i. We relate the two influences in the *signal-to-noise ratio* $\|X\boldsymbol{\beta}\|_2/\|\boldsymbol{u}\|_2$. (But note that the signal-to-noise ratio is typically unknown in practice.)

And finally, estimation and support recovery become easier with increasing differences among the predictors. The reason for this is that the relationships of the outcome with similar predictors are hard to disentangle. This is not necessarily a problem for prediction, where we consider the relationship of the outcome with the collection of all predictors (▶ Chap. 6). But for estimation and support recovery, where we consider the relationship of the outcome with each predictor individually, this can cause ambiguity (▶ Chap. 7).

Since the predictors and their relationships play an important role in linear regression, we establish here some vocabulary and first insights. Predictor vectors are typically *normalized*, which means that they are scaled to Euclidean lengths equal to, say, the square-root of the sample size: $\|\boldsymbol{x}_i\|_2 = \sqrt{n}$. The differences among the predictors are then captured by their relative spatial orientations, that is, the angle $\angle_{\boldsymbol{x}_i,\boldsymbol{x}_j}$ between any two predictors $\boldsymbol{x}_i$, $\boldsymbol{x}_j$. We call the cosines of these angles the *correlations*:

$$\mathrm{cor}[\boldsymbol{x}_i, \boldsymbol{x}_j] \;:=\; \cos[\angle_{\boldsymbol{x}_i,\boldsymbol{x}_j}] \;=\; \frac{\langle \boldsymbol{x}_i,\, \boldsymbol{x}_j\rangle}{\|\boldsymbol{x}_i\|_2\|\boldsymbol{x}_j\|_2} \;\in\; [0, 1]\,.$$

Correlations are symmetric: $\mathrm{cor}[\boldsymbol{x}_i, \boldsymbol{x}_j] = \mathrm{cor}[\boldsymbol{x}_j, \boldsymbol{x}_i]$. Small correlations (that is, large angles) indicate that the corresponding predictors are different; large correlations (small angles) indicate that the predictors are similar. We speak of a *highly correlated design* if "many" of these correlations are large ($\mathrm{cor}[\boldsymbol{x}_i, \boldsymbol{x}_j] \approx 1$ for many $i \neq j$), a *weakly correlated design* if "most" of these correlations are small ($\mathrm{cor}[\boldsymbol{x}_i, \boldsymbol{x}_j] \approx 0$ for most $i \neq j$), and a *scaled orthogonal design* or just *orthogonal design*[2] if there are no correlations and the predictors are normalized ($\mathrm{cor}[\boldsymbol{x}_i, \boldsymbol{x}_j] = 0$ for all $i \neq j$ and $\|\boldsymbol{x}_i\|_2 = \sqrt{n}$ for all i).

(scaled) orthogonal design

The predictors are the columns of the design matrix $X = (\boldsymbol{x}_1, \ldots, \boldsymbol{x}_p)$, so that

$$\begin{aligned}
(X^\top X)_{ij} &= \sum_{k=1}^{n} X^\top_{ik} X_{kj} && \text{definition of matrix–matrix multiplications}\\
&= \sum_{k=1}^{n} X_{ki} X_{kj} && \text{Definition B.2.1 of matrix transposes}\\
&= \sum_{k=1}^{n} (\boldsymbol{x}_i)_k (\boldsymbol{x}_j)_k && \text{above formulation of } X\\
&= \langle \boldsymbol{x}_i,\, \boldsymbol{x}_j\rangle && \text{definition of the standard inner product}
\end{aligned}$$

for all $i, j \in \{1, \ldots, p\}$. Hence, the diagonal elements of the Gram matrix $X^\top X$ are the squared Euclidean lengths of the predictors: $(X^\top X)_{ii} = \langle \boldsymbol{x}_i, \boldsymbol{x}_i \rangle = \|\boldsymbol{x}_i\|_2^2$. And the off-diagonal elements of the Gram matrix are related to the correlations between predictors: $(X^\top X)_{ij} = \operatorname{cor}[\boldsymbol{x}_i, \boldsymbol{x}_j]\|\boldsymbol{x}_i\|_2\|\boldsymbol{x}_j\|_2$. This means that for normalized designs, the scaled Gram matrix $X^\top X/n$ is

$$\frac{X^\top X}{n} = \begin{pmatrix} 1 & \operatorname{cor}[\boldsymbol{x}_1, \boldsymbol{x}_2] & \cdots & \operatorname{cor}[\boldsymbol{x}_1, \boldsymbol{x}_p] \\ \operatorname{cor}[\boldsymbol{x}_2, \boldsymbol{x}_1] & 1 & & \vdots \\ \vdots & & \ddots & \operatorname{cor}[\boldsymbol{x}_{p-1}, \boldsymbol{x}_p] \\ \operatorname{cor}[\boldsymbol{x}_p, \boldsymbol{x}_1] & \cdots & \operatorname{cor}[\boldsymbol{x}_p, \boldsymbol{x}_{p-1}] & 1 \end{pmatrix}.$$

Thus, the scaled Gram matrix conveniently summarizes the correlations. In particular, $X^\top X/n = \mathrm{I}_{p\times p}$ for orthogonal designs, and more generally, the larger the magnitudes of the off-diagonal entries of $X^\top X/n$, the larger the correlations.

We now proceed as follows: We introduce regularized least-squares estimators in ▶ Sect. 2.2 and post-processing strategies for them in ▶ Sect. 2.3. The two following sections then form the mathematical basis for the remainder of this book, for example, for deriving guarantees of those high-dimensional estimators in terms of prediction: In ▶ Sect. 2.4, we establish the Hölder inequality (Theorem 2.4.1), which will allow us to transform basic inequalities into prediction bounds (▶ Sect. 6.3). In ▶ Sect. 2.5, we establish KKT conditions (Example 2.5.3), which will allow us to derive some basic inequalities in the first place (▶ Sect. 6.2).

2.2 Sparsity-Inducing Prior Functions

In the previous chapter, we have shown that classical estimators can deteriorate rapidly in performance with increasing number of model parameters. This deterioration can manifest in a phenomenon called *overfitting*—see ◘ Fig. 2.1: the estimators miss the essential structure of the data-generating process over the peculiarities of the data at hand. The culprit is the noise, because it masks the essential structure; the larger the noise, the higher the risk of overfitting—cf. (1.5). Overfitting can be avoided by complementing the bare measurements with additional information. Such information can stem from previous

overfitting

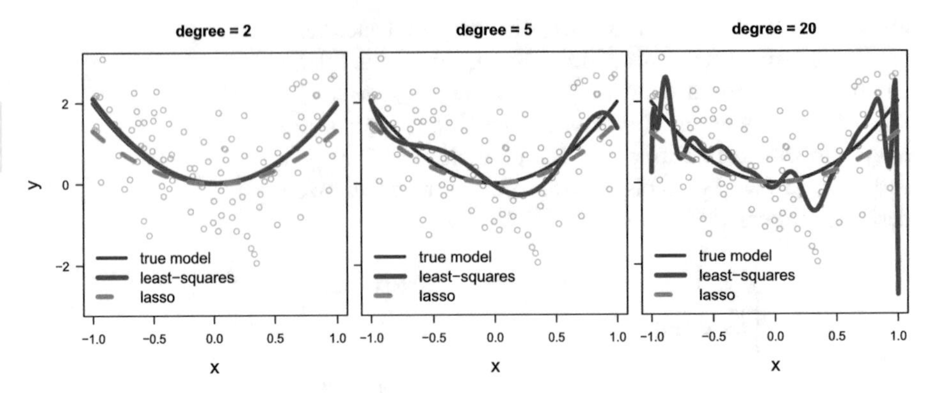

Fig. 2.1 This illustration of overfitting involves noisy observations (gray circles) of a simple quadratic function (red, solid curves) for fitting polynomials with the least-squares (blue, solid lines) and the lasso (green, dashed lines). The polynomials used in the estimations have degrees 2, 5, 20 (panels from left to right). The larger the degree of these polynomials, that is, the larger the number of irrelevant predictors (the degree of the true data-generating polynomial is 2), the less the least-squares estimates capture the shape of the underlying function; we call this overfitting. The lasso (with a cross-validated tuning parameter), on the other hand, simply disregards those additional predictors, and therefore, does not suffer from overfitting in this example. This is the case because the lasso assumes correctly that the underlying model is simple. See the lab for details

studies, the experimental design, physical laws, and other sources. Prior functions formulate this information mathematically and funnel it into the statistical analysis.

The type of information that is most frequently encountered in high-dimensional statistics is *sparsity*. A linear regression model of the form (2.1) is called sparse if only a small number of its model parameters are different from zero: $|\{j : \beta_j \neq 0\}| \ll n, p$. Similarly, an estimator $\widehat{\boldsymbol{\beta}} \in \mathbb{R}^p$ for the regression parameter $\boldsymbol{\beta}$ is called sparse if it produces a sparse model: $|\{j : \widehat{\beta}_j \neq 0\}| \ll n, p$; and more generally, a vector $\boldsymbol{\alpha} \in \mathbb{R}^p$ is called sparse if it contains only a small number of non-zero-valued coordinates as compared to the model dimensions: $|\{j : \alpha_j \neq 0\}| \ll n, p$.

best-subset selection

The first attempt to leverage sparsity is the *best-subset selection estimator*

$$\widehat{\boldsymbol{\beta}}_{\text{subset}} \in \underset{\boldsymbol{\alpha}\in\mathbb{R}^p}{\arg\min} \left\{ \|\boldsymbol{y} - X\boldsymbol{\alpha}\|_2^2 + r\|\boldsymbol{\alpha}\|_0 \right\},$$

where $r \in [0, \infty)$ is a tuning parameter and $\|\boldsymbol{\alpha}\|_0 = \#\{j \in \{1, \ldots, p\} : \alpha_j \neq 0\}$ counts the number of non-zero-valued coordinates in $\boldsymbol{\alpha}$. The least-squares term $\|\boldsymbol{y} - X\boldsymbol{\alpha}\|_2^2$ ensures a good fit to the data, while the ℓ_0-prior term favors regression vectors that have only a small number of non-zero-valued coordinates.

The ℓ_0-prior is a non-convex, non-linear, "combinatorial" function, which makes the objective function $\boldsymbol{a} \mapsto \|\boldsymbol{y} - X\boldsymbol{a}\|_2^2 + r\|\boldsymbol{a}\|_0$ hard to optimize—especially for large p. One approach to reducing this computational burden is to mimic $\|\boldsymbol{\alpha}\|_0$ through $\|\boldsymbol{\alpha}\|_q := (\sum_{j=1}^{p} |\alpha_j|^q)^{1/q}$ for some $q \in (0, \infty)$.[3] Especially interesting are $q \in [1, \infty)$, because these values lead to convex objective functions (see ▶ Sect. 2.5), for which there are standard optimization algorithms. We have already seen a corresponding estimator in the previous chapter: the ridge estimator, where $q = 2$. The ridge estimator is particularly easy to compute (it even has an explicit solution), but it does not yield sparse models—see ◘ Fig. 2.2. A closer mimic of the best-subset selection estimator is the *lasso estimator*,[4] where $q = 1$:

lasso

$$\widehat{\boldsymbol{\beta}}_{\text{lasso}} \in \operatorname*{arg\,min}_{\boldsymbol{\alpha} \in \mathbb{R}^p} \left\{ \|\boldsymbol{y} - X\boldsymbol{\alpha}\|_2^2 + r\|\boldsymbol{\alpha}\|_1 \right\}. \tag{2.2}$$

The lasso has the best of two worlds: its objective function is convex and produces sparse solutions; in fact, $q = 1$ is the only choice that ensures both convexity and sparsity—see again ◘ Fig. 2.2.

Refinements of the simple notion of sparsity above are called *structured sparsity*. For example, structured sparsity in the form of *group sparsity* describes group-wise behaviors: Consider a partition of the index set $\{1, \dots, p\}$, that is, a collection of disjoint, non-empty sets $\mathcal{A}_1, \dots, \mathcal{A}_k \subset \{1, \dots, p\}$ that satisfy $\cup_{j=1}^{k} \mathcal{A}_j = \{1, \dots, p\}$. Sparsity means that only a small number of *individual* coordinates are not equal to zero: $|\{j : \beta_j \neq 0\}| \ll n, p$; in contrast, group sparsity now means that only a small number of *groups* of coordinates as indexed by the sets $\mathcal{A}_j$ are not equal to zero: $|\{j : \boldsymbol{\beta}_{\mathcal{A}_j} \neq \mathbf{0}_{|\mathcal{A}_j|}\}| \ll n, p$. An estimator that leverages this type of structured sparsity is the *group-lasso estimator*:[5]

structured sparsity

group lasso

$$\widehat{\boldsymbol{\beta}}_{\text{group}} \in \operatorname*{arg\,min}_{\boldsymbol{\alpha} \in \mathbb{R}^p} \left\{ \|\boldsymbol{y} - X\boldsymbol{\alpha}\|_2^2 + r\sum_{j=1}^{k} \|\boldsymbol{\alpha}_{\mathcal{A}_j}\|_2 \right\}. \tag{2.3}$$

The group lasso can be thought of as an intermediate between the lasso and ridge estimators: The group lasso coincides with the lasso when $k = p$ and $\mathcal{A}_j = \{j\}$ and, more generally, inherits the sparsity of the lasso in the sense that it sets entire subvectors $\boldsymbol{\alpha}_{\mathcal{A}_j}$ to zero. The group lasso coincides with the ridge estimator (or the

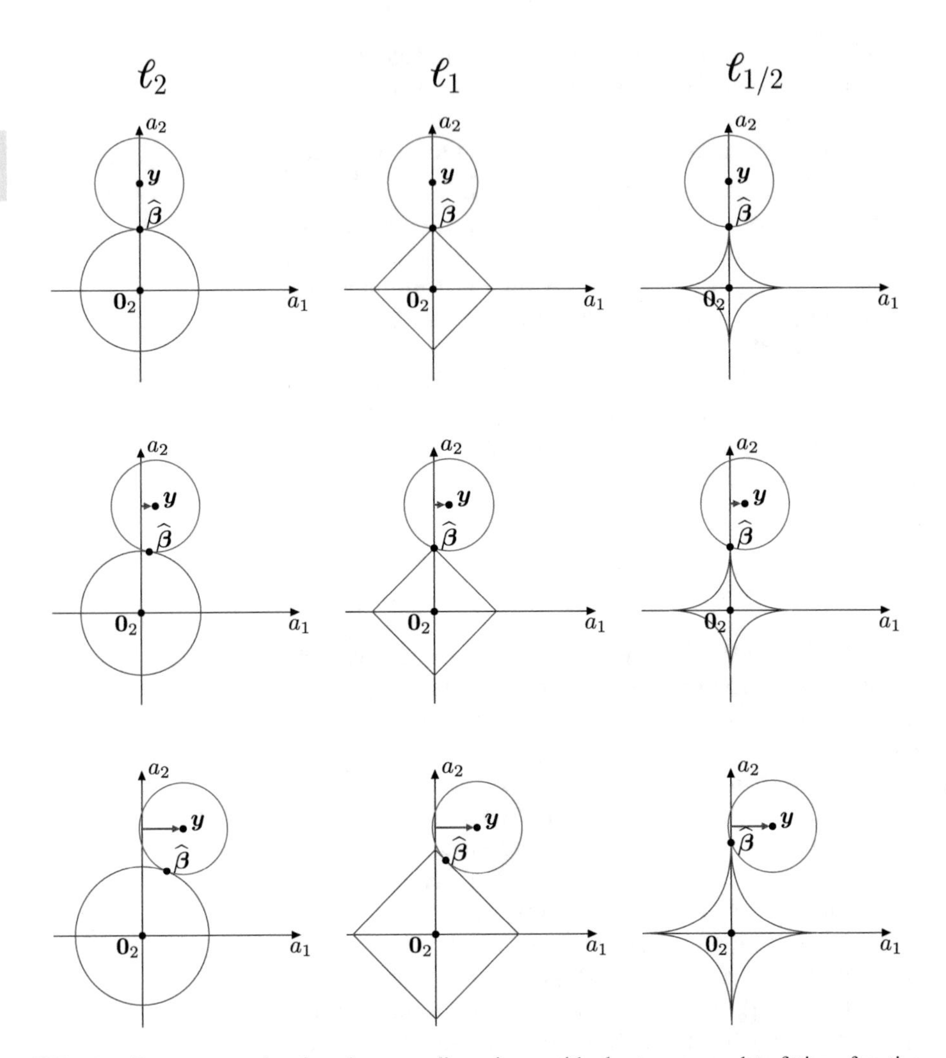

Fig. 2.2 Parameter estimation in two dimensions with least-squares data-fitting function $a \mapsto \|y - Xa\|_2^2$ and ℓ_2- (ridge), ℓ_1- (lasso), and $\ell_{1/2}$-prior function. The design is $X = I_{2\times 2}$ throughout, while the outcome $y \in \mathbb{R}^2$ is altered from top to bottom. The tuning parameters are chosen such that all estimators' fits are equal: $\|y - X\widehat{\beta}\|_2^2 = b$ for some constant $b \in (0, \infty)$; the blue circles denote the corresponding level sets $\{a \in \mathbb{R}^2 : \|y - Xa\|_2^2 = b\}$. Since the estimators minimize a weighted sum of the data-fitting function and the prior function, they are found where a blue level set of the least-squares function "touches" a level set of the prior function; those latter level sets are drawn in red. The different touching points illustrate that the ridge estimator yields zero-valued coordinates only in very special cases (in the first column, $\widehat{\beta}_1 = 0$ only on the top), while zero-valued coordinates are more common for the lasso estimator and especially for the estimator with the $\ell_{1/2}$-prior function ($\widehat{\beta}_1 = 0$ on the top and middle of the second column and across all of the third column). The shapes of the red level sets also indicate that the ℓ_2- and ℓ_1-prior functions lead to convex objective functions, while the $\ell_{1/2}$-prior function does not—see see ▶ Sect. 2.5 for details. The ℓ_1-regularizer is a sweet spot in that it typically yields sparse solutions (in contrast to ℓ_q with $q > 1$) and, at the same time, makes the objective function amenable to convex optimization (in contrast to ℓ_q with $q < 1$)

Euclidean distance ridge estimator)[6] when $k = 1$ and $\mathscr{A}_1 = \{1, \ldots, p\}$, and more generally, acts like the ridge within the groups in the sense that the objective function is invariant under orthogonal transformations within groups and that if $\|\boldsymbol{\alpha}_{\mathscr{A}_j}\|_2 \neq 0$, then typically *all* coordinates of that subvector are non-zero-valued.

Estimators can also comprise combinations of several prior functions. A popular example is the *elastic net estimator*[7]

elastic net

$$\widehat{\boldsymbol{\beta}}_{\text{elastic}} \in \underset{\boldsymbol{\alpha} \in \mathbb{R}^p}{\arg\min} \left\{ \|\boldsymbol{y} - X\boldsymbol{\alpha}\|_2^2 + r\big(w\|\boldsymbol{\alpha}\|_1 + (1-w)\|\boldsymbol{\alpha}\|_2^2\big) \right\},$$

which interpolates between the lasso ($w = 1$) and the ridge ($w = 0$). The elastic net with an intermediate value $w \in (0, 1)$ inherits properties from both of the two base estimators: On the one hand, the resulting estimator is similar to the lasso in the sense that it tends to be sparse; on the other hand, the resulting estimator is much unlike the lasso but instead similar to the ridge in the sense that it is always unique and tends to select whole groups of highly correlated predictors rather than just one representative among them.[8] The value of w is often fixed based on subjective reasonings beforehand, because a fully data-driven calibration of both tuning parameters $r \in [0, \infty)$ and $w \in [0, 1]$ is conceptually and computationally challenging. In general, combining prior functions always involves the problem of having to deal with multiple tuning parameters.

2.3 Post-Processing Methods

Prior functions push estimators in the directions indicated by the prior information. This can improve estimation in high dimensions, but it can also generate a bias. This bias is the target of *post-processing methods*. A first method, least-squares refitting, applies a least-squares estimator to the support of the estimator. This uses the fact that the least-squares estimator is unbiased in low dimensions. A second method, thresholding, simply sets small elements of the estimator to zero. This reinforces the effect of sparsity-inducing priors and, thereby, can decrease the amount of regularization that is needed in the first place. Both methods should, however, be applied with care: least-squares refitting can sometimes even increase estimation errors, and thresholding introduces yet another tuning parameter.

The ℓ_0-function favors solutions with many zero-valued coordinates, but it completely disregards parameter values otherwise: for example, $\|\boldsymbol{\alpha}\|_0 = 1$ whether $\boldsymbol{\alpha} = (1, 0, \ldots, 0)^\top$ or $\boldsymbol{\alpha} = (100, 0, \ldots, 0)^\top$. In contrast, the discussed replacements of that function keep increasing in the magnitudes of the parameter values: for example, $\|\boldsymbol{\alpha}\|_1 = 1$ for $\boldsymbol{\alpha} = (1, 0, \ldots, 0)^\top$ but $\|\boldsymbol{\alpha}\|_1 = 100$ for $\boldsymbol{\alpha} = (100, 0, \ldots, 0)^\top$. In addition to setting a fraction of the model parameters exactly to zero as intended, this general favoring of small model parameters can introduce an unwanted *overall* shrinkage of the estimates. To remove such biases, *least-squares refitting*[9] complements high-dimensional estimators $\widehat{\boldsymbol{\beta}}$ with subsequent least-squares estimation on its support:

least-squares refitting

$$\widehat{\boldsymbol{\beta}}_{\mathrm{ls}}[\widehat{\boldsymbol{\beta}}] \in \underset{\substack{\boldsymbol{\alpha}\in\mathbb{R}^p \\ \mathrm{supp}[\boldsymbol{\alpha}]\subset\mathrm{supp}[\widehat{\boldsymbol{\beta}}]}}{\arg\min} \|\boldsymbol{y} - X\boldsymbol{\alpha}\|_2^2 .$$

In other words, the initial estimator is used only for a screening for non-zero-valued coordinates, while the corresponding parameter values are determined entirely by the subsequent least-squares. The rationale is that the least-squares is an accurate and unbiased estimator in low-dimensional and correctly specified models (see ▶ Sect. 1.3); hence, the two-stage approach presumes that the initial estimator is sparse, which means here $|\mathrm{supp}[\widehat{\boldsymbol{\beta}}]| \ll n$, and that the initial estimator provides accurate support recovery, that is, $\mathrm{supp}[\widehat{\boldsymbol{\beta}}]$ is a good approximation of the true support $\mathrm{supp}[\boldsymbol{\beta}]$. In the ideal case $\mathrm{supp}[\widehat{\boldsymbol{\beta}}] = \mathrm{supp}[\boldsymbol{\beta}]$, the least-squares refitted estimator possesses the *strong oracle property*, which means that the refitted estimator $\widehat{\boldsymbol{\beta}}_{\mathrm{ls}}[\widehat{\boldsymbol{\beta}}]$ equals the oracle "estimator"

$$\widehat{\boldsymbol{\beta}}_{\mathrm{ls}}[\boldsymbol{\beta}] \in \underset{\substack{\boldsymbol{\alpha}\in\mathbb{R}^p \\ \mathrm{supp}[\boldsymbol{\alpha}]\subset\mathrm{supp}[\boldsymbol{\beta}]}}{\arg\min} \|\boldsymbol{y} - X\boldsymbol{\alpha}\|_2^2 ,$$

which knows the true support beforehand; in particular, $\widehat{\boldsymbol{\beta}}_{\mathrm{ls}}[\boldsymbol{\beta}]$ is unbiased (see ▶ Sect. 1.3). But in practice, exact support recovery $\mathrm{supp}[\widehat{\boldsymbol{\beta}}] = \mathrm{supp}[\boldsymbol{\beta}]$ is often unrealistic and, in any case, unverifiable (see ▶ Sect. 7.4 for a discussion about support recovery).[10,11]

To a varying extent, least-squares refitting is already integrated in many estimators. For example, least-squares refitting leaves best-subset selection completely

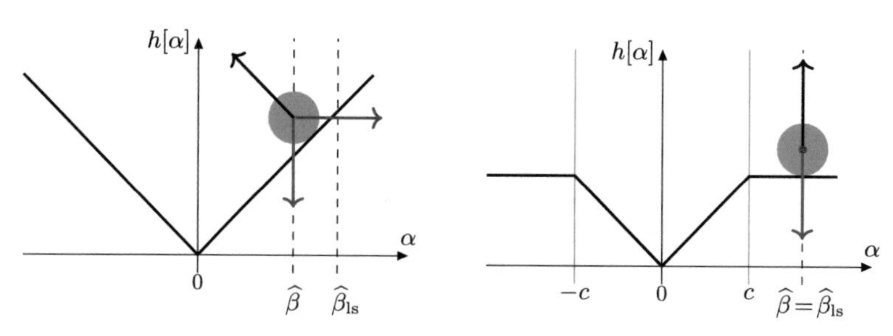

Fig. 2.3 A physics analogy for how capping a prior function can avoid bias in large parameter estimates. The toy estimator is $\widehat{\beta} \in \arg\min_{\alpha \in \mathbb{R}}\{\|\boldsymbol{y} - \alpha \boldsymbol{x}\|_2^2 + rh[\alpha]\}$, where $\boldsymbol{x} \in \mathbb{R}^n$ is the only predictor and $r \in (0, \infty)$ a fixed tuning parameter. On the left, $h[a] := |a|$ is the usual ℓ_1-prior in $\mathbb{R}$; on the right, $h[a] := \min\{|a|, c\}$ is a capped version with $c \in (0, \infty)$ defining the transition point. One can think of the estimator's objective function as a physical potential for an iron ball at α that is subject to three forces: 1. a "magnetic force" (red) that is generated by the magnitude of the least-squares function at that point; this force pulls the ball horizontally to the least-squares solution $\widehat{\beta}_{\text{ls}} = \boldsymbol{x}^\top \boldsymbol{y}/\|\boldsymbol{x}\|_2^2$; 2. a "gravitational force" (blue) that is generated by the magnitude of the prior function; this force pulls the ball vertically downwards; 3. a "normal force" (black) that is generated by the slope of the prior function; this force pushes the ball upwards perpendicular to the surface. The three forces are in equilibrium at $\widehat{\beta}$. For the ℓ_1-prior on the left, the inclined surface allows the gravitational force, more precisely, its component parallel to the surface, to pull the estimate away from the (typically unbiased) least-squares solution. For the capped prior on the right, this is still the case if $|\widehat{\beta}_{\text{ls}}| < c$. If $|\widehat{\beta}_{\text{ls}}| \geq c$, on the other hand, the gravitational force is perpendicular to the surface and, therefore, cannot work against the magnetic force anymore. The magnetic force then moves the ball all the way to the least-squares solution, which is the minimum of the magnetic potential (and, consequently, the magnetic force is zero there). This means that our toy estimator can coincide with a least-squares solution even though regularization is imposed

unchanged, that is, $\widehat{\boldsymbol{f}}_{\text{ls}}[\widehat{\boldsymbol{\beta}}_{\text{subset}}] = \widehat{\boldsymbol{\beta}}_{\text{subset}}$. This means that adding least-squares refitting to the best-subset selection estimator would be redundant. Other examples are least-squares with variants of the capped ℓ_1-norm as prior. The capped ℓ_1-norm with cutoff $c \in [0, \infty]$, is the map $\boldsymbol{a} \mapsto \sum_{j=1}^{p} \min\{|a_j|, c\}$. The boundary cases for least-squares with this prior are classical least-squares (for $c = 0$, the prior is zero) and lasso (for $c = \infty$, the prior is the ℓ_1-function); more generally, c is the value below which model parameters are pulled toward zero—see Fig. 2.3. Smooth versions of the capped ℓ_1-norm are used in the *scad* and *mcp* estimators, for example.[12] Such estimators have been shown to satisfy the strong oracle property if $\text{supp}[\widehat{\boldsymbol{\beta}}] = \text{supp}[\boldsymbol{\beta}]$.[13] However, (i) exact support recovery remains a strict and unverifiable assumption; (ii) capped ℓ_1-norms render the objective functions non-convex, which can make computations challenging; and (iii) the prior functions involve one or more additional

scad and mcp

tuning parameters, such as a in the vanilla case of capped ℓ_1-regularization, that need to be calibrated.[14] In practice, these difficulties have to be weighted against a potential gain in accuracy.

thresholding

Thresholding sets small estimates to zero. Given a *cut-off* $c \in [0, \infty]$, we define the hard-thresholded version $\widehat{\boldsymbol{\beta}}^c$ of an estimator $\widehat{\boldsymbol{\beta}}$ via

$$(\widehat{\beta}^c)_j := \begin{cases} 0 & \text{if } |\widehat{\beta}_j| \leq c \\ \widehat{\beta}_j & \text{otherwise} \end{cases} \tag{2.4}$$

for $j \in \{1, \ldots, p\}$. While $\widehat{\boldsymbol{\beta}}^0 = \widehat{\boldsymbol{\beta}}$, thresholding with $c > 0$ sets small coordinate values of $\widehat{\boldsymbol{\beta}}$ to zero. This means that thresholding promotes sparsity further, with the effect that the estimator $\widehat{\boldsymbol{\beta}}$ can use a smaller tuning parameter—and, therefore, can have smaller bias—and still lead to a sparse output. However, thresholding requires calibration of both the original tuning parameter and of the cutoff c; see ► Sect. 7.4 for details.

One can also combine least-squares refitting and thresholding—at the expense of an even more complex pipeline. In general, we recommend using post-processing methods cautiously.

2.4 Hölder Inequality*

The analysis of regularized least-squares estimators centers around inner products of the form $\langle X^\top \boldsymbol{u}, \boldsymbol{a}\rangle$ with $\boldsymbol{a} \in \mathbb{R}^p$. In particular, such inner products determine good tuning parameters—see ► Chaps. 4, 6, and 7. Our main tool for working with these inner products is the *Hölder inequality*. The classical version of Hölder inequality bounds inner products in terms of ℓ_q-norms and their duals. In this section, we establish a generalized version and use it to connect inner products to prior information and regularization.

(Hölder) dual function

The essential ingredients of the Hölder inequality are dual functions.

Definition 2.4.1

Dual Functions Given a function $\hbar : \mathbb{R}^p \to \mathbb{R}$, we define $\overline{\hbar} : \mathbb{R}^p \to [-\infty, \infty]$ through

$$\overline{\hbar} : \boldsymbol{a} \mapsto \sup\left\{ \langle \boldsymbol{a}, \boldsymbol{c} \rangle : \boldsymbol{c} \in \mathbb{R}^p, \hbar[\boldsymbol{c}] \leq 1 \right\},$$

where $\langle \boldsymbol{a}, \boldsymbol{c} \rangle = \sum_{j=1}^{p} a_j c_j$ is the standard inner product. As a convention, we set the supremum over the empty set to $-\infty$. We call $\overline{\hbar}$ the *Hölder dual function* of $\hbar$ or simply the *dual function* of $\hbar$.

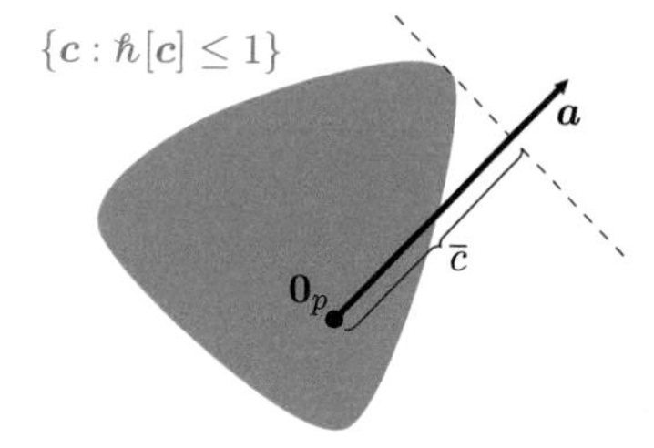

In the illustration to the right, the red area depicts the unit "ball" with respect to some $\hbar$, namely $\{\boldsymbol{c} : \hbar[\boldsymbol{c}] \leq 1\}$. The solid line depicts the 1-dimensional space spanned by the vector $\boldsymbol{a}$, and the dashed line depicts the $(p-1)$-dimensional hyperplane that is orthogonal to this space and the furthest into the direction of $\boldsymbol{a}$ while still touching the unit ball. The quantity $\overline{c}$ then denotes the distance[15] of the origin to this hyperplane; in other words, $\overline{c}$ measures the size of the unit ball in direction $\boldsymbol{a}$. The value of the dual function at $\boldsymbol{a}$ is finally the product of this quantity $\overline{c}$ and the Euclidean length of $\boldsymbol{a}$, that is, $\overline{\hbar}[\boldsymbol{a}] = \overline{c}\|\boldsymbol{a}\|_2$. Thus, the scaled version $\boldsymbol{a} \mapsto \overline{\hbar}[\boldsymbol{a}]/\|\boldsymbol{a}\|_2$ of the dual function describes the shape of the unit ball that is generated by $\hbar$.

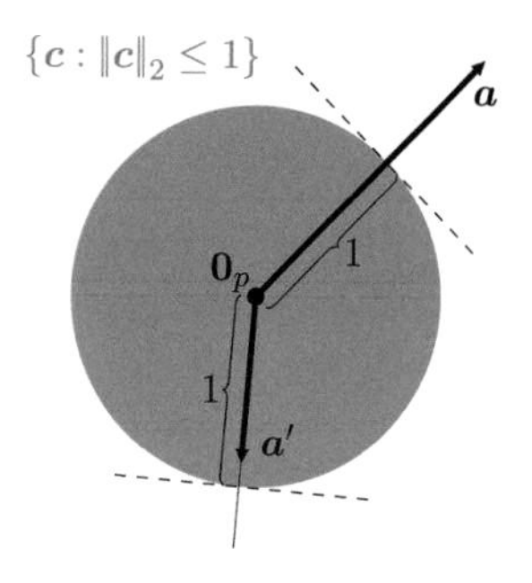

The unit ball of the Euclidean norm $\hbar : \boldsymbol{a} \mapsto \|\boldsymbol{a}\|_2$, for example, is "round" in the sense that it is invariant under rotations. Hence, the distance $\overline{c}$ is always equal to 1—see the illustration. This means that the dual function of the Euclidean norm is again the Euclidean norm (see also 3. of Exercise 2.2), that is, $\overline{\hbar} : \boldsymbol{a} \mapsto \overline{c}\|\boldsymbol{a}\|_2 = \|\boldsymbol{a}\|_2$.

Exercise 2.3 states a number of properties of dual functions. But important here is that dual functions allow us to bound inner products through the Hölder inequality.

Hölder inequality

Theorem 2.4.1

General Hölder Inequality Let $\hbar : \mathbb{R}^p \to [0, \infty]$ be a non-negative function that satisfies

1. (positive definiteness) $\hbar[\boldsymbol{a}] = 0$ if and only if $\boldsymbol{a} = \mathbf{0}_p$;
2. (scalability) $\hbar[\boldsymbol{a}/\hbar[\boldsymbol{a}]] \le 1$ for all $\boldsymbol{a} \in \mathbb{R}^p \setminus \{\mathbf{0}_p\}$.

Then, also the dual function $\overline{\hbar}$ of $\hbar$ is positive definite and

$$\langle \boldsymbol{a}, \boldsymbol{b} \rangle \le \overline{\hbar}[\boldsymbol{a}]\hbar[\boldsymbol{b}] \qquad \text{for all } \boldsymbol{a}, \boldsymbol{b} \in \mathbb{R}^p . \tag{2.5}$$

The algebra rules on the extended real line $[-\infty, \infty]$ are summarized on Page X. The scalability stipulates some sort of linearity; in particular, every linear function (and similarly, every absolute homogeneous function) is scalable.[16] The positive definiteness essentially avoids dividing by zero. Both conditions are satisfied by every norm. Finally, since both the dual function and the original function are positive definite (according to the first claim of the theorem and by assumption, respectively), the right-hand side of Inequality (2.5) is always non-negative.

A typical first step in the analysis of a regularized least-squares estimator $\widehat{\boldsymbol{\beta}}$ is the decomposition of its objective function (▶ Sect. 6.2):

$$\begin{aligned}\|\boldsymbol{y} - X\boldsymbol{\alpha}\|_2^2 + r\hbar[\boldsymbol{\alpha}] &= \|X\boldsymbol{\beta} - X\boldsymbol{\alpha}\|_2^2 + 2\langle X^\top \boldsymbol{u}, \boldsymbol{\beta} - \boldsymbol{\alpha}\rangle \\ &\quad + \|\boldsymbol{u}\|_2^2 + r\hbar[\boldsymbol{\alpha}] ,\end{aligned}$$

where we have used the linear regression model $\boldsymbol{y} = X\boldsymbol{\beta} + \boldsymbol{u}$ in (2.1). The next step is then to control the inner product $2\langle X^\top \boldsymbol{u}, \boldsymbol{\beta} - \boldsymbol{\alpha}\rangle$ (▶ Sect. 6.3). Elementary trigonometry teaches us that $\langle \boldsymbol{a}, \boldsymbol{b}\rangle = \cos[\angle_{\boldsymbol{a},\boldsymbol{b}}]\|\boldsymbol{a}\|_2\|\boldsymbol{b}\|_2$ for every pair of vectors $\boldsymbol{a}, \boldsymbol{b} \in \mathbb{R}^p$, where $\angle_{\boldsymbol{a},\boldsymbol{b}}$ is the angle between $\boldsymbol{a}$ and $\boldsymbol{b}$. To avoid working with angles, we can use the estimate $|\cos[\angle_{\boldsymbol{a},\boldsymbol{b}}]| \le 1$, which leads to the bound $\langle X^\top \boldsymbol{u}, \boldsymbol{\beta} - \boldsymbol{\alpha}\rangle \le \|X^\top \boldsymbol{u}\|_2 \|\boldsymbol{\beta} - \boldsymbol{\alpha}\|_2$. This bound nicely separates the model parameters $\boldsymbol{\alpha}, \boldsymbol{\beta}$ from the rest of the problem, but it does not relate to the prior term $r\hbar[\boldsymbol{\alpha}]$. To bring the separation in accordance with $r\hbar[\boldsymbol{\alpha}]$, we instead apply the Hölder inequality, which yields $\langle X^\top \boldsymbol{u}, \boldsymbol{\beta} - \boldsymbol{\alpha}\rangle \le \overline{\hbar}[X^\top \boldsymbol{u}]\hbar[\boldsymbol{\beta} - \boldsymbol{\alpha}]$. This separates $\boldsymbol{\alpha}, \boldsymbol{\beta}$ from the rest (which we will identify later as the effective noise of regularized estimators) in a way that makes appear the prior function $\hbar$. In this sense, the Hölder inequality allows us to connect inner products to prior information and regularization.

This property makes the Hölder inequality indispensable for high-dimensional statistics, but the inequality is also important in mathematics more generally. Mostly, it is stated in its classical form:

► Example 2.4.1

Classical Hölder Inequality In this example, we show that Theorem 2.4.1 implies the classical Hölder inequality. The classical version reads

$$\langle \boldsymbol{a}, \boldsymbol{b} \rangle \leq \|\boldsymbol{a}\|_l \|\boldsymbol{b}\|_m \tag{2.6}$$

for $\boldsymbol{a}, \boldsymbol{b} \in \mathbb{R}^p$ and $l, m \in [1, \infty]$ such that $1/l + 1/m = 1$ (where $1/\infty = 0$ by convention—see Page X). The special case $l = m = 2$ is called *Cauchy–Schwarz inequality*.

One can check that $\hbar : \boldsymbol{a} \mapsto \|\boldsymbol{a}\|_m$ satisfies both conditions in Theorem 2.4.1, which means that we can apply the theorem to $\hbar = \|\cdot\|_m$. The dual of that function is $\overline{\hbar} = \|\cdot\|_l$ (see 3. in Exercise 2.2). Hence, Inequality (2.5) in the theorem applied to $\hbar = \|\cdot\|_m$ coincides with the above classical version of the Hölder inequality.◄

We conclude this section by proving the Hölder inequality.

Proof of Theorem 2.4.1 The proof is based on the definition of dual functions and on the linearity of inner products. A subtlety is the calculus with infinite values.

We first prove that $\overline{\hbar}$ is positive definite under the stated assumptions. We observe that

$$\begin{aligned}
\overline{\hbar}[\mathbf{0}_p] &= \sup\left\{ \langle \mathbf{0}_p, \boldsymbol{c} \rangle \,:\, \boldsymbol{c} \in \mathbb{R}^p,\, \hbar[\boldsymbol{c}] \leq 1 \right\} && \text{Definition 2.4.1 (dual functions)}\\
&= \sup\left\{ 0 \,:\, \boldsymbol{c} \in \mathbb{R}^p,\, \hbar[\boldsymbol{c}] \leq 1 \right\} && \text{linearity of inner products}\\
&= 0\,. && \text{Assumption 1. ensures that } \{\boldsymbol{c} \in \mathbb{R}^p : \hbar[\boldsymbol{c}] \leq 1\} \supset \{\mathbf{0}_p\} \neq \varnothing
\end{aligned}$$

Next, it holds for all $\boldsymbol{a} \neq \mathbf{0}_p$ that

$$\sup\left\{ \langle \boldsymbol{a}, \boldsymbol{c} \rangle \,:\, \boldsymbol{c} \in \mathbb{R}^p,\, \hbar[\boldsymbol{c}] \leq 1 \right\} \geq \langle \boldsymbol{a}, \boldsymbol{a}/\hbar[\boldsymbol{a}] \rangle\,.$$

To see this, set $\boldsymbol{c} = \boldsymbol{a}/\hbar[\boldsymbol{a}]$ on the left-hand side, noting that $\hbar[\boldsymbol{a}] > 0$ by the 1. assumption (positive definiteness of $\hbar$) and $\hbar[\boldsymbol{a}/\hbar[\boldsymbol{a}]] \leq 1$ by the 2. assumption (scalability of $\hbar$).

This observation allows us to derive for every $\boldsymbol{a} \neq \mathbf{0}_p$

$$\begin{aligned}
\overline{\hbar}[\boldsymbol{a}] &= \sup\left\{ \langle \boldsymbol{a}, \boldsymbol{c} \rangle \,:\, \boldsymbol{c} \in \mathbb{R}^p, \hbar[\boldsymbol{c}] \leq 1 \right\} && \text{definition of the dual function } \overline{\hbar} \\
&\geq \langle \boldsymbol{a}, \boldsymbol{a}/\hbar[\boldsymbol{a}] \rangle && \text{above observation} \\
&= \frac{\langle \boldsymbol{a}, \boldsymbol{a} \rangle}{\hbar[\boldsymbol{a}]} && \text{linearity of inner products} \\
&> 0\,. && \langle \boldsymbol{a}, \boldsymbol{a} \rangle = \|\boldsymbol{a}\|_2^2 > 0 \text{ for all } \boldsymbol{a} \neq \mathbf{0}_p;\ \hbar[\boldsymbol{a}] > 0 \text{ by 1. (positive definiteness of } \hbar)
\end{aligned}$$

Details

Since a/∞ is well-defined for all $a \in \mathbb{R}$—see Page X—this derivation holds irrespective of whether $\hbar[\boldsymbol{a}]$ is finite or not.

Hence, $\overline{\hbar}[\boldsymbol{a}] \geq 0$ with equality if and only if $\boldsymbol{a} = \mathbf{0}_p$, which means that $\overline{\hbar}$ is positive definite, as desired.

The proof of Inequality (2.5) is divided into three cases.

Case 1 $\hbar[\boldsymbol{b}] = 0$. The left-hand side of the inequality in question then equals

$$\begin{aligned}
\langle \boldsymbol{a}, \boldsymbol{b} \rangle &= \langle \boldsymbol{a}, \mathbf{0}_p \rangle && \hbar[\boldsymbol{b}] = 0 \Rightarrow \boldsymbol{b} = 0_p \text{ by 1. (positive definiteness of } \hbar) \\
&= 0\,. && \text{linearity of inner products}
\end{aligned}$$

The right-hand side of the inequality in question satisfies

$$\begin{aligned}
\overline{\hbar}[\boldsymbol{a}]\hbar[\boldsymbol{b}] &= \overline{\hbar}[\boldsymbol{a}] \cdot 0 && \hbar[\boldsymbol{b}] = 0 \text{ by assumption} \\
&= 0\,. && \infty \cdot 0 = 0 \text{ by the conventions on Page X}
\end{aligned}$$

Combining the displays yields $\langle \boldsymbol{a}, \boldsymbol{b} \rangle = \overline{\hbar}[\boldsymbol{a}]\hbar[\boldsymbol{b}]$, which implies the desired inequality (2.5).

Case 2 $\hbar[\boldsymbol{b}] \neq 0$, $\hbar[\boldsymbol{b}] \neq \infty$. We find

$$\begin{aligned}
&\langle \boldsymbol{a},\, \boldsymbol{b}\rangle \\
&= \langle \boldsymbol{a},\, \boldsymbol{b} \cdot \frac{\hbar[\boldsymbol{b}]}{\hbar[\boldsymbol{b}]}\rangle && \hbar[\boldsymbol{b}] \notin \{0, \infty\} \text{ by assumption} \\
&= \langle \boldsymbol{a},\, \boldsymbol{b}/\hbar[\boldsymbol{b}]\rangle \cdot \hbar[\boldsymbol{b}]\,. && \text{linearity of inner products}
\end{aligned}$$

Since $\hbar$ is non-negative by assumption, we are left with showing that $\langle \boldsymbol{a},\, \boldsymbol{b}/\hbar[\boldsymbol{b}]\rangle \leq \overline{\hbar}[\boldsymbol{a}]$.

The scalability of $\hbar$ assumed in 2. ensures that

$$\hbar\left[\frac{\boldsymbol{b}}{\hbar[\boldsymbol{b}]}\right] \leq 1\,.$$

Therefore,

$$\begin{aligned}
&\langle \boldsymbol{a},\, \boldsymbol{b}/\hbar[\boldsymbol{b}]\rangle \\
&\leq \sup\left\{\langle \boldsymbol{a},\, \boldsymbol{c}\rangle \;:\; \boldsymbol{c} \in \mathbb{R}^p,\; \hbar[\boldsymbol{c}] \leq 1\right\} && \text{considering } \boldsymbol{c} = \boldsymbol{b}/\hbar[\boldsymbol{b}];\ \hbar[\boldsymbol{b}/\hbar[\boldsymbol{b}]] \leq 1 \text{ by the previous display} \\
&= \overline{\hbar}[\boldsymbol{a}]\,, && \text{definition of the dual function } \overline{\hbar}
\end{aligned}$$

as desired.

Case 3 $\hbar[\boldsymbol{b}] = \infty$. If $\overline{\hbar}[\boldsymbol{a}] \neq 0$, the right-hand side of the desired inequality is infinite—see the conventions on Page X and recall that $\overline{\hbar} \geq 0$ according to above. This then means that the inequality holds irrespective of the left-hand side.

If $\overline{\hbar}[\boldsymbol{a}] = 0$, the right-hand side of the desired inequality is zero—see again the conventions on Page X. However, since $\overline{\hbar}$ is positive definite as shown above, it then also holds that $\boldsymbol{a} = \mathbf{0}_p$, and therefore, using the linearity of inner products, $\langle \boldsymbol{a},\, \boldsymbol{b}\rangle = 0$. Thus, $\langle \boldsymbol{a},\, \boldsymbol{b}\rangle = \overline{\hbar}[\boldsymbol{a}]\hbar[\boldsymbol{b}] = 0$, which is commensurate with Inequality (2.5).

This concludes the proof of Theorem 2.4.1. □

2.5 Optimality Conditions*

Many high-dimensional estimators are minimizers of a convex objective function. Some of these objective functions are also differentiable: For example, the ridge estimator (1.7) is the minimizer of the objective function $f_{\text{ridge}} : \boldsymbol{a} \mapsto \|\boldsymbol{y} - X\boldsymbol{a}\|_2^2 + r\|\boldsymbol{a}\|_2^2$, which is both (strictly) convex and differentiable. In ▶ Sect. 1.4, we have exploited the differentiability of the ridge estimator's objective function to derive an explicit formulation for the estimator. Our strategy for this was to set the gradient of the objective function to zero and then solve for the estimator. On the other hand, objective functions of high-dimensional estimators are not always differentiable, and, therefore, there might not be a gradient to start with: for example, the lasso estimator (2.2) is the minimizer of $f_{\text{lasso}} : \boldsymbol{a} \mapsto \|\boldsymbol{y} - X\boldsymbol{a}\|_2^2 + r\|\boldsymbol{a}\|_1$, which is still convex (see Example 2.5.1 below) but not differentiable. However, as long as objective functions are convex, they can be equipped with *generalized* gradients called subgradients (see Definition 2.5.2 below). Setting these subgradients to zero does not necessarily provide explicit formulations as in the case of the ridge estimator and, therefore, does not necessarily provide a direct way to compute the estimators, but the equations characterize the estimators in a way that is very useful in developing algorithms and mathematical guarantees (see ▶ Sects. 6.2 and 7.3, for example). We call these characterizations optimality conditions or, in the special case of regularized least-squares estimators, KKT conditions.

convex function

The crucial concept in this section is convexity. A function is *convex* if its graph[17] is on or below the closed line segment[18] between any two points in the graph; a function is *strictly convex* if its graph is strictly below the open line segment between any two points in the graph. The two concepts are illustrated in ◘ Fig. 2.4 and recorded in the following definition:

Definition 2.5.1

Convex Functions A function $f : \mathbb{R}^p \to \mathbb{R}$ is *convex*[19] if and only if

$$f[w\boldsymbol{a} + (1-w)\boldsymbol{b}] \leq wf[\boldsymbol{a}] + (1-w)f[\boldsymbol{b}] \qquad \text{for all } w \in [0,1];\ \boldsymbol{a}, \boldsymbol{b} \in \mathbb{R}^p .$$

The function f is also *strictly convex* if

$$f[w\boldsymbol{a} + (1-w)\boldsymbol{b}] < wf[\boldsymbol{a}] + (1-w)f[\boldsymbol{b}] \qquad \text{for all } w \in (0,1);\ \boldsymbol{a}, \boldsymbol{b} \in \mathbb{R}^p, \boldsymbol{a} \neq \boldsymbol{b} .$$

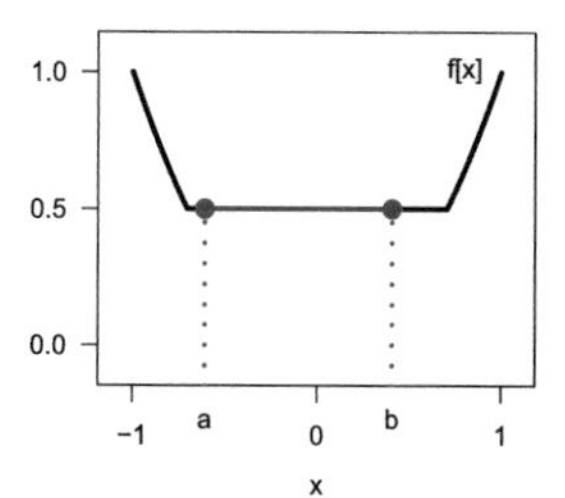

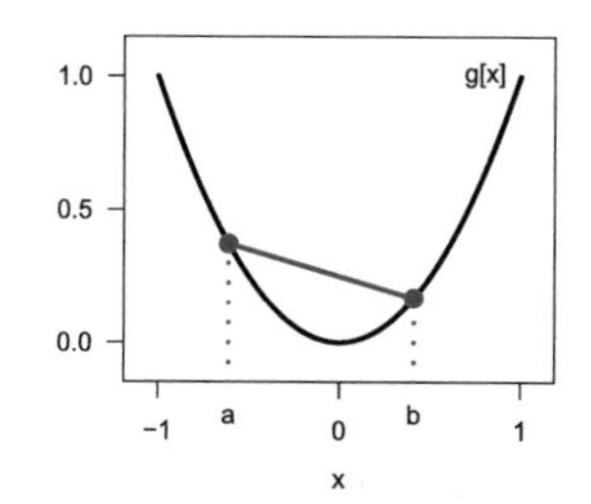

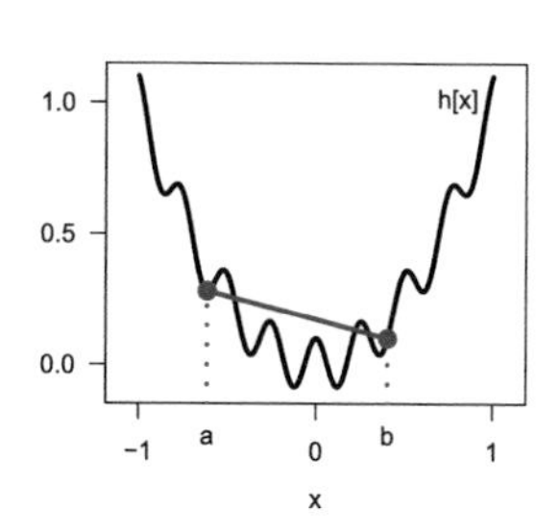

Fig. 2.4 The function $f : x \mapsto \max\{x^2, 0.5\}$ displayed on the left-hand side is convex: between every given $a, b \in \mathbb{R}$, the points on the graph (black line) are on or below the closed line segment between a and b (blue line including the end points). The function $g : x \mapsto x^2$ displayed in the middle is strictly convex: between every given $a, b \in \mathbb{R}$, $a \neq b$, the points on the graph are strictly below the open line segment between a and b (blue line excluding the end points). The function $h : x \mapsto x^2 + 0.1\cos(25x)$ displayed on the right-hand side is not convex: the graph is sometimes above the line segment

Hence, every strictly convex function is convex. A main convenience in working with convex and strictly convex functions is that there is no ambiguity between local and global minima: every local minimum of a convex/strictly convex function is also a global minimum—see Exercise 2.6 for details.

Another property of convexity that will be very helpful in our analyses is that non-negative combinations of convex functions remain convex:

Lemma 2.5.1

Convexity of Non-negative Combinations If the functions $f, g : \mathbb{R}^p \to \mathbb{R}$ are convex and $u, v \in [0, \infty)$, then the function $uf + vg$ is also convex.

If, additionally, f is strictly convex and $u \neq 0$, then the function $uf + vg$ is also strictly convex.

The objective functions of many high-dimensional estimators are of the form (see Display (1.6) in ▶ Chap. 1)

$$f_{\text{hd}} \; : \; \boldsymbol{a} \mapsto \; \text{DataFitting}[Z, \boldsymbol{a}] + r\,\text{Prior}[\boldsymbol{a}]\,.$$

Lemma 2.5.1 ensures that such f_{hd} are convex as long as the data-fitting and prior functions are convex and the tuning parameter is non-negative.

Proof of Lemma 2.5.1 The proof is a short calculation based on the formulation of convexity in Definition 2.5.1.

If $f, g : \mathbb{R}^p \to \mathbb{R}$ are convex and $u, v \in [0, \infty)$, it holds for all $w \in [0, 1]$ and $\boldsymbol{a}, \boldsymbol{b} \in \mathbb{R}^p$ that

$$
\begin{aligned}
&(uf + vg)[w\boldsymbol{a} + (1 - w)\boldsymbol{b}] \\
&= uf[w\boldsymbol{a} + (1 - w)\boldsymbol{b}] + vg[w\boldsymbol{a} + (1 - w)\boldsymbol{b}] && \text{evaluating the function } uf + vg \\
&\leq uwf[\boldsymbol{a}] + u(1 - w)f[\boldsymbol{b}] + vwg[\boldsymbol{a}] + v(1 - w)g[\boldsymbol{b}] && \text{assumed convexity of } f, g \\
&= w(uf[\boldsymbol{a}] + vg[\boldsymbol{a}]) + (1 - w)(uf[\boldsymbol{b}] + vg[\boldsymbol{b}]) && \text{summarizing terms} \\
&= w(uf + vg)[\boldsymbol{a}] + (1 - w)(uf + vg)[\boldsymbol{b}]\,, && \text{adding up the functions}
\end{aligned}
$$

which means in view of Definition 2.5.1 that $uf + vg$ is convex.

The statement about strict convexity can be proved along the same lines. □

▶ **Example 2.5.1**

Convexity of the Lasso's Objective Function In this exercise, we show that the lasso's objective function in (2.2)

$$
f_{\text{lasso}} : \boldsymbol{a} \mapsto \|\boldsymbol{y} - X\boldsymbol{a}\|_2^2 + r\|\boldsymbol{a}\|_1
$$

is convex. In view of the above Lemma 2.5.1, a sufficient condition for the convexity of f_{lasso} is that $r \in [0, \infty)$ and that the least-squares function and the ℓ_1-norm are convex individually.

Convexity of the least-squares function has been shown in 1. of Exercise 1.4.

Convexity of the ℓ_1-norm follows from the formulation of convexity in Definition 2.5.1 and from

$$
\begin{aligned}
&\|w\boldsymbol{a} + (1 - w)\boldsymbol{b}\|_1 \\
&\leq \|w\boldsymbol{a}\|_1 + \|(1 - w)\boldsymbol{b}\|_1 && \text{norms satisfy the triangle inequality (see Page IX)} \\
&= |w|\|\boldsymbol{a}\|_1 + |1 - w|\|\boldsymbol{b}\|_1 && \text{norms are absolute homogeneous (see Page IX)} \\
&= w\|\boldsymbol{a}\|_1 + (1 - w)\|\boldsymbol{b}\|_1 && w \in [0, 1]
\end{aligned}
$$

for all $w \in [0, 1]$ and $\boldsymbol{a}, \boldsymbol{b} \in \mathbb{R}^p$. The same calculation applies to *every* norm, that is, norms are convex in general.

We conclude that the lasso's objective function, as well as the least-squares data-fitting function complemented with any norm prior, is convex. ◀

Our main motivation for studying convex functions, however, is that they permit the formulation of *subgradients*, which are generalized gradients that do not require differentiability. Setting these subgradients to zero will allow us to characterize the minima of every convex objective function.

subgradient

Definition 2.5.2

Subgradients and Subdifferentials Consider a convex function $f : \mathbb{R}^p \to \mathbb{R}$ and a vector $\boldsymbol{a} \in \mathbb{R}^p$. A vector $\boldsymbol{b} \in \mathbb{R}^p$ is a *subgradient* of f at $\boldsymbol{a}$ if

$$f[\boldsymbol{c}] \geq f[\boldsymbol{a}] + \langle \boldsymbol{b}, \boldsymbol{c} - \boldsymbol{a} \rangle \qquad \text{for all } \boldsymbol{c} \in \mathbb{R}^p .$$

The *subdifferential* of f at $\boldsymbol{a}$ is the set

$$\partial f[\boldsymbol{a}] := \{\boldsymbol{b} \in \mathbb{R}^p \ : \ \boldsymbol{b} \text{ is a subgradient of } f \text{ at } \boldsymbol{a}\} .$$

It can be shown that subdifferentials are not empty.[20]

For differentiable functions, subgradients simplify to standard gradients:

Lemma 2.5.2

Differentiable Functions If $f : \mathbb{R}^p \to \mathbb{R}$ is convex and differentiable at $\boldsymbol{a}$ with gradient $\nabla f[\boldsymbol{a}]$, it holds that $\partial f[\boldsymbol{a}] = \{\nabla f[\boldsymbol{a}]\}$.

Hence, the subdifferentials of a differentiable function each contain exactly one element. The subdifferentials of a general convex function, in contrast, can be uncountably infinite.

Proof of Lemma 2.5.2 We presume two facts without proof: Fact 1 is that, as mentioned before, subdifferentials of convex functions are never empty. Fact 2 is the basic calculus result that $\boldsymbol{b}$ is the gradient of a differentiable function f at $\boldsymbol{a}$ (that is, $\boldsymbol{b} = \nabla f[\boldsymbol{a}]$) if and only if

$$\langle \boldsymbol{b},\, \boldsymbol{d}\rangle \;=\; \lim_{t\to 0^+} \frac{f[\boldsymbol{a}+t\boldsymbol{d}] - f[\boldsymbol{a}]}{t} \qquad \text{for all } \boldsymbol{d} \in \mathbb{R}^p\,.$$

In light of Facts 1 and 2, we need to show that

$$\boldsymbol{b} \in \partial f[\boldsymbol{a}] \quad\Rightarrow\quad \langle \boldsymbol{b},\, \boldsymbol{d}\rangle \;=\; \lim_{t\to 0^+} \frac{f[\boldsymbol{a}+t\boldsymbol{d}] - f[\boldsymbol{a}]}{t} \quad \text{for all } \boldsymbol{d} \in \mathbb{R}^p\,.$$

The assumption $\boldsymbol{b} \in \partial f[\boldsymbol{a}]$ implies via the Definition 2.5.2 of subgradients that

$$f[\boldsymbol{c}] \;\ge\; f[\boldsymbol{a}] + \langle \boldsymbol{b},\, \boldsymbol{c}-\boldsymbol{a}\rangle \qquad \text{for all } \boldsymbol{c} \in \mathbb{R}^p\,.$$

Setting in this inequality $\boldsymbol{c} = \boldsymbol{a} + t\boldsymbol{d}$ for arbitrary $t \in \mathbb{R}$ and $\boldsymbol{d} \in \mathbb{R}^p$ gives

$$f[\boldsymbol{a}+t\boldsymbol{d}] \;\ge\; f[\boldsymbol{a}] + \langle \boldsymbol{b},\, (\boldsymbol{a}+t\boldsymbol{d})-\boldsymbol{a}\rangle\,.$$

Simplifying and using the linearity of inner products, we can deduce from the inequality that

$$f[\boldsymbol{a}+t\boldsymbol{d}] \;\ge\; f[\boldsymbol{a}] + t\langle \boldsymbol{b},\, \boldsymbol{d}\rangle\,.$$

Rearranging further, we find for every $t \neq 0$ that

$$\langle \boldsymbol{b},\, \boldsymbol{d}\rangle \;\le\; \frac{f[\boldsymbol{a}+t\boldsymbol{d}] - f[\boldsymbol{a}]}{t}\,.$$

Also, making the replacements $t \mapsto -t$ and $\boldsymbol{d} \mapsto -\boldsymbol{d}$ (both t and $\boldsymbol{d}$ were arbitrary except for $t \neq 0$), we find readily

$$\langle \boldsymbol{b},\, \boldsymbol{d}\rangle \;\ge\; \frac{f[\boldsymbol{a}+t\boldsymbol{d}] - f[\boldsymbol{a}]}{t}\,.$$

Taken together, the two previous displays yield

$$\boldsymbol{b} \in \partial f[\boldsymbol{a}] \quad\Rightarrow\quad \langle \boldsymbol{b},\, \boldsymbol{d}\rangle \;=\; \frac{f[\boldsymbol{a}+t\boldsymbol{d}] - f[\boldsymbol{a}]}{t} \quad \text{for all } t \in \mathbb{R}\backslash\{0\},\, \boldsymbol{d} \in \mathbb{R}^p\,.$$

We can conclude by taking the limit in t on the right-hand side. □

Another important property of subdifferentials is that they are linear in the following sense:

Lemma 2.5.3

Non-negative Combinations of Functions Let $f, g : \mathbb{R}^p \to \mathbb{R}$ be convex functions and $u, v \in [0, \infty)$ non-negative constants. Then, it holds for every $\boldsymbol{a} \in \mathbb{R}^p$ that

$$\partial\big(uf[\boldsymbol{a}] + vg[\boldsymbol{a}]\big) = u\partial f[\boldsymbol{a}] + u\partial g[\boldsymbol{a}]\,,$$

where $u\partial f[\boldsymbol{a}] + v\partial g[\boldsymbol{a}] := \{u\boldsymbol{c}^1 + v\boldsymbol{c}^2 : \boldsymbol{c}^1 \in \partial f[\boldsymbol{a}],\ \boldsymbol{c}^2 \in \partial g[\boldsymbol{a}]\}$ by Page IX.

We omit the proof.[21]

► Example 2.5.2

Subdifferentials of the Lasso In this exercise, we derive the subdifferentials of the lasso's objective function in (2.2):

$$f_{\text{lasso}} : \boldsymbol{a} \mapsto \|\boldsymbol{y} - X\boldsymbol{a}\|_2^2 + r\|\boldsymbol{a}\|_1\,.$$

This function is not differentiable if $r > 0$, but it is still convex according to Example 2.5.1 above.

The least-squares function $f_{\text{ls}} : \boldsymbol{a} \mapsto \|\boldsymbol{y} - X\boldsymbol{a}\|_2^2$ is convex (see 1. in Exercise 1.4) and differentiable with gradient $\nabla f_{\text{ls}} : \boldsymbol{a} \mapsto -2X^\top(\boldsymbol{y} - X\boldsymbol{a})$ (see Page 6). The subdifferentials of the least-squares function are, therefore, (see Lemma 2.5.2 about subdifferentials of differentiable functions)

$$\partial f_{\text{ls}}[\boldsymbol{a}] = \big\{\nabla f_{\text{ls}}[\boldsymbol{a}]\big\} = \big\{-2X^\top(\boldsymbol{y} - X\boldsymbol{a})\big\}\,.$$

The prior function $f_{\ell_1} : \boldsymbol{a} \mapsto \|\boldsymbol{a}\|_1$ can be written as $f_{\ell_1}[\boldsymbol{a}] = \sum_{j=1}^p |a_j| = \sum_{j=1}^p f_{\ell_1}^j[\boldsymbol{a}]$, where $f_{\ell_1}^j : \boldsymbol{a} \mapsto |a_j|$ is convex (see 2. in Exercise 2.7). The subdifferential of f_{ℓ_1} is, therefore, the sum of the subdifferentials of the $f_{\ell_1}^j$'s (see Lemma 2.5.3 about subdifferentials of non-negative combinations of functions).

Each function $f_{\ell_1}^j$ is differentiable as long as $a_j \neq 0$, and the coordinates of the gradient are $(\nabla f_{\ell_1}^j)[\boldsymbol{a}]_j = \text{sign}[a_j]$, where $\text{sign} : a \mapsto \mathbb{1}\{a \geq 0\} - \mathbb{1}\{a \leq 0\}$ is the signum function, and $(\nabla f^j_{\ell_1})[\boldsymbol{a}]_i = 0$ for all $i \in \{1,\ldots,p\}$, $i \neq j$. Hence, if $a_j \neq 0$, (see Lemma 2.5.2 about the subdifferentials of differentiable functions)

$$\partial f^j_{\ell_1}[\boldsymbol{a}] = \big\{\boldsymbol{b} \in \mathbb{R}^p : b_j = \text{sign}[a_j] \text{ and } b_i = 0 \text{ for } i \in \{1,\ldots,p\}, i \neq j\big\}.$$

For the case $a_j = 0$, we invoke the formulation of subgradients directly. The corresponding Definition 2.5.2 applied to the function $f^j_{\ell_1}$ yields, since $f^j_{\ell_1}[\boldsymbol{a}] = 0$ in this case, and since $f^j_{\ell_1}[\boldsymbol{c}] = |c_j|$ in general, that $\boldsymbol{b} \in \partial f^j_{\ell_1}[\boldsymbol{a}]$ if and only if

$$|c_j| \geq \langle \boldsymbol{b},\ \boldsymbol{c} - \boldsymbol{a}\rangle \qquad \text{for all } \boldsymbol{c} \in \mathbb{R}^p .$$

Writing the inner product out, we can formulate the condition in the form (note that $a_j = 0$)

$$|c_j| \geq b_j c_j + \sum_{\substack{i=1\\ i\neq j}}^{p} b_i(c_i - a_i) \qquad \text{for all } \boldsymbol{c} \in \mathbb{R}^p .$$

This condition must be true for *all* $\boldsymbol{c} \in \mathbb{R}^p$. For $\boldsymbol{c} \in \mathbb{R}^p$ such that $c_j = 0$ and $c_i = b_i + a_i$ for $i \neq j$, it becomes

$$0 \geq \sum_{\substack{i=1\\ i\neq j}}^{p} b_i^2 ,$$

which means that $b_i = 0$ for all $i \neq j$. The condition on $\boldsymbol{b}$, therefore, can be written as

$$|c_j| \geq b_j c_j \text{ for all } c_j \in \mathbb{R} \quad \text{and} \quad b_i = 0 \text{ for } i \neq j .$$

The first part of this condition, as one can check readily, is satisfied if and only if $|b_j| \leq 1$. Therefore, we get for $a_j = 0$ that

$$\partial f^j_{\ell_1}[\boldsymbol{a}] = \big\{\boldsymbol{b} \in \mathbb{R}^p : |b_j| \leq 1 \text{ and } b_i = 0 \text{ for } i \in \{1,\ldots,p\}, i \neq j\big\}.$$

Combining the subdifferentials of the $f^j_{\ell_1}$'s according to Lemma 2.5.3 yields ($\|\boldsymbol{a}\|_1 = f_{\ell_1}[\boldsymbol{a}] = \sum_{j=1}^{p} f^j_{\ell_1}[\boldsymbol{b}]$)

$$\partial\|\boldsymbol{a}\|_1 = \big\{\boldsymbol{b} \in \mathbb{R}^p : \|\boldsymbol{b}\|_\infty \leq 1 \text{ and } b_j = \text{sign}[a_j] \text{ for all } j \in \{1,\ldots,p\} \text{ such that } a_j \neq 0\big\},$$

and combining with the subdifferentials of ℓ (using that $\ell_{\text{lasso}} = \ell_{\text{ls}} + r\ell_{\ell_1}$ and that r is non-negative by assumption) finally gives us the subdifferentials of the lasso objective function:

$$\partial\ell_{\text{lasso}}[\boldsymbol{a}] = \Big\{ -2X^\top(\boldsymbol{y} - X\boldsymbol{a}) + r\boldsymbol{b} \in \mathbb{R}^p : \|\boldsymbol{b}\|_\infty \leq 1 \text{ and } b_j = \text{sign}[a_j] \text{ for all } j \in \{1, \ldots, p\} \text{ such that } a_j \neq 0 \Big\}.$$

The subdifferentials of the lasso objective consist of exactly one point if and only if the function argument has no zero-valued coordinates, that is, $a_1, \ldots, a_p \neq 0$. In general, the subdifferential is a $(p - \|\boldsymbol{a}\|_0)$-dimensional cube. the plots below depict examples for $p = 2$ (see Exercise 2.9): Plot A corresponds to $a_1, a_2 \neq 0$; Plot B corresponds to $a_1 = 0, a_2 \neq 0$; Plot C corresponds to $a_1 = a_2 = 0$. The subdifferential $\partial\ell_{\text{lasso}}[\boldsymbol{a}]$ is depicted by the blue point/line/square; the vector $\boldsymbol{v} = (v_1, v_2)^\top := -2X^\top(\boldsymbol{y}-X\boldsymbol{a})+r(\text{sign}[a_1], \text{sign}[a_2])^\top \in \mathbb{R}^2$, where $\text{sign}[b] = \mathbb{1}\{b \geq 0\} - \mathbb{1}\{b \leq 0\}$ for $b \in \mathbb{R}$, used as an orientation point has different values in each plot.◀

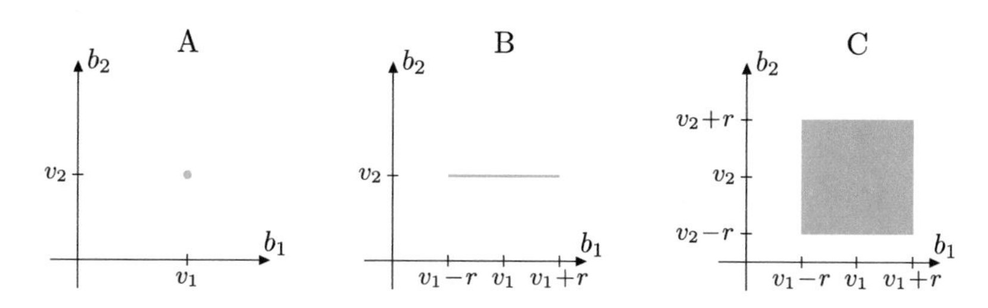

Having established the notions of convexity and subdifferentials, we can finally characterize minima of convex functions.

Theorem 2.5.1

Minima of Convex Functions Consider a convex function $\ell : \mathbb{R}^p \to \mathbb{R}$. A vector $\boldsymbol{a} \in \mathbb{R}^p$ is a minimizer of ℓ if and only if $\boldsymbol{b} = \boldsymbol{0}_p$ is in the subdifferential of ℓ at $\boldsymbol{a}$, that is,

$$\ell[\boldsymbol{c}] \geq \ell[\boldsymbol{a}] \text{ for all } \boldsymbol{c} \in \mathbb{R}^p \quad \Leftrightarrow \quad \boldsymbol{0}_p \in \partial\ell[\boldsymbol{a}].$$

We refer to these sufficient and necessary conditions for minima as *optimality conditions*.

Lemma 2.5.2 states that $\partial f[\boldsymbol{a}] = \{\nabla f[\boldsymbol{a}]\}$ for every convex function f that is differentiable; the theorem here implies, therefore, the classical result that $\boldsymbol{a} \in \mathbb{R}^p$ is a minimum of a convex and differentiable function f if and only if $\nabla f[\boldsymbol{a}] = \mathbf{0}_p$. However, the optimality conditions in the theorem apply to *every* convex function, and consequently Theorem 2.5.1 generalizes that classical result to convex but not necessarily differentiable functions.

Proof of Theorem 2.5.1 The proof relies on Definition 2.5.2 of subdifferentials and the fact that, by linearity of the inner product, $\langle \mathbf{0}_p, \boldsymbol{d}\rangle = 0$ for all $\boldsymbol{d} \in \mathbb{R}^p$.

Step 1: Necessity We first prove that

$$f[\boldsymbol{c}] \geq f[\boldsymbol{a}] \text{ for all } \boldsymbol{c} \in \mathbb{R}^p \qquad \Rightarrow \qquad \mathbf{0}_p \in \partial f[\boldsymbol{a}]\,.$$

If $f[\boldsymbol{c}] \geq f[\boldsymbol{a}]$ for all $\boldsymbol{c} \in \mathbb{R}^p$, we get by linearity of inner products

$$f[\boldsymbol{c}] \geq f[\boldsymbol{a}] + \langle \mathbf{0}_p, \boldsymbol{c} - \boldsymbol{a}\rangle \qquad \text{for all } \boldsymbol{c} \in \mathbb{R}^p\,.$$

By Definition 2.5.2 of the subdifferential, this means that $\mathbf{0}_p \in \partial f[\boldsymbol{a}]$, as desired.

Step 2: Sufficiency We now prove that

$$\mathbf{0}_p \in \partial f[\boldsymbol{a}] \qquad \Rightarrow \qquad f[\boldsymbol{c}] \geq f[\boldsymbol{a}] \text{ for all } \boldsymbol{c} \in \mathbb{R}^p\,.$$

If $\mathbf{0}_p \in \partial f[\boldsymbol{a}]$, Definition 2.5.2 of the subdifferential yields

$$f[\boldsymbol{c}] \geq f[\boldsymbol{a}] + \langle \mathbf{0}_p, \boldsymbol{c} - \boldsymbol{a}\rangle \qquad \text{for all } \boldsymbol{c} \in \mathbb{R}^p\,.$$

By linearity of inner products, this inequality includes

$$f[\boldsymbol{c}] \geq f[\boldsymbol{a}] \qquad \text{for all } \boldsymbol{c} \in \mathbb{R}^p\,,$$

as desired. □

► Example 2.5.3

KKT Conditions for Regularized Least-Squares In this example, we establish optimality conditions that are customized for high-dimensional least-squares estimators. We call these conditions *KKT conditions*.[22] We first consider the lasso's objective function in (2.2):

$$f_{\text{lasso}} \; : \; \boldsymbol{a} \mapsto \; \|\boldsymbol{y} - X\boldsymbol{a}\|_2^2 + r\|\boldsymbol{a}\|_1 \, .$$

The function f_{lasso} is convex according to Example 2.5.1; therefore, in view of Theorem 2.5.1, $\widehat{\boldsymbol{\beta}}_{\text{lasso}} \in \mathbb{R}^p$ is a lasso estimator if and only if $\mathbf{0}_p \in \partial f_{\text{lasso}}[\widehat{\boldsymbol{\beta}}_{\text{lasso}}]$. The latter condition is—see Example 2.5.2—equivalent to $-2X^\top(\boldsymbol{y} - X\widehat{\boldsymbol{\beta}}_{\text{lasso}}) + r\widehat{\boldsymbol{\kappa}} = \mathbf{0}_p$ for a vector $\widehat{\boldsymbol{\kappa}} \in \partial\|\widehat{\boldsymbol{\beta}}_{\text{lasso}}\|_1 = \{\boldsymbol{b} \in \mathbb{R}^p : \|\boldsymbol{b}\|_\infty \le 1 \text{ and } b_j = \text{sign}[(\widehat{\beta}_{\text{lasso}})_j] \text{ if } (\widehat{\beta}_{\text{lasso}})_j \neq 0\}$. These conditions are the KKT conditions for the lasso.

Now, generalizing the ℓ_1-prior function to an arbitrary convex function $h : \mathbb{R}^p \to \mathbb{R}$ simply changes the subdifferential in which $\widehat{\boldsymbol{\kappa}}$ is

$$\begin{gathered}
\widehat{\boldsymbol{\beta}} \in \operatorname*{arg\,min}_{\boldsymbol{\alpha} \in \mathbb{R}^p} \left\{ \|\boldsymbol{y} - X\boldsymbol{\alpha}\|_2^2 + r h[\boldsymbol{\alpha}] \right\} \\
\Updownarrow \\
-2X^\top(\boldsymbol{y} - X\widehat{\boldsymbol{\beta}}) + r\widehat{\boldsymbol{\kappa}} = \mathbf{0}_p \quad \text{for a } \widehat{\boldsymbol{\kappa}} \in \partial h[\widehat{\boldsymbol{\beta}}] \, .
\end{gathered} \tag{2.7}$$

This specific form of the optimality conditions are the KKT conditions for the corresponding high-dimensional estimator. The KKT conditions are a starting point for obtaining a more detailed understanding of lasso-type estimators in special cases (see Exercises 2.10 and 2.11), for interpreting the debiasing approach in inference (see ► Chap. 5 and especially Exercise 5.3), and for deriving guarantees for high-dimensional estimators (see ► Chaps. 6 and 7).◄

2.6 Exercises

2.6.1 Exercises for ► Sect. 2.2

Exercise 2.1 ♦♦ In this exercise, we illustrate that additional predictors typically increase the complexity of least-squares estimates. We consider data $(\boldsymbol{y}, X)$ from the linear regression model in ► Sect. 2.2 and an augmented version of these data $(\boldsymbol{y}, X')$ with $X' := (X, \boldsymbol{x}) \in \mathbb{R}^{n\times(p+1)}$ for a vector $\boldsymbol{x} \in \mathbb{R}^n$. We denote the corresponding least-squares estimators by $\widehat{\boldsymbol{\beta}}_{\text{ls}}$ and $(\widehat{\boldsymbol{\beta}}_{\text{ls}})'$, respectively. Note that $\widehat{\boldsymbol{\beta}}_{\text{ls}} \in \mathbb{R}^p$, whereas $(\widehat{\boldsymbol{\beta}}_{\text{ls}})' \in \mathbb{R}^{p+1}$.

1. Show that

$$\min_{\boldsymbol{\alpha}' \in \mathbb{R}^{p+1}} \|\boldsymbol{y} - X'\boldsymbol{\alpha}'\|_2^2 \le \min_{\boldsymbol{\alpha} \in \mathbb{R}^p} \|\boldsymbol{y} - X\boldsymbol{\alpha}\|_2^2 .$$

2. Show that if the additional predictor $\boldsymbol{x}$ and the residual $\boldsymbol{y} - X\widehat{\boldsymbol{\beta}}_{\text{ls}}$ are not orthogonal, that is, $\langle \boldsymbol{y} - X\widehat{\boldsymbol{\beta}}_{\text{ls}}, \boldsymbol{x}\rangle \neq 0$, it holds that

$$\min_{\boldsymbol{\alpha}' \in \mathbb{R}^{p+1}} \|\boldsymbol{y} - X'\boldsymbol{\alpha}'\|_2^2 < \min_{\boldsymbol{\alpha} \in \mathbb{R}^p} \|\boldsymbol{y} - X\boldsymbol{\alpha}\|_2^2 .$$

3. Show that the strict inequality in the above display is a sufficient condition for $(\widehat{\boldsymbol{\beta}}_{\text{ls}})'_{p+1} \neq 0$.
4. Show that if $\text{rank}[X] \ge n$, it holds that

$$\min_{\boldsymbol{\alpha}' \in \mathbb{R}^{p+1}} \|\boldsymbol{y} - X'\boldsymbol{\alpha}'\|_2^2 = \min_{\boldsymbol{\alpha} \in \mathbb{R}^p} \|\boldsymbol{y} - X\boldsymbol{\alpha}\|_2^2 .$$

5. Show that $\text{rank}[X] \ge n$ is nevertheless a sufficient condition for the existence of a least-squares solution with $(\widehat{\boldsymbol{\beta}}_{\text{ls}})'_{p+1} \neq 0$.

This proves that both $\langle \boldsymbol{y} - X\widehat{\boldsymbol{\beta}}_{\text{ls}}, \boldsymbol{x}\rangle \neq 0$ (cf. Claims 2 and 3) and $\text{rank}[X] \ge n$ (cf. Claim 5) are sufficient conditions for a least-squares estimator assigning non-zero weight to the additional predictor $\boldsymbol{x}$. Since these conditions seem likely to be satisfied in high-dimensional settings, our results suggest that least-squares estimation typically uses every additionally provided predictor—irrespective of whether that predictor is actually relevant or not.

2.6.2 Exercises for ▶ Sect. 2.4

Exercise 2.2 ◇◇ In this exercise, we review three basic properties of the ℓ_q-functions defined on Page IX.

1. Show that for $q \in [1, \infty]$, the ℓ_q-functions are norms on $\mathbb{R}^p$.
2. Show that for $q \in [0, 1)$, the ℓ_q-functions are not norms.
3. Show that for $q, k \in [1, \infty]$ such that $1/q + 1/k = 1$, the dual function of $\mathbf{a} \mapsto \|\mathbf{a}\|_q$ is $\mathbf{a} \mapsto \|\mathbf{a}\|_k$, that is, $\overline{\|\cdot\|}_q = \|\cdot\|_k$. Conclude that $\overline{\|\cdot\|}_q$ is a norm on $\mathbb{R}^p$.

Exercise 2.3 ♦♦ In this exercise, we establish some properties of dual functions. According to Definition 2.4.1, the dual function $\overline{\hbar} : \mathbb{R}^p \to [-\infty, \infty]$ of a function $\hbar : \mathbb{R}^p \to [-\infty, \infty]$ is defined via

$$\overline{\hbar}[\boldsymbol{a}] = \sup\big\{ \langle \boldsymbol{a}, \boldsymbol{c}\rangle : \boldsymbol{c} \in \mathbb{R}^p,\ \hbar[\boldsymbol{c}] \le 1 \big\} \qquad \text{for all } \boldsymbol{a} \in \mathbb{R}^p ,$$

where the supremum over the empty set is defined as $-\infty$.

1. (Triangle Inequality) Show that

$$\overline{\hbar}[\boldsymbol{a}+\boldsymbol{b}] \le \overline{\hbar}[\boldsymbol{a}] + \overline{\hbar}[\boldsymbol{b}] \qquad \text{for all } \boldsymbol{a}, \boldsymbol{b} \in \mathbb{R}^p .$$

2. (Absolute Semi-Homogeneity) Show that

$$\overline{\hbar}[a\boldsymbol{b}] = |a|\overline{\hbar}\big[\operatorname{sign}[a]\boldsymbol{b}\big] \qquad \text{for all } a \in \mathbb{R},\ \boldsymbol{b} \in \mathbb{R}^p .$$

   This implies in particular that $\overline{\hbar}[\boldsymbol{0}_p] = 0$ (set $a = 0$ and keep in mind the convention $0 \cdot (\pm\infty) = 0$—see Page X).

3. (Absolute Homogeneity) Show that if $\hbar[a\boldsymbol{b}] = |a|\hbar[\boldsymbol{b}]$ for all $a \in \mathbb{R}$, $\boldsymbol{b} \in \mathbb{R}^p$, then also

$$\overline{\hbar}[a\boldsymbol{b}] = |a|\overline{\hbar}\big[\boldsymbol{b}\big] \qquad \text{for all } a \in \mathbb{R},\ \boldsymbol{b} \in \mathbb{R}^p .$$

4. (Non-negativity) Show that if $\hbar[\boldsymbol{0}_p] \le 1$, then

$$\overline{\hbar}[\boldsymbol{a}] \ge 0 \qquad \text{for all } \boldsymbol{a} \in \mathbb{R}^p .$$

5. (Symmetry) Show that if $\hbar[\boldsymbol{a}] = \hbar[-\boldsymbol{a}]$ for all $\boldsymbol{a} \in \mathbb{R}^p$, then also

$$\overline{\hbar}[\boldsymbol{a}] = \overline{\hbar}[-\boldsymbol{a}] \qquad \text{for all } \boldsymbol{a} \in \mathbb{R}^p .$$

6. (Norms) Show that if $\hbar$ is a norm, then $\overline{\hbar}$ is also a norm.
7. (Convexity) Show that

$$\overline{\hbar}\big[w\boldsymbol{a} + (1-w)\boldsymbol{b}\big] \le w\overline{\hbar}[\boldsymbol{a}] + (1-w)\overline{\hbar}[\boldsymbol{b}] \qquad \text{for all } \boldsymbol{a}, \boldsymbol{b} \in \mathbb{R}^p,\ w \in [0, 1] .$$

8. Bonus: Give an example function $\hbar$ for which $\overline{\overline{\hbar}} = \hbar$ (that is, the dual function of the dual function is the function itself) and an example function for which this does not hold.

9. Bonus: Give an example function $\hbar$ that is not a norm but whose dual function is a norm.

This exercise shows especially that dual functions inherit many properties from their basis functions and are equipped with some other properties "automatically."

Exercise 2.4 ◊◊ In this example, we study the Hölder inequality in Theorem 2.4.1 for typical $\hbar$. Give the specific forms (including $\overline{\hbar}$) of Inequality (2.5) for the following functions $\hbar$—or argue why Theorem 2.4.1 does not apply.

1. Best-subset selection prior function:

$$\hbar \, : \, \boldsymbol{a} \mapsto \|\boldsymbol{a}\|_0 \, .$$

2. Group-lasso prior function without overlap:

$$\hbar \, : \, \boldsymbol{a} \mapsto \sum_{j=1}^{k} \|\boldsymbol{a}_{\mathcal{A}_j}\|_2 \, ,$$

where $\mathcal{A}_1, \ldots, \mathcal{A}_k$ is a partition of $\{1, \ldots, p\}$, that is, $\cup_{j=1}^{k} \mathcal{A}_j = \{1, \ldots, p\}$, $\mathcal{A}_j \neq \varnothing$ for all j, and $\mathcal{A}_i \cap \mathcal{A}_j = \varnothing$ for all $i \neq j$.

3. The group-lasso prior function with overlap:

$$\hbar \, : \, \boldsymbol{a} \mapsto \sum_{j=1}^{k} \|\boldsymbol{a}_{\mathcal{A}_j}\|_2 \, ,$$

where $\mathcal{A}_1, \ldots, \mathcal{A}_k \subset \{1, \ldots, p\}$ such that $\cup_{j=1}^{k} \mathcal{A}_j = \{1, \ldots, p\}$ and $\mathcal{A}_i \cap \mathcal{A}_j \neq \varnothing$ for a pair (i, j), $i \neq j$.

4. The incomplete group-lasso prior function without overlap:

$$\hbar \, : \, \boldsymbol{a} \mapsto \sum_{j=1}^{k} \|\boldsymbol{a}_{\mathcal{A}_j}\|_2 \, ,$$

where $\mathcal{A}_1, \ldots, \mathcal{A}_k \subset \{1, \ldots, p\}$ such that $\cup_{j=1}^{k} \mathcal{A}_j \neq \{1, \ldots, p\}$ and $\mathcal{A}_i \cap \mathcal{A}_j = \varnothing$ for all $i \neq j$.

5. The non-negativity constraint:

$$\hbar : \boldsymbol{a} \mapsto \infty \cdot \mathbb{1}\{a_1, \ldots, a_p < 0\} \, .$$

6. The ridge prior function:

$$h : \boldsymbol{a} \mapsto \|\boldsymbol{a}\|_2^2 .$$

7. The edr prior function:

$$h : \boldsymbol{a} \mapsto \|\boldsymbol{a}\|_2 .$$

The theories derived in ▶ Chaps. 6 and 7 apply essentially to the regularized least-squares estimators whose prior functions are amenable to the Hölder inequality. The exercise here demonstrates that this includes a variety of regularized least-squares estimators—but not all of them.

2.6.3 Exercises for ▶ Sect. 2.5

Exercise 2.5 ♦♦ In this exercise, we derive the *Jensen inequality*.

1. Consider a convex function $f : \mathbb{R}^d \to \mathbb{R}$. Show that for all $a_1, \ldots, a_k \in [0, 1]$ such that $a_1 + \cdots + a_k = 1$, and for all $\boldsymbol{b}^1, \ldots, \boldsymbol{b}^k \in \mathbb{R}^d$, the function f satisfies the Jensen inequality

$$f\Bigl[\sum_{j=1}^{k} a_j \boldsymbol{b}^j\Bigr] \leq \sum_{j=1}^{k} a_j f[\boldsymbol{b}^j] .$$

The Jensen inequality in the above form is essentially just a reformulation of convexity. Indeed, in the special case $k = 2$, the inequality above equals the one in Definition 2.5.1 of convexity ($d = p$; $a_1 = 1 - a_2 = w$; $\boldsymbol{b}^1 = \boldsymbol{a}$; $\boldsymbol{b}^2 = \boldsymbol{b}$); therefore, a function satisfies the Jensen inequality if and only if it is convex.

Exercise 2.6 ◊◊◊ In this exercise, we study the local and global minima of the functions f, g, and h of ◘ Fig. 2.4 and of convex and non-convex functions more generally. A point $\boldsymbol{a} \in \mathbb{R}^p$ is a *local minimum* of a function $k : \mathbb{R}^p \to \mathbb{R}$ if for some $c \in (0, \infty)$,

local minimum

$$k[\boldsymbol{a}] \leq k[\boldsymbol{b}] \quad \text{for all } \boldsymbol{b} \in \mathbb{R}^p \text{ that satisfy } \|\boldsymbol{a} - \boldsymbol{b}\|_2 \leq c .$$

It is also a *global minimum* (or just *minimum*) of k if

global minimum

$$k[\boldsymbol{a}] \leq k[\boldsymbol{b}] \quad \text{for all } \boldsymbol{b} \in \mathbb{R}^p .$$

1. Compute the local minima of $\mathscr{f}$, $\mathscr{g}$, and $\mathscr{h}$. How many minima are there for each of these three functions? Hint: You may use the fact that if $\mathscr{k} : \mathbb{R} \to \mathbb{R}$ is differentiable, (i) $\mathscr{k}'[a] = 0$ for every local minimum $a \in \mathbb{R}$, and (ii) $\mathscr{k}'[a] = 0$ and $\mathscr{k}''[a] > 0$ together imply that $a \in \mathbb{R}$ is a local minimum.
2. Compute the global minima of $\mathscr{f}$, $\mathscr{g}$, and $\mathscr{h}$.
3. More generally, show that every local minimum of a convex function $\mathscr{k} : \mathbb{R}^p \to \mathbb{R}$ is also a global minimum of $\mathscr{k}$.
4. Show also that every strictly convex function $\mathscr{k} : \mathbb{R}^p \to \mathbb{R}$ has at most one local and one global minimum, and show that—if they exist—these two points coincide. Bonus: Can you state a strictly convex function $\mathscr{k} : \mathbb{R}^p \to \mathbb{R}$ that has neither a local nor a global minimum?
5. Conclude from 1. and 2. that neither of the previous two statements is necessarily true for non-convex functions.

Exercise 2.7 ◊◊ In this exercise, we study the convexity of some prior functions.

Prove or refute that the convexity of the following functions $\mathscr{h} : \mathbb{R}^p \to \mathbb{R}$ defined as:

1. $\mathscr{h} : \boldsymbol{a} \mapsto \|\boldsymbol{a}\|_0$;
2. $\boldsymbol{a} \mapsto |a_j|$ for $j \in \{1, \ldots, p\}$;
3. $\mathscr{h} : \boldsymbol{a} \mapsto \|\boldsymbol{a}\|_1$;
4. $\mathscr{h} : \boldsymbol{a} \mapsto \min\{a_j, b\}$ for $j \in \{1, \ldots, p\}$ and $b \in (0, \infty)$.

Hint: For 4., you can use the fact that $\min\{a, b\} = (a + b)/2 - |a - b|/2$ for all $a, b \in \mathbb{R}$.

Exercise 2.8 ◊◊ In this exercise, we extend Lemma 2.5.3 about the subdifferentials of combinations of functions. For a given index set $\mathscr{A} \subset \{1, \ldots, p\}$, consider two convex functions $\mathscr{h}_1 : \mathbb{R}^{|\mathscr{A}|} \to \mathbb{R}$ and $\mathscr{h}_2 : \mathbb{R}^{|\mathscr{A}^\complement|} \to \mathbb{R}$ and their combination $\mathscr{h} : \mathbb{R}^p \to \mathbb{R}$ defined as $\mathscr{h}[\boldsymbol{a}] := \mathscr{h}_1[\boldsymbol{a}_{\mathscr{A}}] + \mathscr{h}_2[\boldsymbol{a}_{\mathscr{A}^\complement}]$ for $\boldsymbol{a} \in \mathbb{R}^p$. Use Lemma 2.5.3 to show that

$$\partial\mathscr{h}[\boldsymbol{a}] = \left\{\boldsymbol{b} \in \mathbb{R}^p \ : \ \boldsymbol{b}_{\mathscr{A}} \in \partial\mathscr{h}_1[\boldsymbol{a}_{\mathscr{A}}] \text{ and } \boldsymbol{b}_{\mathscr{A}^\complement} \in \partial\mathscr{h}_2[\boldsymbol{a}_{\mathscr{A}^\complement}]\right\}.$$

Exercise 2.9 ◊◊ In this exercise, we corroborate the plots in Example 2.5.2 (subdifferentials of the lasso estimator).

Consider the lasso estimator's objective function

$$\ell_{\text{lasso}} \;:\; \boldsymbol{a} \mapsto \|\boldsymbol{y} - X\boldsymbol{a}\|_2^2 + r\|\boldsymbol{a}\|_1$$

in $p = 2$ dimensions. Compute $\partial \ell_{\text{lasso}}[\boldsymbol{a}]$ as a function of $\boldsymbol{y}, X, r, \boldsymbol{a}$ for the following three cases:
1. $a_1, a_2 \neq 0$;
2. $a_1 = 0, a_2 \neq 0$;
3. $a_1 = a_2 = 0$.

Compare the Plots A, B, and C in the example.

Exercise 2.10 ♦♦ In this exercise, we compute the lasso estimator (2.2) for orthogonal design.

Prove the following three results under the assumption of orthogonality, that is, $X^\top X = n\mathrm{I}_{p\times p}$. You may use the KKT conditions for the lasso established in Example 2.5.3.
1. Show that the KKT conditions are in the case of orthogonal design

$$\widehat{\boldsymbol{\beta}}_{\text{lasso}} = \frac{X^\top \boldsymbol{y}}{n} - \frac{r\widehat{\boldsymbol{\kappa}}}{2n}$$

   for a vector $\widehat{\boldsymbol{\kappa}} \in \partial \|\widehat{\boldsymbol{\beta}}_{\text{lasso}}\|_1$.
2. Use 1. to show that for all $j \in \{1, \ldots, p\}$, it holds that

$$\begin{aligned}
\big|(X^\top \boldsymbol{y})_j\big| &\leq \frac{r}{2} &\quad\Leftrightarrow\quad& (\widehat{\beta}_{\text{lasso}})_j = 0\,;\\
(X^\top \boldsymbol{y})_j &> \frac{r}{2} &\quad\Leftrightarrow\quad& (\widehat{\beta}_{\text{lasso}})_j > 0\,;\\
(X^\top \boldsymbol{y})_j &< -\frac{r}{2} &\quad\Leftrightarrow\quad& (\widehat{\beta}_{\text{lasso}})_j < 0\,.
\end{aligned}$$

3. Use 1. and 2. to show that for all $j \in \{1, \ldots, p\}$, it holds that

$$(\widehat{\beta}_{\text{lasso}})_j = \operatorname{sign}\left[(X^\top \boldsymbol{y})_j\right]\left(\frac{\big|(X^\top \boldsymbol{y})_j\big|}{n} - \frac{r}{2n}\right)_+, \tag{2.8}$$

   where the *positive part* $(a)_+$ of a number $a \in \mathbb{R}$ is defined as $(a)_+ := a$ if $a > 0$ and $(a)_+ := 0$ otherwise. This means that the lasso problem has a unique and explicit solution.

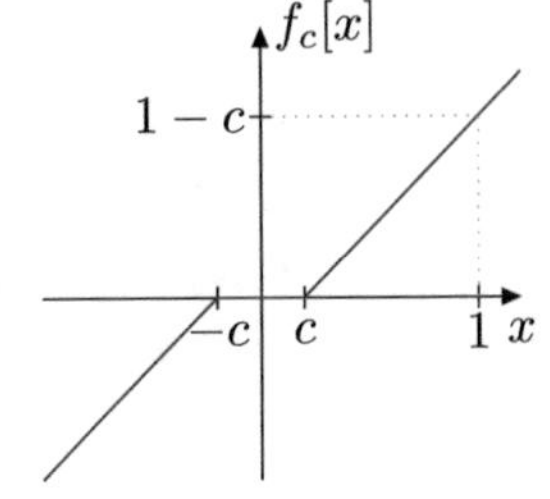

We conclude that for orthogonal design, the coordinates of the lasso estimator are $(\widehat{\beta}_{\text{lasso}})_j = f_{r/2}[(X^\top y)_j]/n, j \in \{1, \ldots, p\}$, where f_c is the *soft-thresholding operator*

$$
\begin{aligned}
f_c \,:\, \mathbb{R} &\to \mathbb{R}\\
x &\mapsto \operatorname{sign}[x]\big(|x| - c\big)_+
\end{aligned}
$$

for a given cutoff $c \in [0, \infty]$. Hence, in the orthogonal case, the lasso estimator is a soft-thresholded version of the least-squares estimator $\widehat{\boldsymbol{\beta}}_{\text{ls}} = (X^\top X)^{-1} X^\top \boldsymbol{y} = X^\top \boldsymbol{y}$.

Exercise 2.11 ♦♦ In this exercise, we derive further properties of the lasso estimator

$$\widehat{\boldsymbol{\beta}}_{\text{lasso}}[r] \in \underset{\boldsymbol{\alpha} \in \mathbb{R}^p}{\arg\min} \left\{ \|\boldsymbol{y} - X\boldsymbol{\alpha}\|_2^2 + r\|\boldsymbol{\alpha}\|_1 \right\}$$

for certain tuning parameters r.

First, we establish another relationship between the lasso and the least-squares estimator. We can use again the lasso's KKT conditions from Example 2.5.3.

1. Show that if the Gram matrix $X^\top X$ is invertible and $r \in [0, \infty)$, the lasso estimator's KKT conditions are

$$\widehat{\boldsymbol{\beta}}_{\text{lasso}}[r] = \widehat{\boldsymbol{\beta}}_{\text{ls}} - \frac{r}{2}(X^\top X)^{-1}\widehat{\boldsymbol{\kappa}}$$

for a $\widehat{\boldsymbol{\kappa}} \in \partial\|\widehat{\boldsymbol{\beta}}_{\text{lasso}}[r]\|_1$.

2. Show that then

$$\|X\widehat{\boldsymbol{\beta}}_{\text{lasso}}[r] - X\widehat{\boldsymbol{\beta}}_{\text{ls}}\|_2^2 \le \frac{r^2 p}{4m_1},$$

where m_1 is the smallest eigenvalue of the Gram matrix $X^\top X$ (see ► Sect. B.2).

In view of Eq. (1.5), this means that if the lasso's tuning parameter is sufficiently small, say $r \ll 2\sqrt{m_1}\sigma$, the lasso and the least-squares estimator are about equal in terms of prediction.

Second, we identify—now for arbitrary X—the range of tuning parameters that set the lasso to zero.

3. Show that $\widehat{\boldsymbol{\beta}}_{\text{lasso}}[r] = \mathbf{0}_p$ is a lasso solution if and only if $r \ge 2\|X^\top \boldsymbol{y}\|_\infty$.
4. Show that $\widehat{\boldsymbol{\beta}}_{\text{lasso}}[r] = \mathbf{0}_p$ is the *unique* lasso solution if $r \ge 2\|X^\top \boldsymbol{y}\|_\infty$ *and* $r > 0$.

5. If $r = 2\|X^\top \mathbf{y}\|_\infty = 0$, the vector $\widehat{\boldsymbol{\beta}}_{\text{lasso}}[r]$ is a lasso solution if and only if $X\widehat{\boldsymbol{\beta}}_{\text{lasso}}[r] = \mathbf{0}_n$.

This implies in particular that in practice, it is usually sufficient to consider tuning parameters smaller or equal to $2\|X^\top \mathbf{y}\|_\infty$.

2.7 R Lab: Overfitting

In this lab, we illustrate the overfitting phenomenon. For this, we generate data according to a linear regression model with standard polynomial basis functions as predictors. The model parameters are set to zero except for the quadratic term. We then compare the least-squares and the lasso in estimating the corresponding curve from the noisy data. We do not assume that it is known that the underlying function is quadratic beforehand; instead, we only assume that it is known that the function is a polynomial, and we assume as given an upper bound for the degree of that polynomial. In addition, we assume that it is known that the model is sparse, that is, that only a small (but otherwise unknown) number of polynomial terms are relevant, which motivates the application of ℓ_1-regularization. We find that an increase in the number of such predictors can get least-squares estimation completely off course, while the lasso remains largely unimpressed.

As always, your task is to replace the keyword `REPLACE` with suitable code and to answer the questions in the text.

2.7.1 Generating Data

We consider data from the linear regression model

$$y_i = \beta_0 + \beta_1 x_i + \beta_2 (x_i)^2 + \cdots + \beta_d (x_i)^d + u_i \quad \text{for all } i \in \{1, \ldots, n\}$$

with regression vector $\boldsymbol{\beta} = (0, 0, 2, 0, \ldots, 0)^\top \in \mathbb{R}^{d+1}$ and independently distributed measurements $x_i \sim \text{Unif}[-1, 1]$ and noise $u_i \sim \mathcal{N}[0, 1]$. This means that the outcomes y_i are noisy observations of the quadratic function $x \mapsto 2x^2$, but since $\boldsymbol{\beta}$ is unknown, the data analyst does not know this relationship beforehand.

Set the degree of the polynomial to $d = 20$, and generate $n = 100$ independent samples according to the above model. The function `runif()` might be helpful to sample from the uniform distribution, and the function `rnorm()` to sample from the Gauss distribution. Summarize the outcomes in a vector $\boldsymbol{y} := (y_1, \ldots, y_n)^\top \in \mathbb{R}^n$ and the predictors in a matrix $X \in \mathbb{R}^{n\times(d+1)}$ with coordinates $X_{ij} = (x_i)^j$. Including the intercept, the number of predictors is $p = d + 1$.

```
set.seed(87)
PolynomialDesign <- function(x.vector, d)
{
  REPLACE
}
n <- 100; d <- 20
X <- PolynomialDesign(REPLACE, d)
regression.vector <- c(0, 0, 2, rep(0, d - 2))
y <- REPLACE
cbind(y, X)[1:4, 1:5]
```

```
##              [,1] [,2]       [,3]      [,4]        [,5]
## [1,] 1.319628    1 -0.9678621 0.9367571 -0.90665165
## [2,] 1.839104    1 -0.4171889 0.1740466 -0.07261032
## [3,] 3.089433    1 -0.9150774 0.8373667 -0.76625536
## [4,] 1.657062    1  0.7153142 0.5116745  0.36600803
```

2.7.2 Implementing the Estimators

Implement a least-squares estimator and a lasso estimator. For the latter, use the `cv.glmnet()` function from the `glmnet` package with the flag `intercept=FALSE`. The `coef()` function might be helpful in extracting the estimated regression vector from the `glmnet` object (note that the first coordinate of the resulting vector needs to be removed in our case, since that coordinate contains a placeholder for an additional intercept).

```
library(glmnet)
set.seed(98)  # glmnet uses randomized cross-validation routines
LsEstimator <- function(y, X)
{
  return(REPLACE)
}
LassoEstimator <- function(y, X)
{
  return(REPLACE)
}
cbind(LsEstimator(y, X[, 1:3]), LassoEstimator(y, X[, 1:3])) # a quick check
```

```
##                  [,1]     [,2]
## [1,]  0.02221062 0.000000
## [2,] -0.07859756 0.000000
## [3,]  2.00685799 1.310734
```

Detail: We set `intercept=FALSE`, because otherwise, `glmnet` would estimate an additional *unregularized* intercept. However, `glmnet` also disregards the first column of X (cf. Line 2156 in the file `glmnet5.f90` on https://github.com/cran/glmnet; this line is executed even if `standardize=FALSE`). Hence, strictly speaking, our lasso implementation has a tiny advantage over the least-squares, as it is not tempted to fit an intercept. As a bonus, you can explore the subtleties.

2.7.3 Computing and Visualizing the Results

We now compute and visualize the results for varying degree $d \in \{2, 5, 20\}$. The estimators are fed with (subsets of) the above generated data: the outputs y are the values stored in `y`, and the designs X are the first $d + 1$ columns of the values stored in `X`. The estimated functions are then evaluated on a fine grid called `x.plot` to obtain smooth graphs.

```
FunctionOutputs <- function(FUN, d, x.plot)
{
  return(REPLACE)
}
PlotLsLasso <- function(d, first.plot)
{
  x.plot <- seq(from=-1, to=1, by=0.01)
  if (first.plot == TRUE) ylab <- "y" else ylab <- ""  # y label only for first plot
  plot(x        = X[, 2],
       y        = y,  # samples
       xlim     = c(-1, 1),
       ylim     = c(-3, 3),
       col      = "gray68",
       xlab     = "x",
       cex.lab = 1.5,
       yaxt     = "n",
       ylab     = ylab,
       main     = paste0("degree = ", d))
  axis(side   = 2,
       labels = first.plot,
       las    = 1,
       yaxp   = c(-2, 2, 2))
  lines(x   = x.plot,
        y   = 2*x.plot^2,  # true model
        lwd = 3,
        col = "red")
  lines(x   = x.plot,
        y   = FunctionOutputs(FUN=LsEstimator, d, x.plot),  # least-squares estimates
        lwd = 4,
        col = "blue")
  lines(x   = x.plot,
        y   = FunctionOutputs(FUN=LassoEstimator, d, x.plot),  # lasso estimates
        lty = 2,
        lwd = 4,
        col = "seagreen3")
  legend("bottomleft",
         legend = c("true model", "least-squares", "lasso"),
         lty    = c(1, 1, 2),
         lwd    = c(3, 4, 4),
```

```
        col     = c("red", "blue", "seagreen3"),
        bty     = "n",   # no box
        cex     = 1.3)
}
par(mfrow=c(1, 3),  # three plots side-by-side
    oma = c(3, 3, 0, 0),   # outer margins
    mar = c(3, 1, 3, 0),   # inner margins
    mgp = c(3, 1, 0),   # location of the labels
    xpd = NA)  # allows the plots to overlap
PlotLsLasso(2, TRUE)
PlotLsLasso(5, FALSE)
PlotLsLasso(20, FALSE)
```

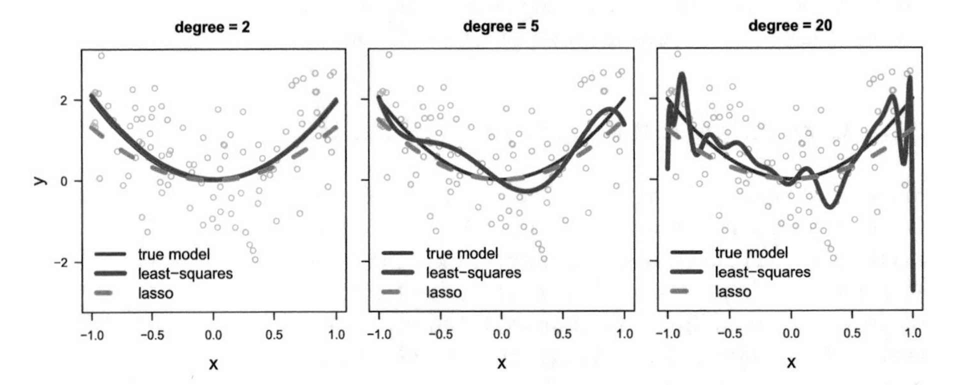

What can you conclude from the plots?

2.7.4 Further Illustrations

We now provide further illustrations of the above overfitting phenomenon. For this, we compare the least-squares and the lasso in four types of metrics: (i) data-fitting error $\|\boldsymbol{y} - X\widehat{\boldsymbol{\beta}}\|_2^2/n$, (ii) average prediction error $\|X\boldsymbol{\beta} - X\widehat{\boldsymbol{\beta}}\|_2^2/n$, (iii) estimation error $\|\boldsymbol{\beta} - \widehat{\boldsymbol{\beta}}\|_2$, and (iv) number of non-zero-valued coordinates $\|\widehat{\boldsymbol{\beta}}\|_0$—all as functions of the number of predictors/the degree of the assumed polynomial.

```
set.seed(68)
Metrics <- function(FUN, p.max, type)
{
  REPLACE
}
plot(x        = 3:(d + 1),  # starting from degree two = three predictors
     y        = Metrics(LsEstimator, d + 1, "fitting"),
     pch      = 1,
     ylim     = c(0, 1.2),
     yaxp     = c(0, 1, 2),
     col      = "blue",
     xlab     = "Number of predictors",
     ylab     = "Data-fitting error",
     las      = 1)
points(x   = 3:(d + 1),
       y   = Metrics(LassoEstimator, d + 1, "fitting"),
       pch = 0,
```

```
        col = "seagreen3")
legend("bottomleft",
       legend = c("least-squares", "lasso"),
       pch    = c(1, 0),
       lty    = 0,
       col    = c("blue", "seagreen3"),
       bty    = "n")  # no box
```

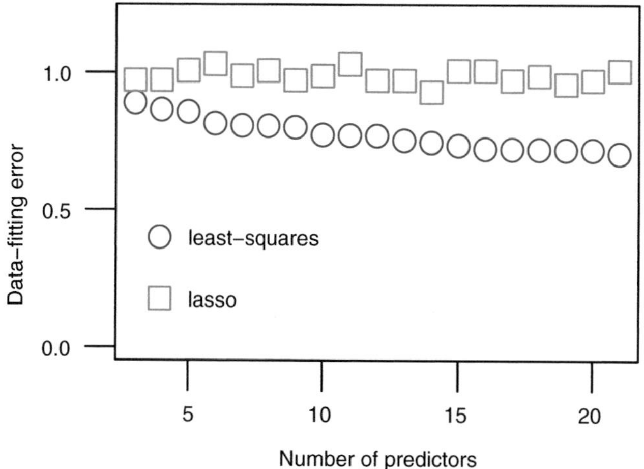

While for the least-squares, more predictors mean a better fit, the cross-validated lasso does not follow such a trend.

```
REPLACE  # generate the second plot
```

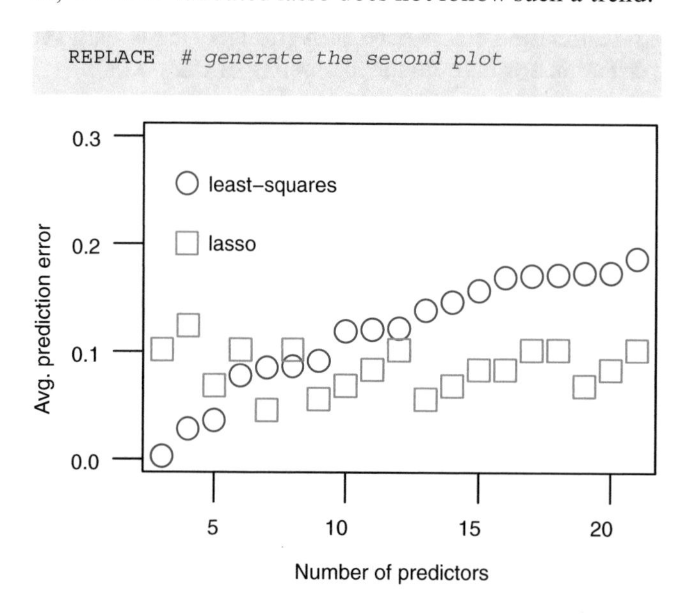

The prediction error of the least-squares increases as more predictors become available, while again, the lasso remains relatively stable. This is commensurate with the results of ► Sect. 1.2, which state a linear increase for the least-squares and only a logarithmic increase for the lasso. The data-fitting error above and the prediction error here are closely related to training and validation errors, which we will discuss in the context of cross-validation in ► Chap. 4.

```
REPLACE   # generate the third plot
```

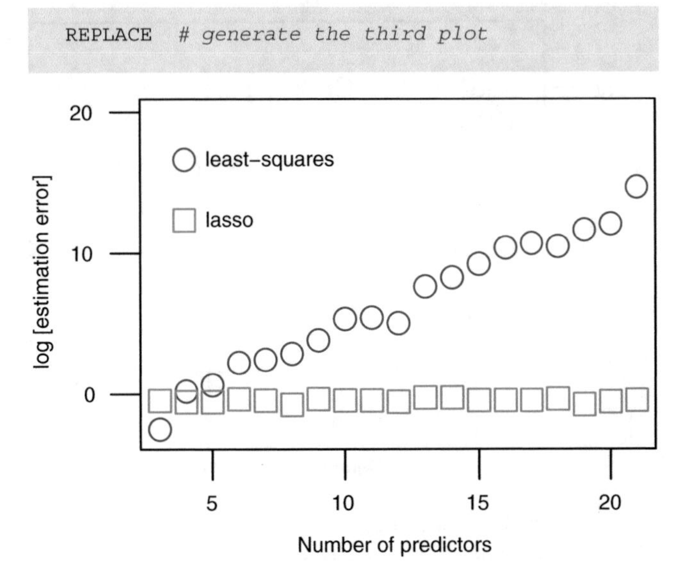

The estimation errors have even stronger trends than the prediction errors (note the log-scaling of the y-axis).

```
REPLACE   # generate the fourth plot
```

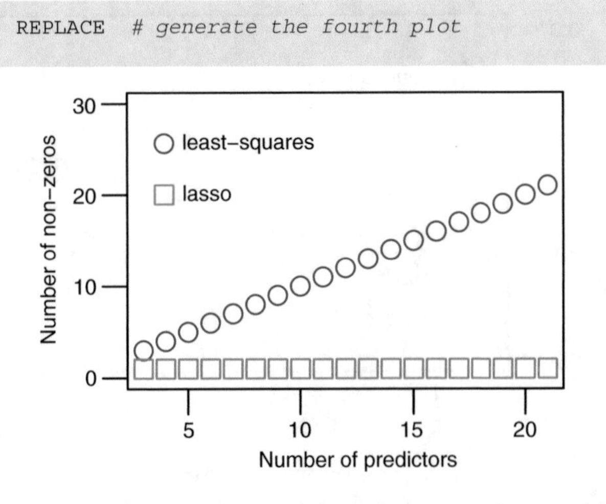

The lasso estimator always picks only one predictor, while the least-squares estimator picks all available ones. Ambiguities among those predictors can make the least-squares numerically and statistically instable. Since the polynomial layout generates strong dependencies among the predictors, these instabilities are expressed particularly strongly in the estimation errors.

2.8 Notes and References

1 More formally: a linear regression model is a combination of a probability space $(\mathscr{A}, \mathfrak{A}, \mathbb{P})$, random quantities $\boldsymbol{y} : (\mathscr{A}, \mathfrak{A}) \to (\mathbb{R}^n, \mathscr{B}^n)$, $X : (\mathscr{A}, \mathfrak{A}) \to (\mathbb{R}^{n\times p}, \mathscr{B}^{n\times p})$, and $\boldsymbol{u} : (\mathscr{A}, \mathfrak{A}) \to (\mathbb{R}^n, \mathscr{B}^n)$, where $\mathscr{B}^n, \mathscr{B}^{n\times p}$ denote the appropriate Borel σ-algebras, and a fixed vector $\boldsymbol{\beta} \in \mathbb{R}^p$ such that $\mathbb{P}\{\boldsymbol{y} - X\boldsymbol{\beta} - \boldsymbol{u} = \boldsymbol{0}_n\} = 1$.

2 A sufficient condition for (scaled) orthogonal design is that $X/\sqrt{n}$ is an orthogonal matrix—see Definition B.2.8. But this condition requires $p = n$, which we do not assume in general.

3 Frank and Friedman (1993, Equation (54) on p. 124) introduce least-squares regression with general ℓ_q-prior functions, $q \in [0, \infty]$; these estimators were later termed *bridge estimators*. The paper also motivates these priors from a Bayes perspective; we have adopted this viewpoint in Exercise 1.3. Bridge estimators with $q \in [1, 2]$ can be seen as interpolations between the lasso and the ridge; however, in contrast to the elastic net estimator, which is another such interpolation introduced in the main text, these estimators are sparse only if $q = 1$—see ◘ Fig. 2.2.

4 The lasso has been introduced in Tibshirani (1996). Its fast penetration into the sciences was also due to the rapid development of corresponding algorithms, such as in Osborne et al. (2000) and Efron et al. (2004).

5 Least-squares regression with a grouped ℓ_1-prior was first considered in Bakin (1999, Equation (2.7) on p. 22). Yuan and Lin (2006, Equation (2.1) on p. 51) introduce the more general prior function $\sum_{j=1}^{k} \sqrt{\boldsymbol{\alpha}_{\mathscr{A}_j}^\top K_j \boldsymbol{\alpha}_{\mathscr{A}_j}}$, where $K_j \in \mathbb{R}^{|\mathscr{A}_j|\times|\mathscr{A}_j|}$, and those authors coined the term group-lasso estimator for least-squares estimators with such priors. To facilitate the calibration of the tuning parameter r, Bunea et al. (2014, Definition (4) on p. 1314) combined the group lasso with the square-root lasso (6.2) to the *square-root group-lasso estimator*

$$\widehat{\boldsymbol{\beta}}_{\sqrt{\text{group}}} \in \underset{\boldsymbol{\alpha}\in\mathbb{R}^p}{\arg\min} \left\{ \|\boldsymbol{y} - X\boldsymbol{\alpha}\|_2 + r \sum_{j=1}^{k} \sqrt{\boldsymbol{\alpha}_{\mathscr{A}_j}^\top K_j \boldsymbol{\alpha}_{\mathscr{A}_j}} \right\}. \qquad (2.9)$$

Both Yuan and Lin (2006) and Bunea et al. (2014) suggest $K_j := |\mathscr{A}_j| \mathrm{I}_{|\mathscr{A}_j|\times|\mathscr{A}_j|}$ if the predictors are orthogonal within groups (in fact, the predictors can be orthogonalized within groups without loss of generality). The factor $|\mathscr{A}_j|$ balances the selection of small and large groups and can be motivated by empirical process theory: van de Geer and Bühlmann (2011, Lemma 8.1 on p. 254) and Bunea et al. (2014, Lemma 2.1 on p. 1316) show for the original case and for the square-root case, respectively, that the mentioned choice of K_j can allow for a suitable regularization of all groups simultaneously if the noise is i.i.d. Gauss-distributed. The *sparse group-lasso estimator* of Simon et al. (2013, Equation (3) on p. 232) complements the group regularization with an additional ℓ_1-prior to obtain sparsity also within groups. Finally, overlapping groups have been studied in Obozinski et al. (2011) and others.

6 Huang et al. (2019) have studied the estimator

$$\widehat{\boldsymbol{\beta}}_{\text{edr}} \in \underset{\boldsymbol{\alpha} \in \mathbb{R}^p}{\arg\min} \left\{ \|\boldsymbol{y} - X\boldsymbol{\alpha}\|_2^2 + r\|\boldsymbol{\alpha}\|_2 \right\}$$

and termed it *Euclidean distance ridge (edr) estimator*. For every $r \in [0, \infty]$, there is a (data-dependent) tuning parameter r' such that $r\|\boldsymbol{\alpha}\|_2^2$- and $r'\|\boldsymbol{\alpha}\|_2$-regularization are equivalent, and, for every $r \in [0, \infty]$, there is a tuning parameter r' such that $r\|\boldsymbol{\alpha}\|_2$- and $r'\|\boldsymbol{\alpha}\|_2^2$-regularization are equivalent (Huang et al., 2019, Chapter 3). Hence, swapping the ℓ_2^2-prior for the ℓ_2-functions is essentially a change of tuning.

7 The elastic net was introduced in Zou and Hastie (2005, Equation (3) on p. 303).

8 Lemma 2 on p. 306 in Zou and Hastie (2005) supports our earlier statement about the different selection tendencies of the ridge estimator/elastic net and the lasso: On the one hand, every least-squares estimator with *strictly* convex prior terms (such as the elastic net with $w \in [0, 1)$) assigns the same coordinate estimates $\widehat{\beta}_i = \widehat{\beta}_j$ to two equal predictors $\boldsymbol{x}_{[i]} = \boldsymbol{x}_j$; on the other hand, there is always one solution of the lasso estimator that sets one of those coordinate estimates to zero. Thus, the elastic net selects or disregards perfectly correlated predictors as a group, while the lasso selects at most one representative among such predictors. More generally, Theorem 1 in that paper shows that two coordinate estimates of the elastic net converge as (i) the corresponding predictors become more correlated or (ii) the tuning parameter $(1 - w)r$ increases. Further observations in this direction are made in Bien and Wegkamp (2013).

9 Least-squares refitting for the *lars estimator*, a sibling of the lasso estimator, has been proposed by Efron et al. (2004, p. 421) under the name *lars-ols hybrid.* Meinshausen (2007, Definition 1 on p. 376) introduced the *relaxed lasso*: a lasso on the support of an initial lasso, where the tuning parameter for the second stage lasso is chosen smaller than the one for the first stage.

10 Settings where the standard least-squares refitting described in our text increases the lasso's accuracy are described in Belloni and Chernozhukov (2013); settings where least-squares refitting decreases the lasso's accuracy are described in Lederer (2013). As a rule of thumb, least-squares refitting can render estimations even more accurate in "easy" settings, but it can add considerable error in "difficult" settings.

11 A weaker version of the strong oracle property is the *weak oracle property*, which states that an estimator has (approximately) the same accuracy as the oracle estimator. In the case of linear regression models with Gauss-distributed noise, this latter property basically refers to bounds that do not involve the lasso's $\log p$-terms. Still, the requirements for those inequalities are usually strict and unverifiable in practice.

12 The scad (smoothly clipped absolute deviation) regularizer was introduced in Fan and Li (2001, Display (2.7) on p. 1350); the mcp (minimax concave penalty) in Zhang (2010, Display (2.2) on p. 897).
13 As two examples among many such results, Zhang and Zhang (2012, Theorem 1 on p. 584) and Kim et al. (2008, Theorem 3 on p. 1668) provide sufficient conditions for such estimators satisfying weak and strong oracle properties, respectively. However, these conditions are strict: For example, they imply $p \leq n$ in the latter result (see their subsequent remark).
14 Note that ℓ_q-regularization, $q \in (0, 1)$, also renders least-squares estimation non-convex, but it is otherwise very different from capped ℓ_1-regularization: First, ℓ_q-priors change the regularization landscape of the entire *vector* of parameters, while the capped ℓ_1-prior consists of sums over regularizers for each individual *coordinate*. Second, capped ℓ_1-norms are bounded, while ℓ_q-functions are absolute homogenous, that is, linearly increasing in their function argument; this means in particular that ℓ_q-regularization (without additional steps such as refitting) does not satisfy the strong oracle property. Third, the (sub-)gradients of the capped ℓ_1-norms are bounded everywhere, while the (sub-)gradients of ℓ_q-functions go to infinity as the function argument goes to zero; this divergence at zero can lead to numerical instabilities.
15 In fact, it is a "signed" distance: $\overline{c}$ is negative if the hyperplane is on the side of the origin opposite to $\boldsymbol{a}$. Another subtlety is that $\overline{c}$ might not exist (this is why the definition has a supremum rather than a maximum), but one can always approximate it to an arbitrary precision. For details, we refer to Hiriart-Urruty and Lemaréchal (2004, Section C.2.1 on pp. 134ff): This contains an illustration for *support functions*, for which our dual functions are a special case.
16 The reverse statement is not true: $\mathscr{h} : \boldsymbol{a} \mapsto 1$ is scalable but not absolute homogenous.
17 The *graph of a function* $\mathscr{f} : \mathbb{R}^p \to \mathbb{R}$ is the set $\{(\boldsymbol{a}, \mathscr{f}[\boldsymbol{a}]) : \boldsymbol{a} \in \mathbb{R}^p\}$. It should not be confused with the graphs that we discuss in ▸ Chap. 3 on graphical models.
18 The *closed line segment* between two points $\boldsymbol{a}, \boldsymbol{b} \in \mathbb{R}^p$ is the set of points $\{w\boldsymbol{a} + (1 - w)\boldsymbol{b} \in \mathbb{R}^p : w \in [0, 1]\}$. The *open line segment* between two points $\boldsymbol{a}, \boldsymbol{b} \in \mathbb{R}^p$, $\boldsymbol{a} \neq \boldsymbol{b}$, is the set of points $\{w\boldsymbol{a} + (1 - w)\boldsymbol{b} \in \mathbb{R}^p : w \in (0, 1)\}$.
19 Similarly, we call a function $\mathscr{f}$ *(strictly) concave* if $-\mathscr{f}$ is (strictly) convex.
20 See Hiriart-Urruty and Lemaréchal (2004, Section VI.1.4 on pp. 247ff) for different approaches to proving the existence of a subgradient.
21 See Hiriart-Urruty and Lemaréchal (2004, Theorem 4.1 on p. 183), for example. The result is sometimes referred to as *Moreau–Rockafellar theorem*.
22 The name KKT refers to the authors of Karush (1939) and Kuhn and Tucker (1951).

Graphical Models

Contents

J. Lederer, *Fundamentals of High-Dimensional Statistics*, Springer Texts in Statistics,
https://doi.org/10.1007/978-3-030-73792-4_3

The beginning of this book illustrates that linear regression models can describe the relationships between the genes' copy numbers and a biomarker. However, those models do not provide information about the relationships among the copy numbers themselves. To describe such relationships, we use a different type of models, called graphical models. We neglect the biomarker and summarize the measured copy numbers in vector-valued observations, where each vector corresponds to a specific subject and each coordinate of these vectors to a specific gene (in the linear regression model, these vectors are the rows of the design matrix). Graphical models then formulate the relationships among the copy numbers as conditional dependence networks among the coordinates of the vector-valued observations. If the observations follow a multivariate Gauss distribution, we speak of Gaussian graphical models. This is the most common class of graphical models and, therefore, the focus of this chapter.

3.1 Overview

Natural and artificial phenomena often consist of many parts that depend on each other in a complex manner. Consider biology, for example: cells feature hundreds of biochemical processes that affect each other through various metabolic pathways; the human gut accommodates thousands of different species that feed off each other or interact in other ways; the human brain contains several billions of neurons that communicate through trillions of synapses. Our goal is to develop mathematical models for those network structures to unravel the underpinning biological, physical, or mechanical principles.

There are a number of different types of mathematical network models, among them *differential equations, Boolean networks,* and *graphical models.*[1] In recent years, graphical models have become the dominant type in a number of fields, because they summarize dependence structures in comprehensive, yet concise graphical representations that lend themselves naturally to scientific interpretation.[2] The basic concept of graphical models is *conditional dependence.* Consider the two events `bike`= "you bike to work" and `dog` = "neighbor walks dog". The events `bike` and `dog` are not independent, as sunshine might make you feel tempted to use your bike as well as it might motivate the neighbor to go outside and walk the dog:

$$\texttt{bike} \not\perp \texttt{dog} \qquad \text{"}\texttt{bike}\text{ is not independent of }\texttt{dog}\text{"}.$$

However, the events bike and dog are not congruent either, as you might ride the bike even in hard rain in guilt over a big meal you had the night before, which on the other hand has no influence on the neighbor's inclination to walk her dog. Stating the above dependence relation alone thus conceals that there is a common trigger for both events (sunshine) as well as independent triggers for each of the two events (such as your big meal the night before). We can unravel this structure by adding a third event sun = "sun is shining": the events bike and dog are dependent, but they are independent *after adjusting* for the influence of sun. We call the latter statement *conditional independence*,[3] indicated in speech by adding the word *given* together with the event we adjust for:

conditional independence

$$\texttt{bike} \perp \texttt{dog} \mid \texttt{sun} \qquad \text{"given }\texttt{sun}\text{, }\texttt{bike}\text{ is independent of }\texttt{dog}\text{"}.$$

Hence, conditional dependence allows for a more detailed description of the relationships than traditional dependence.

We now can visualize these relationships by using graphs. The basic elements of the graph are the events bike, dog, and sun. We call them *nodes* (or *vertices*). Thinking in terms of independence, two nodes are directly connected if and only if the corresponding events are dependent—see the left panel of ◘ Fig. 3.1. Thinking in terms of conditional independence, two nodes are directly connected if and only if the corresponding events are conditional dependent given all other events—see the right panel of ◘ Fig. 3.1. In any case, we call these

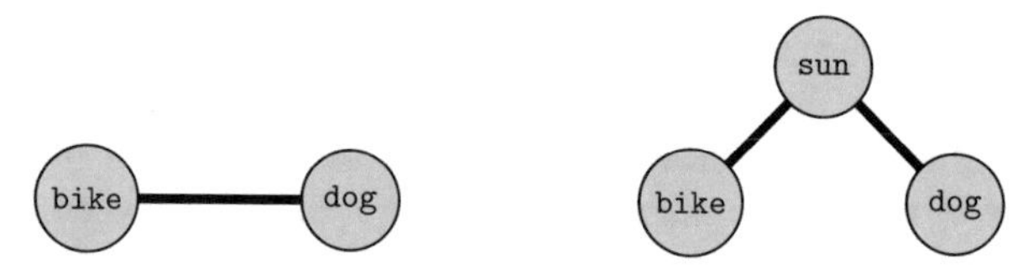

◘ **Fig. 3.1** The graph on the left-hand side depicts that bike and dog are dependent; the graph in the middle depicts the more granular statement that bike and dog are dependent but conditionally independent, that is, independent *given* sun

connections *edges*, and a pair $\mathcal{G} = (\mathcal{I}, \mathcal{E})$ of a set of nodes $\mathcal{I}$ and a corresponding set of edges $\mathcal{E}$ a *graph*. The graph on the left-hand side of ◘ Fig. 3.1 describes the dependence relation between `bike` and `dog`: the nodes are `bike` and `dog`, and the edge is between `bike` and `dog`. The graph on the right-hand side of ◘ Fig. 3.1 describes the dependence relation between `bike`, `dog`, and `sun`: the nodes are `bike`, `dog`, and `sun`, and the edges are between `bike` and `sun` and between `dog` and `sun`.

In more realistic examples, the nodes are not necessarily simple events but rather real-valued random variables such as the expression levels of genes or the activity levels of neurons. The edges then describe the (conditional) dependencies among those random variables. We denote the random variables by $z_1, \ldots, z_d$ and summarize them in the vector $z := (z_1, \ldots, z_d)^\top \in \mathbb{R}^d$. Now, a pair $(z, \mathcal{G})$ of such a random vector z and a graph $\mathcal{G}$ that encapsulates the *conditional* dependence relationships of the random variables that form the vector is called a *graphical model*.[4] For ease of notation, we identify the nodes with the indexes of the random variables: $\mathcal{I} = \{1, \ldots, p\}$; accordingly, we denote an edge between z_i and z_j by the unordered pair (i, j), where unordered means that (i, j) and (j, i) are the same edge.

graphical model

In practice, we do not know the conditional dependence relationships among the variables. Consequently, our goal for this chapter is to derive the corresponding graph from data. Such data consist of n snapshots of the network's state, that is, n realizations $z_1, \ldots, z_n \in \mathbb{R}^d$ of the random vector z. For example, if the graphical model $(z, \mathcal{G})$ concerns the genes' coactivation network in a certain type of tissue, then z_i could comprise the expression levels of the d genes under consideration in the ith tissue sample. In contrast to linear regression, data for graphical models do not contain separate outcomes y and designs X; instead, the data vectors $z_1, \ldots, z_n$ are now both outcome and design simultaneously—see especially ▶ Sect. 3.4. This double role also increases the model complexities: In linear regression, the number of model parameters equals the number of predictors; in graphical modeling, the number of model parameters equals the number of potential connections among the nodes and, therefore, quadratic in the number of nodes. More precisely, the number of potential connections, that is, the maximal size of the edge set, is $d(d-1)/2$; accordingly, a graphical model is low-dimensional only if $d(d-1)/2 \ll n$ and high-dimensional whenever $d(d-1)/2 \approx n$ or even $d(d-1)/2 \gg n$.

We focus on the most popular type of graphical models: Gaussian graphical models (▶ Sect. 3.2). The name indicates that the observations are from a Gauss distribution. We introduce two approaches to learning the corresponding graph: Maximum likelihood (▶ Sect. 3.3) and neighborhood selection (▶ Sect. 3.4). The two approaches coincide in low dimensions (Exercise 3.4), but they differ in how they include prior information (regularizing all edges collectively versus regularizing each node's neighborhood individually).

3.2 Gaussian Graphical Models

Gaussian graphical models are graphical models whose random vectors follow a multivariate Gauss distribution. Gaussian graphical models are the most popular type of graphical models, because they are especially easy to handle; in particular, their conditional and unconditional dependence structures are fully determined by the inverse of the covariance matrix of the distribution at hand, and the estimation of the covariance matrix is amenable to standard methodology such as maximum (regularized) likelihood. Hence, observations that are not Gauss-distributed, such as copy number counts of genes, are often transformed to fit a Gauss distribution at least approximately.[5]

Gaussian graphical model

In mathematical terms, a *Gaussian graphical model* is a pair $(z, \mathcal{G})$ that consists of a Gauss vector $z \sim \mathcal{N}_d[\boldsymbol{\mu}, \Sigma]$ for an arbitrary mean vector $\boldsymbol{\mu} \in \mathbb{R}^d$ and a symmetric and positive definite *covariance matrix* $\Sigma \in \mathbb{R}^{d \times d}$ and of a corresponding conditional independence graph $\mathcal{G}$. In such models, the graph $\mathcal{G}$ and the inverse of the covariance matrix, the *precision matrix* $\Theta := \Sigma^{-1}$, are intimately related:[6]

covariance and precision matrices

Theorem 3.2.1

Hammersley–Clifford, Part I Given a Gaussian graphical model $(z, \mathscr{G})$ with precision matrix Θ, it holds for all pairs of indexes $i, j \in \{1, \ldots, d\}$, $i \neq j$, that

$$z_i \perp z_j \mid z_{\{1,\ldots,d\}\setminus\{i,j\}} \quad \Leftrightarrow \quad \Theta_{ij} = 0\,,$$

that is, the edge set of the graph is $\mathscr{E} = \{(i, j) \in \mathscr{I} \times \mathscr{I} : i \neq j, \Theta_{ij} \neq 0\}$.

The same graph $\mathscr{G}$ also describes the unconditional dependencies among the coordinates of z:

Theorem 3.2.2

Hammersley–Clifford, Part II Given a Gaussian graphical model $(z, \mathscr{G})$ with precision matrix Θ, it holds for all pairs of indexes $i, j \in \{1, \ldots, d\}$, $i \neq j$, that

$$z_i \perp z_j \quad \Leftrightarrow$$
$$\nexists k \in \{1, 2, \ldots\},\ l_1, \ldots, l_k \in \{1, \ldots, d\} : \Theta_{il_1}\Theta_{l_1l_2}\cdots\Theta_{l_kj} \neq 0\,,$$

that is, two coordinates z_i and z_j are independent if and only if there is no path of edges $(i, l_1), (l_1, l_2), \ldots, (l_k, j) \in \mathscr{E}$ between them.

(We omit the proofs.[7]) For example, if $\Theta_{ij} \neq 0$, that is, $(i, j) \in \mathscr{E}$, then z_i and z_j are neither conditional independent (given any set of coordinates) nor unconditionally independent.

The covariance matrix Σ is symmetric and positive definite by definition and also invertible according to 1. in Lemma B.2.5. Hence, also the precision matrix Θ is symmetric according to 2. in Lemma B.2.6, positive definite according to 2. in Lemma B.2.5, and invertible according to 1. in Lemma B.2.5.

In summary, the non-zero pattern of the precision matrix captures the entire dependence structure of the Gauss-distributed vector z; ◘ Fig. 3.2 contains an illustration. Hence, our goal is to estimate Θ (rather than Σ), and we call the elements of Θ the *model parameters* of Gaussian graphical models.

$$\Theta = \begin{pmatrix} 1.2 & -0.2 & 0 & 0 \\ -0.2 & 1.5 & 0 & 0.3 \\ 0 & 0 & 1 & 0 \\ 0 & 0.3 & 0 & 0.5 \end{pmatrix}$$

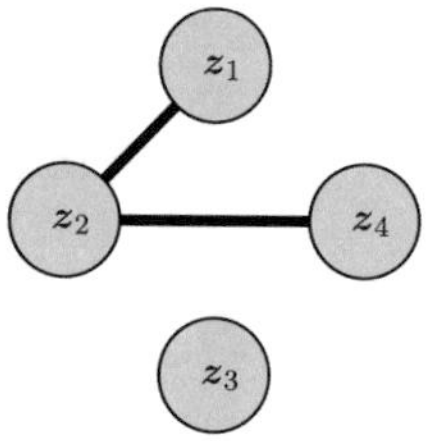

Fig. 3.2 The right panel contains an example of a precision matrix Θ of a Gauss-distributed vector z. Since $\Theta_{14} = 0$ but $\Theta_{12}\Theta_{24} \neq 0$, the coordinates z_1 and z_4 are conditionally independent given the other coordinates but not unconditionally independent. This is illustrated also in the corresponding dependence graph $\mathscr{G}$ on the right: $(1, 4) \notin \mathscr{E}$ but $(1, 2), (2, 4) \in \mathscr{E}$

3.3 Maximum Regularized Likelihood Estimation

Having discussed the concept of Gaussian graphical models, we now turn to estimating its parameters. We first think of the models as parameterized by the coordinates of the inverse covariance matrix, which indeed specifies the entire distribution of the observations. The proposed estimators for these parameters are maximum likelihood in low-dimensional settings and regularized variants of it in high-dimensional settings. We then focus in on the elements of the underpinning edge set, which, in view of the Hammersley–Clifford theorem, specifies the conditional dependence network. Since the edge set corresponds to the non-zero-valued entries of the inverse covariance matrix, it can be estimated by simply thresholding the estimate of the inverse covariance matrix.

The density of a single Gauss vector $z \sim \mathscr{N}_d[\gamma, \Omega^{-1}]$ is

$$\mathscr{f}[z] = \frac{1}{\sqrt{(2\pi)^d \det[\Omega^{-1}]}} e^{-(z-\gamma)^\top \Omega (z-\gamma)/2} .$$

(A brief review of determinants can be found in ▶ Sect. B.2 in the Appendix.) The density of n independent random vectors $z_1, \ldots, z_n \sim \mathscr{N}_d[\gamma, \Omega^{-1}]$ is, therefore,

$$\mathscr{f}[z_1, \ldots, z_n] = \prod_{i=1}^{n} \frac{1}{\sqrt{(2\pi)^d \det[\Omega^{-1}]}} e^{-(z_i-\gamma)^\top \Omega (z_i-\gamma)/2} .$$

The logarithm of this density as a function of the model parameters is called the *likelihood function* $\ell : \mathbb{R}^d \times \mathbb{R}^{d\times d} \to \mathbb{R}$. We find

$$\ell[\gamma, \Omega] = \log\left[\prod_{i=1}^{n} \frac{1}{\sqrt{(2\pi)^d \det[\Omega^{-1}]}} e^{-(z_i-\gamma)^\top\Omega(z_i-\gamma)/2}\right]$$

preceding display

$$= \sum_{i=1}^{n} \Big(- d\log[2\pi]/2 + \log\big[\det[\Omega]\big]/2$$

$$- (z_i-\gamma)^\top\Omega(z_i-\gamma)/2\Big)$$

$\log[ab] = \log[a] + \log[b]$; $\log[a^b] = b\log[a]$; $\det[A] = 1/\det[A^{-1}]$

$$\hat{=} \frac{1}{n}\sum_{i=1}^{n}\Big(\log\big[\det[\Omega]\big] - (z_i-\gamma)^\top\Omega(z_i-\gamma)\Big)$$

$\max_{\boldsymbol{a}} f[\boldsymbol{a}] = \max_{\boldsymbol{a}} b(f[\boldsymbol{a}] + c)$ for $b \in (0,\infty)$, $c \in \mathbb{R}$ constant: here $b = 2/n$, $c = d\log[2\pi]/2$

$$\hat{=} -\frac{1}{n}\sum_{i=1}^{n}\Big((z_i-\gamma)^\top\Omega(z_i-\gamma) - \log\big[\det[\Omega]\big]\Big)$$

$\max_{\boldsymbol{a}} f[\boldsymbol{a}] = \min_{\boldsymbol{a}} -f[\boldsymbol{a}]$

$$= -\frac{1}{n}\sum_{i=1}^{n}(z_i-\gamma)^\top\Omega(z_i-\gamma) + \log\big[\det[\Omega]\big]$$

linearity of sums

$$= -\frac{1}{n}\sum_{i=1}^{n}\operatorname{trace}\big[(z_i-\gamma)^\top\Omega(z_i-\gamma)\big] + \log\big[\det[\Omega]\big]$$

$a = \operatorname{trace}[a]$ for $a \in \mathbb{R}$ by Definition B.2.6

$$= -\frac{1}{n}\sum_{i=1}^{n}\operatorname{trace}\big[(z_i-\gamma)(z_i-\gamma)^\top\Omega\big] + \log\big[\det[\Omega]\big]$$

the trace function is symmetric according to Lemma B.2.7

$$= -\operatorname{trace}\left[\frac{1}{n}\sum_{i=1}^{n}(z_i-\gamma)(z_i-\gamma)^\top\Omega\right] + \log\big[\det[\Omega]\big].$$

the trace function is linear according to Lemma B.2.7

Given data, that is, concrete values for $z_1, \ldots, z_n$, the maximum of the likelihood function ℓ, or equivalently, the minimum of the negative likelihood function $-\ell$, is called the *maximum likelihood estimator*. In our case, the optimization is over $\mathbb{R}^d$ and $\mathcal{S}_d^+$, the set of symmetric and positive definite matrices in $\mathbb{R}^{d\times d}$:

$$(\widehat{\boldsymbol{\mu}}_{\mathrm{ml}}, \widehat{\Theta}_{\mathrm{ml}}) \in \underset{\boldsymbol{\gamma}\in\mathbb{R}^d,\, \Omega\in\mathcal{S}_d^+}{\arg\min} \left\{ \operatorname{trace}\left[\frac{1}{n}\sum_{i=1}^{n}(z_i-\boldsymbol{\gamma})(z_i-\boldsymbol{\gamma})^\top\Omega\right] - \log[\det[\Omega]] \right\}.$$

For practical and computational convenience, however, we typically transform the data first. One option is to *center* the data according to $(z_i)_j \mapsto (z_i)_j - \sum_{k=1}^{n}(z_k)_j/n$ for all $i \in \{1,\ldots,n\}$ and $j \in \{1,\ldots,d\}$. Centering allows us to work with centered Gauss distributions ($\boldsymbol{\mu} = \mathbf{0}_d$) and, therefore, to avoid intercepts. Another option is to *standardize* the data according to

standardizing data

$$(z_i)_j \mapsto \frac{(z_i)_j - \sum_{k=1}^{n}(z_k)_j/n}{\sqrt{\sum_{l=1}^{n}\left((z_l)_j - \sum_{k=1}^{n}(z_k)_j/n\right)^2/(n-1)}} \tag{3.1}$$

for all $i \in \{1,\ldots,n\}$ and $j \in \{1,\ldots,d\}$. Standardizing additionally homogenizes the variances, which can avoid complications in regularizing and computing the estimators. After either transformation, we can fix the true mean vector to $\boldsymbol{\mu} = \mathbf{0}_d$, which simplifies the maximum likelihood estimator to

maximum likelihood estimator

$$\widehat{\Theta}_{\mathrm{ml}} = \underset{\Omega\in\mathcal{S}_d^+}{\arg\min} \left\{ \operatorname{trace}\left[\frac{1}{n}\sum_{i=1}^{n} z_i z_i^\top \Omega\right] - \log\left[\det[\Omega]\right] \right\}. \tag{3.2}$$

The maximum likelihood estimator can be effective in estimating the inverse covariance matrix in low-dimensional settings, where the number of samples is much larger than the number of model parameters: $n \gg d(d-1)/2$. In particular, if $n \geq d$, the maximum likelihood estimator (3.2) exists, is unique, and is equal to

$$\widehat{\Theta}_{\mathrm{ml}} = \left(\frac{1}{n}\sum_{i=1}^{n} z_i z_i^\top\right)^{-1}, \tag{3.3}$$

all with probability 1—see 5. in Exercise 3.3. The matrix $\sum_{i=1}^{n} z_i z_i^\top/n$ is called the *empirical covariance matrix*.

In high-dimensional settings, the likelihood function is complemented with a prior function. Given such a function $\mathcal{h} : \mathcal{S}_d^+ \to \mathbb{R}$ and a tuning parameter $r \in [0, \infty)$, this yields the *maximum regularized likelihood estimator*

$$\widehat{\Theta}_{\text{mrl}} \in \underset{\Omega \in \mathcal{S}_d^+}{\arg\min} \left\{ \text{trace}\left[\frac{1}{n}\sum_{i=1}^{n} z_i z_i^\top \Omega\right] - \log\left[\det[\Omega]\right] + r\mathcal{h}[\Omega] \right\}. \quad (3.4)$$

graphical lasso

The most popular example is the *graphical lasso estimator*,[8] where $\mathcal{h}[\Omega] = \sum_{i,j=1}^{d} |\Omega_{ij}|$ or $\mathcal{h}[\Omega] = \sum_{\substack{i,j=1\\ i\neq j}}^{d} |\Omega_{ij}|$. Similarly as the lasso in linear regression, the graphical lasso estimator leverages sparsity, which means for Gaussian graphical models that the precision matrix Ω has only a small number of non-zero-valued entries: $|\{(i,j) : \Omega_{ij} \neq 0\}| \ll n, d(d-1)/2$. The graphical lasso estimator does not have a general closed-form solution but still can be computed efficiently—see 2. in Exercise 3.3.

Graph estimates can finally be obtained through *thresholding* the estimated precision matrix, similarly as in ► Sect. 2.3 for linear regression. We define $\widehat{\mathcal{G}} = (\mathcal{I}, \widehat{\mathcal{E}})$ from estimates $\widehat{\Theta} \in \mathbb{R}^{d\times d}$ of the precision matrix, $\widehat{\Theta} \in \{\widehat{\Theta}_{\text{ml}}, \widehat{\Theta}_{\text{mrl}}\}$, through (cf. ► Sect. 7.4)

$$\widehat{\mathcal{E}} := \left\{(i,j) \in \mathcal{I} \times \mathcal{I} : i \neq j,\ |\widehat{\Theta}_{ij}| > c\right\}, \quad (3.5)$$

where $c \in [0, \infty]$ is a cutoff—cf. (2.4). The discussed estimators $\widehat{\Theta}_{\text{ml}}, \widehat{\Theta}_{\text{mrl}}$ are symmetric by construction and, therefore, generate symmetric edge sets: $(i,j) \in \widehat{\mathcal{E}}$ if and only if $(j,i) \in \widehat{\mathcal{E}}$. The cutoff c regulates how conservative the graph estimate is: the larger c, the less likely are false positives but the more likely are false negatives (cf. Theorem 7.4.1). In the case of sparse estimators such as the graphical lasso, one may take $c = 0$, that is, the estimated edges are the ones that have non-zero-valued entries in the estimated precision matrix. This choice avoids the introduction of yet another tuning parameter.[9] In the case of unregularized maximum likelihood estimation, however, $c = 0$ almost always leads to a full graph. To remove spurious dependencies, a suggested cutoff is then $c = \sqrt{\log[d]/n}$. The size of this cutoff is related to the size of tuning parameters r in front of ℓ_1-prior terms—cf. ► Sect. 4.2.

3.4 Neighborhood Selection

Neighborhood selection is an alternative approach to estimating the elements of the precision matrix and the corresponding graphs. It exploits the fact that the coordinates of Gauss random vectors are connected via standard linear regression models with the entries of the inverse covariance matrix forming the corresponding regression vectors. This transforms the estimation of the inverse covariance matrix into multiple regressions, which are amenable to the techniques of the previous chapter.

The following result states that the coordinates of Gauss-distributed vectors are connected via linear regressions.

Lemma 3.4.1

Neighborhood Selection Given a Gauss random vector $z \sim \mathcal{N}_d[\boldsymbol{\mu}, \Theta^{-1}]$, it holds for all indexes $j \in \{1, \ldots, d\}$ that

$$z_j = \mu_j + \Theta_{j\{j\}^\complement} \boldsymbol{\mu}_{\{j\}^\complement} / \Theta_{jj} + z_{\{j\}^\complement}^\top \boldsymbol{\beta}^j + u_j ,$$

where $\{j\}^\complement := \{1, \ldots, d\} \setminus \{j\}$, $\boldsymbol{\beta}^j := -(\Theta_{j\{j\}^\complement})^\top / \Theta_{jj} \in \mathbb{R}^{d-1}$, and $u_j \sim \mathcal{N}_1[0, 1/\Theta_{jj}]$ is independent of $z_{\{j\}^\complement}$.

Note that $\Theta_{jj} \neq 0$ by 3. in Lemma B.2.5. The lemma states that the entries of the precision matrix form the regression vectors for regressing one coordinate of a Gauss-distributed random vector onto the others. In the following, we assume again that the data is centered or standardized and fix $\boldsymbol{\mu} = \mathbf{0}_d$ (see Page 89). This means in particular that we can neglect the intercepts: $\mu_j + \Theta_{j\{j\}^\complement} \boldsymbol{\mu}_{\{j\}^\complement} / \Theta_{jj} = 0$.

Proof of Lemma 3.4.1 We assume $\boldsymbol{\mu} = \mathbf{0}_d$ without loss of generality but otherwise prove a more general statement: Consider a Gauss-distributed vector $z \sim \mathcal{N}_d[\mathbf{0}_d, \Theta^{-1}]$ with a precision matrix that we write as

$$\Theta = \begin{pmatrix} \Theta_{\mathcal{A}\mathcal{A}} & \Theta_{\mathcal{A}\mathcal{B}} \\ \Theta_{\mathcal{B}\mathcal{A}} & \Theta_{\mathcal{B}\mathcal{B}} \end{pmatrix},$$

where $\mathcal{A} := \{1, \ldots, k\}$, $\mathcal{B} := \{k+1, \ldots, d\}$ for a fixed integer $k \in \{1, \ldots, d-1\}$. Then, the conditional distribution of $z_{\mathcal{A}}$ given $z_{\mathcal{B}}$ is $\mathcal{N}_k[-(\Theta_{\mathcal{A}\mathcal{A}})^{-1}\Theta_{\mathcal{A}\mathcal{B}}z_{\mathcal{B}}, (\Theta_{\mathcal{A}\mathcal{A}})^{-1}]$, that is,

$$z_{\mathcal{A}} = -(\Theta_{\mathcal{A}\mathcal{A}})^{-1}\Theta_{\mathcal{A}\mathcal{B}}z_{\mathcal{B}} + \boldsymbol{u}_{\mathcal{A}},$$

where $\boldsymbol{u}_{\mathcal{A}} \sim \mathcal{N}_k[\mathbf{0}_k, (\Theta_{\mathcal{A}\mathcal{A}})^{-1}]$ is independent of $z_{\mathcal{B}}$.

The key ingredient of the proof is Lemma B.2.15, which relates submatrices and inverses of matrices. We also use properties that are specific to Gauss-distributed data; for example, we invoke the fact that marginals of Gauss distributions are again Gauss distributions.

Lemma 3.4.1 follows by setting $k = 1$ (and reshuffling the model parameters if $j \neq 1$).

Writing

$$\Sigma = \begin{pmatrix} \Sigma_{\mathcal{A}\mathcal{A}} & \Sigma_{\mathcal{A}\mathcal{B}} \\ \Sigma_{\mathcal{B}\mathcal{A}} & \Sigma_{\mathcal{B}\mathcal{B}} \end{pmatrix},$$

Lemma B.2.15 (with $M = \Sigma$ and $M^{-1} = \Theta$) yields

$$\text{(i)}\ (\Sigma_{\mathcal{B}\mathcal{B}})^{-1} = \Theta_{\mathcal{B}\mathcal{B}} - \Theta_{\mathcal{B}\mathcal{A}}(\Theta_{\mathcal{A}\mathcal{A}})^{-1}\Theta_{\mathcal{A}\mathcal{B}} \quad \text{and}$$

$$\text{(ii)}\ \frac{\det[\Sigma_{\mathcal{B}\mathcal{B}}]}{\det[\Sigma]} = \frac{1}{\det[(\Theta_{\mathcal{A}\mathcal{A}})^{-1}]}.$$

We denote the conditional density of $z_{\mathcal{A}}$ given $z_{\mathcal{B}}$ by $f_{\mathcal{A}|\mathcal{B}}[z_{\mathcal{A}} \mid z_{\mathcal{B}}]$ and the marginal densities of z and $z_{\mathcal{B}}$ by $f[z]$ and $f_{\mathcal{B}}[z_{\mathcal{B}}]$, respectively. We then state (without proof) that marginals of Gauss distributions are again Gauss distributions: if $z \sim \mathcal{N}_d[\mathbf{0}_d, \Sigma]$, then $z_{\mathcal{B}} \sim \mathcal{N}_{d-k}[\mathbf{0}_{d-k}, \Sigma_{\mathcal{B}\mathcal{B}}]$. Using this with the two insights above then allows us to derive the following:

$$\begin{aligned}
&f_{\mathcal{A}|\mathcal{B}}[z_{\mathcal{A}} \mid z_{\mathcal{B}}] \\
&= f[z]/f_{\mathcal{B}}[z_{\mathcal{B}}] && \text{Bayes rule} \\
&= \frac{1}{\sqrt{(2\pi)^d \det[\Sigma]}} e^{-z^\top \Theta z/2} \Big/ \frac{1}{\sqrt{(2\pi)^{d-k}\det[\Sigma_{\mathcal{B}\mathcal{B}}]}} e^{-z_{\mathcal{B}}^\top(\Sigma_{\mathcal{B}\mathcal{B}})^{-1}z_{\mathcal{B}}/2} \\
& && \text{above statement about Gaussian marginals} \\
&= \sqrt{\frac{\det[\Sigma_{\mathcal{B}\mathcal{B}}]}{(2\pi)^k \det[\Sigma]}} \\
&\quad \times e^{-z_{\mathcal{A}}^\top\Theta_{\mathcal{A}\mathcal{A}}z_{\mathcal{A}}/2 - z_{\mathcal{B}}^\top\Theta_{\mathcal{B}\mathcal{B}}z_{\mathcal{B}}/2 - z_{\mathcal{A}}^\top\Theta_{\mathcal{A}\mathcal{B}}z_{\mathcal{B}}/2 - z_{\mathcal{B}}^\top\Theta_{\mathcal{B}\mathcal{A}}z_{\mathcal{A}}/2 + z_{\mathcal{B}}^\top(\Sigma_{\mathcal{B}\mathcal{B}})^{-1}z_{\mathcal{B}}/2} \\
& && \text{simplifying; writing out } z^\top\Theta z
\end{aligned}$$

$$= \sqrt{\frac{\det[\Sigma_{\mathscr{B}\mathscr{B}}]}{(2\pi)^k \det[\Sigma]}}$$

$$\times e^{-z_{\mathscr{A}}^\top \Theta_{\mathscr{A}\mathscr{A}} z_{\mathscr{A}}/2 - z_{\mathscr{A}}^\top \Theta_{\mathscr{A}\mathscr{B}} z_{\mathscr{B}}/2 - z_{\mathscr{B}}^\top \Theta_{\mathscr{B}\mathscr{A}} z_{\mathscr{A}}/2 - z_{\mathscr{B}}^\top \Theta_{\mathscr{B}\mathscr{A}} (\Theta_{\mathscr{A}\mathscr{A}})^{-1} \Theta_{\mathscr{A}\mathscr{B}} z_{\mathscr{B}}/2}$$

(i) above

$$= \frac{1}{\sqrt{(2\pi)^k \det\left[(\Theta_{\mathscr{A}\mathscr{A}})^{-1}\right]}}$$

$$\times e^{-(z_{\mathscr{A}} + (\Theta_{\mathscr{A}\mathscr{A}})^{-1}\Theta_{\mathscr{A}\mathscr{B}} z_{\mathscr{B}})^\top \Theta_{\mathscr{A}\mathscr{A}} (z_{\mathscr{A}} + (\Theta_{\mathscr{A}\mathscr{A}})^{-1}\Theta_{\mathscr{A}\mathscr{B}} z_{\mathscr{B}})/2} .$$

(ii) above; summarizing terms in the exponent recalling that $\Theta_{\mathscr{B}\mathscr{A}} = \Theta_{\mathscr{A}\mathscr{B}}$ due to the symmetry of Θ

This is the density of a Gauss distribution with mean $-(\Theta_{\mathscr{A}\mathscr{A}})^{-1}\Theta_{\mathscr{A}\mathscr{B}} z_{\mathscr{B}}$ and covariance matrix $(\Theta_{\mathscr{A}\mathscr{A}})^{-1}$. In other words, the conditional distribution of $z_{\mathscr{A}}$ given $z_{\mathscr{B}}$ is $\mathscr{N}_k[-(\Theta_{\mathscr{A}\mathscr{A}})^{-1}\Theta_{\mathscr{A}\mathscr{B}} z_{\mathscr{B}}, (\Theta_{\mathscr{A}\mathscr{A}})^{-1}]$, as desired. □

We now leverage Lemma 3.4.1 to estimate the parameters of interest. For each $j \in \{1, \ldots, d\}$, we augment the $(d-1)$-dimensional regression vector $\boldsymbol{\beta}^j$ defined in the lemma by inserting a coordinate of value -1 at the jth position, and we denote the resulting d-dimensional vector by $\underline{\boldsymbol{\beta}}^j$; for example, $\underline{\boldsymbol{\beta}}^1 = (-1, (\boldsymbol{\beta}^1)^\top)^\top \in \mathbb{R}^d$. Some algebra yields (see Lemma B.2.16 in the Appendix)

$$\Theta_{ij} = -\frac{\Theta_{ii}(\underline{\boldsymbol{\beta}}^i)_j + \Theta_{jj}(\underline{\boldsymbol{\beta}}^j)_i}{2} \qquad \text{for all } i, j \in \{1, \ldots, d\}.$$

Given independent realizations $z_1, \ldots, z_n$ of the random vector z, we then estimate Θ_{ij} by estimating the four parameters on the right-hand side of the display. We can do this by regressing for each node $j \in \{1, \ldots, d\}$ the vector $\boldsymbol{y}_j := ((z_1)_j, \ldots, (z_n)_j)^\top \in \mathbb{R}^n$ on the matrix $X_{-j} := ((z_1)_{\{j\}^\complement}, \ldots, (z_n)_{\{j\}^\complement})^\top \in \mathbb{R}^{n \times (d-1)}$. We denote the outputs of these regressions by $\widehat{\boldsymbol{\beta}}^j \equiv \widehat{\boldsymbol{\beta}}^j[\boldsymbol{y}_j, X_{-j}] \in \mathbb{R}^{d-1}$ and their augmented versions (again with a coordinate of value -1 inserted at the jth position) by $\underline{\widehat{\boldsymbol{\beta}}}^j \in \mathbb{R}^d$. These outputs yield the estimates $\widehat{\Theta_{jj}} := n/\|\boldsymbol{y}_j - X_{-j}\widehat{\boldsymbol{\beta}}^j\|_2^2$ for the diagonal entries and $\widehat{(\underline{\boldsymbol{\beta}}^j)}_i := (\underline{\widehat{\boldsymbol{\beta}}}^j)_i$ for the coordinates of the regression vectors. Indeed, the above lemma ensures that $n/\|\boldsymbol{y}_j - X_{-j}\boldsymbol{\beta}^j\|_2^2 \sim n/\|\boldsymbol{u}\|_2^2$ with $\boldsymbol{u} \sim \mathscr{N}_n[\boldsymbol{0}_n, \mathrm{I}_{n\times n}/\Theta_{jj}]$, and the law of large numbers that $\|\boldsymbol{u}\|_2^2$ converges to n/Θ_{jj} as $n \to \infty$. Hence, if the $\widehat{\boldsymbol{\beta}}^j$'s are consistently estimating $\boldsymbol{\beta}^j$, also $\widehat{\Theta_{jj}}$ and $\widehat{(\boldsymbol{\beta}^j)_i}$ are consistently estimating their population counterparts.

In summary, the lemma motivates an estimate $\widehat{\Theta}_{\mathrm{ns}}$ of the precision matrix Θ with elements

$$(\widehat{\Theta}_{\mathrm{ns}})_{ij} := -\frac{\frac{n}{\|\boldsymbol{y}_i - X_{-i}\widehat{\boldsymbol{\beta}}^i\|_2^2}(\widehat{\boldsymbol{\beta}}^i)_j + \frac{n}{\|\boldsymbol{y}_j - X_{-j}\widehat{\boldsymbol{\beta}}^j\|_2^2}(\widehat{\boldsymbol{\beta}}^j)_i}{2}$$

$$\text{for all } i, j \in \{1, \ldots, d\}. \quad (3.6)$$

neighborhood selection estimator

neighborhood lasso

We call this the *neighborhood selection estimator*. In the case $d \ll n$, least-squares can be chosen for the initial estimators $\widehat{\boldsymbol{\beta}}^j$; then, in fact, $\widehat{\Theta}_{\mathrm{ns}} = \widehat{\Theta}_{\mathrm{ml}}$—see Exercise 3.4. Otherwise, regularized regression methods can be applied. A particular popular choice is the lasso; we call the corresponding scheme the *neighborhood lasso estimator*.[10]

Finally, graph estimates are obtained again according to the rule (3.5).

Because neighborhood selection can draw on the abundant algorithmic research and software packages for linear regression, it is often faster and easier to implement than the corresponding maximum likelihood approaches. However, regularized neighborhood methods require tuning-parameter calibration for d problems; then again, tuning-parameter calibration is better understood for regression than for other likelihood methods. Overall, there is no clear winner between the two approaches—neither theoretically nor empirically.

A limitation of both approaches is their fundamental dependence on the data being Gauss-distributed. Maximum likelihood invokes Gauss distributions when formulating the likelihoods; neighborhood selection invokes Gauss distributions when splitting the problem into multiple regressions. In contrast, because least-squares—while not necessarily optimal beyond Gauss-distributed data—still works quite generally, the methods for linear regression in the previous chapter do not rely on Gauss-distributed data to such an extent.

3.5 Exercises

3.5.1 Exercises for ▶ Sect. 3.1

Exercise 3.1 ♦♦ Give further examples that show that conditional independence does not necessarily imply independence and vice versa.

3.5.2 Exercises for ▶ Sect. 3.3

Exercise 3.2 ♦♦♦ In this exercise, we show that the function $\Omega \mapsto \text{trace}[A\Omega] - \log\det\Omega$ is strictly convex on $\mathcal{S}_d^+ = \{\Omega \in \mathbb{R}^{d\times d} : \Omega \text{ symmetric and positive definite}\}$ for every $A \in \mathbb{R}^{d\times d}$. This implies in particular that the objective function of the maximum likelihood estimator for the precision matrix Θ in Gaussian graphical models (3.2) is strictly convex.

We first make sure that speaking about convexity makes sense here. A non-empty set of matrices $\mathcal{C} \subset \mathbb{R}^{d\times d}$ is called convex if $wA + (1-w)B \in \mathcal{C}$ for all $w \in [0,1]$ and $A, B \in \mathcal{C}$. In line with Definition 2.5.1, we then call a function $\not{f} : \mathcal{C} \to \mathbb{R}$ for such a $\mathcal{C}$ convex if

$$\not{f}[wA + (1-w)B] \le w\not{f}[A] + (1-w)\not{f}[B] \qquad \text{for all } w \in [0,1];\ A, B \in \mathcal{C}$$

and strictly convex if

$$\not{f}[wA + (1-w)B] < w\not{f}[A] + (1-w)\not{f}[B] \qquad \text{for all } w \in (0,1);\ A, B \in \mathcal{C}, A \neq B.$$

1. Show that the set $\mathcal{S}_d^+$ is convex.

We then consider the trace function $\Omega \mapsto \text{trace}[A\Omega] = \sum_{i=1}^n (A\Omega)_{ii}$.

2. Show that for every $A \in \mathbb{R}^{d\times d}$, this function is convex on the entire space $\mathbb{R}^{d\times d}$ (which is trivially convex), that is, $\text{trace}[A(w\Omega' + (1-w)\Omega'')] \le w\,\text{trace}[A\Omega'] + (1-w)\,\text{trace}[A\Omega'']$ for all $\Omega', \Omega'' \in \mathbb{R}^{d\times d}$ and $w \in [0,1]$. Assure yourself that this implies that the function is convex also on $\mathcal{S}_d^+$.

We now consider the log-determinant function $\Omega \mapsto -\log\det\Omega$.

3. Show that for every matrix $A \in \mathbb{R}^{d\times d}$, it holds that $|\det[A]| = \prod_{j=1}^{d} m_j$, where $m_1, \ldots, m_d$ are the singular values of A. Show similarly that if A is also *symmetric and positive definite*, it holds that $\det[A] = \prod_{j=1}^{d} m_j$, where $m_1, \ldots, m_d > 0$ are the *eigenvalues* of A.

   Hint: You might want to check Lemma B.2.11 (singular value decomposition) and Appendix B.2 more generally.
4. Consider a symmetric and positive definite matrix $\Omega \in \mathcal{S}_d^+$, a symmetric matrix $A \in \mathbb{R}^{d\times d} \setminus \{\mathbf{0}_{d\times d}\}$, and a value $\tilde{t} \equiv \tilde{t}[\Omega, A] > 0$ such that $\Omega + tA$ is symmetric and positive definite for every $t \in [0, \tilde{t}]$. Show by using 3. that the function $t \mapsto -\log\det[\Omega + tA]$ is *strictly* convex on $[0, \tilde{t}]$.

   Bonus: Show that such a $\tilde{t}$ exists in the first place.
5. Show by using 4. that $\Omega \mapsto -\log\det[\Omega]$ is *strictly* convex on $\mathcal{S}_d^+$.

We can finally derive the desired claim.

6. Conclude from 2. and 5. that for every $A \in \mathbb{R}^{d\times d}$, the objective function $\Omega \mapsto \text{trace}[A\Omega] - \log\det[\Omega]$ of the maximum likelihood estimator (3.2) is strictly convex.

Exercise 3.3 ♦♦ In this exercise, we confirm the closed-form solution of the unregularized maximum likelihood estimator stated in ▶ Sect. 3.3.

1. Show that for every given matrix $A \in \mathbb{R}^{d\times d}$, the (matrix-valued) gradient of the trace function $\Omega \mapsto \text{trace}[A\Omega] = \sum_{i=1}^{n} (A\Omega)_{ii}$ on $\mathbb{R}^{d\times d}$ is $A^\top$, that is,

$$\frac{\partial}{\partial\Omega}\text{trace}[A\Omega] = A^\top .$$

2. Show that the (matrix-valued) gradient of the log-determinant function $\Omega \mapsto \log[\det[\Omega]]$ on the invertible matrices in $\mathbb{R}^{d\times d}$ is $(\Omega^{-1})^\top$, that is,

$$\frac{\partial}{\partial\Omega}\log\left[\det[\Omega]\right] = (\Omega^{-1})^\top .$$

   Claims 1 and 2 together with Claim 6 of Exercise 3.2 ensure in particular that the objective function of the maximum likelihood estimator, namely

$\Omega \mapsto \sum_{i=1}^n \operatorname{trace}[z_i z_i^\top \Omega]/n - \log[\det[\Omega]]$ is differentiable and convex. This makes the objective functions of maximum *regularized* likelihood estimators with convex prior functions amenable to a variety of gradient-based methods.[11]

Hint: You might want to use the properties of cofactor matrices in Lemma B.2.12 and the Laplace expansion of determinants in Lemma B.2.13.

3. Conclude that for every given matrix $A \in \mathcal{S}_d^+$, where $\mathcal{S}_d^+$ are the symmetric and invertible matrices in $\mathbb{R}^{d\times d}$, the minimization program

$$\widehat{\Theta} \in \mathop{\arg\min}_{\Omega \in \mathcal{S}_d^+} \Big\{ \operatorname{trace}[A\Omega] - \log\big[\det[\Omega]\big] \Big\}$$

has the unique solution $\widehat{\Theta} = A^{-1}$. Hint: Start from Claim 6 in Exercise 3.2.

4. Show that if $n \geq d$, the empirical covariance matrix $\sum_{i=1}^n z_i z_i^\top/n$ of n independent realizations $z^1, \ldots, z^n$ of $z \sim \mathcal{N}_d[\mathbf{0}_d, \Sigma]$, Σ symmetric and invertible, is symmetric and invertible with probability 1, that is, $\mathbb{P}\{\sum_{i=1}^n z_i z_i^\top/n \in \mathcal{S}_d^+\} = 1$.
5. Conclude that if $n \geq d$, Identity (3.3) on Page 89 holds true with probability one:

$$\mathbb{P}\left\{ \widehat{\Theta}_{\text{ml}} = \left(\frac{1}{n}\sum_{i=1}^n z_i z_i^\top\right)^{-1} \right\} = 1\,.$$

6. Bonus: Compute $(\widehat{\boldsymbol{\mu}}_{\text{ml}}, \widehat{\Theta}_{\text{ml}})$ in the full maximum likelihood approach on Page 89, where the true mean $\boldsymbol{\mu}$ is not assumed to be equal to $\mathbf{0}_d$.

3.5.3 Exercises for ▶ Sect. 3.4

Exercise 3.4 ♦♦♦ In this exercise, we show that the unregularized maximum likelihood estimator and neighborhood selection with the least-squares coincide.

Assume that the empirical covariance matrix $\sum_{i=1}^n z_i z_i^\top/n$ is invertible and denote by $\widehat{\boldsymbol{\beta}}^j \equiv \widehat{\boldsymbol{\beta}}^j[\boldsymbol{y}_j, X_{-j}] \in \mathbb{R}^{d-1}$, $j \in \{1, \ldots, d\}$, the least-squares estimators for regressing $\boldsymbol{y}_j := ((z_1)_j, \ldots, (z_n)_j)^\top \in \mathbb{R}^n$ on $X_{-j} := ((z_1)_{\{j\}^\complement}, \ldots, (z_n)_{\{j\}^\complement})^\top \in \mathbb{R}^{n\times(d-1)}$. The augmented versions (with a coordinate of value -1 inserted at the jth position) of the least-squares estimators are denoted by $\underline{\widehat{\boldsymbol{\beta}}^j} \in \mathbb{R}^d$.

1. Show that for all $j \in \{1, \ldots, d\}$, it holds that

$$\left(\frac{1}{n}\sum_{i=1}^{n} z_i z_i^\top\right)_{\{j\}^\complement\{1,\ldots,d\}} \underline{\widehat{\boldsymbol{\beta}}^j} = \mathbf{0}_{d-1} \,.$$

   This means that the augmented least-squares estimators are in the kernel of a submatrix of the empirical covariance matrix.

2. Show that for all $j \in \{1, \ldots, d\}$, it holds that

$$\left(\frac{1}{n}\sum_{i=1}^{n} z_i z_i^\top\right)_{j\{1,\ldots,d\}} \underline{\widehat{\boldsymbol{\beta}}^j} = -\frac{\|\boldsymbol{y}_j - X_{-j}\widehat{\boldsymbol{\beta}}^j\|_2^2}{n} \,.$$

   This connects the remaining row of the empirical covariance matrix with the augmented least-squares estimators and the least-squares objective function.

3. Show finally that

$$\widehat{\Theta}_{\text{ns}} = \left(\frac{1}{n}\sum_{i=1}^{n} z_i z_i^\top\right)^{-1} .$$

We conclude that the estimates in (3.3) and (3.6) coincide under the stated assumptions.

3.6 R Lab: Estimating a Gene–Gene Coactivation Network

In this lab, we fit gene–gene coactivation networks to gene expression data. The data consists of vector-valued samples, each of them describing the expression levels of genes in a bacterium called *Bacillus subtilis*. Our assumption is that these vectors are independent and identically distributed according to a multivariate Gauss distribution. We describe the dependence structures of the expression levels by using graphs, and since gene expressions measure gene activities, we can interpret these graphs as gene–gene coactivation networks.

As always, your task is to replace the keyword `REPLACE` with suitable code and to answer the questions in the text.

3.6.1 Tests on Synthetic Data

We first test maximum likelihood and neighborhood selection on synthetic data generated from the model in ◘ Fig. 3.2.

3.6.1.1 Generating Data

Generate $n = 200$ independent samples from the Gaussian graphical model in ◘ Fig. 3.2 and summarize these samples in a matrix $Z \in \mathbb{R}^{n \times d}$. You might want to use the `solve()` function to compute the covariance matrix and the `mvrnorm()` function from the `MASS` package to generate the data.

```
library(MASS)
set.seed(3)
invcovariance <- matrix(data=c(1.2, -0.2, 0, 0, -0.2, 1.5, 0, 0.3, 0, 0, 1, 0,
                               0, 0.3, 0, 0.5), nrow=4, ncol=4)
invcovariance
```

```
##      [,1] [,2] [,3] [,4]
## [1,]  1.2 -0.2    0  0.0
## [2,] -0.2  1.5    0  0.3
## [3,]  0.0  0.0    1  0.0
## [4,]  0.0  0.3    0  0.5
```

```
Z <- REPLACE
head(Z)  # displays the first couple of rows of Z
```

```
##             [,1]       [,2]       [,3]       [,4]
## [1,]  1.85932683  1.4249675  1.3323523 -1.0124874
## [2,]  0.84552878  0.3055378 -0.2773236 -0.3242895
## [3,] -0.05897421  1.1439170 -1.0855338  0.7471096
## [4,]  0.66070932 -0.4818663  1.6427185 -1.9616956
## [5,] -0.72279811  0.8543313  0.4571803  0.5120927
## [6,]  0.32338537  1.0411431 -1.4611718  0.3741942
```

Note that $n \gg d$, so that we can apply unregularized estimators for analyzing these data.

3.6.1.2 Parameter Estimation via Maximum Likelihood

We now implement and apply the maximum likelihood estimator. We do this in two steps.

3.6.1.2.1 Estimating the Inverse Covariance Matrix

Recall that the (unregularized) maximum likelihood estimator (3.2) is the inverse of the empirical covariance matrix: in matrix notation, $\widehat{\Theta}_{\text{ml}} = (Z^\top Z/n)^{-1}$. Compute this estimator for the above data and study the stated visualization pipeline.

```
invcovariance.ml <- REPLACE
invcovariance.ml
```

```
##             [,1]        [,2]        [,3]        [,4]
## [1,]  1.23981631 -0.29082882  0.02037997 -0.01386750
## [2,] -0.29082882  1.58948298 -0.01016519  0.27151900
## [3,]  0.02037997 -0.01016519  0.94533132 -0.04109434
## [4,] -0.01386750  0.27151900 -0.04109434  0.49903322
```

Comparing to the true inverse covariance, we find that maximum likelihood estimation is reasonably accurate in our test case.

```
library(igraph)
network.initial <- graph.adjacency(abs(invcovariance.ml), weighted=TRUE,
                                   mode="undirected", diag=FALSE)
network.layout <- layout_in_circle(network.initial, order=c(4, 1, 2, 3))
igraph_options(vertex.size        = 40,
               vertex.color       = "lightskyblue",
               vertex.frame.color = NA,
               vertex.label.cex   = 3,
               vertex.label.color = "black",
               edge.width         = 50 * E(network.initial)$weight,
               edge.color         = "coral1")
plot.igraph(network.initial, layout=network.layout)
```

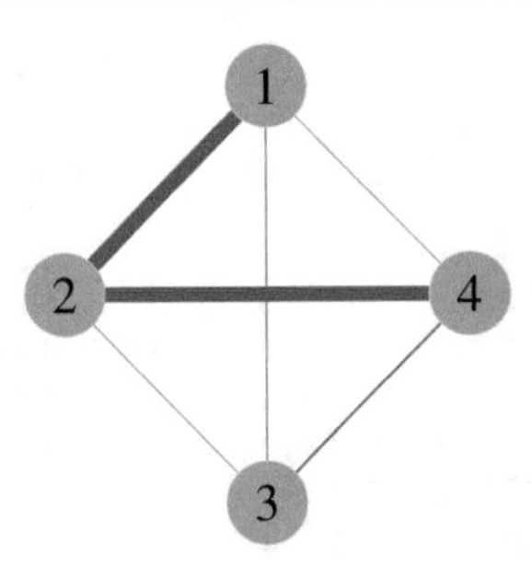

What does this plot visualize?

3.6.1.2.2 Estimating the Graph

Compute the graph estimate (3.5) with cutoff $c = \sqrt{\log[d]/n}$. This estimate should be written in terms of a so-called *adjacency matrix* $\widehat{A} \in \mathbb{R}^{d\times d}$ defined through $\widehat{A}_{ij} := 1$ if $(i, j) \in \widehat{\mathscr{E}}$ and $\widehat{A}_{ij} := 0$ otherwise.

Then, compare the matrix with the adjacency matrix A that captures the true graph: $A_{ij} := 1$ if $(i, j) \in \mathcal{E}$ and $A_{ij} := 0$ otherwise.

Finally, visualize the estimated adjacency matrix as above.

```
adjacencymatrix.ml <- REPLACE  # estimated graph
adjacencymatrix.ml
```

```
##      [,1] [,2] [,3] [,4]
## [1,]    0    1    0    0
## [2,]    1    0    0    1
## [3,]    0    0    0    0
## [4,]    0    1    0    0
```

```
adjacencymatrix <- REPLACE  # true graph
adjacencymatrix
```

```
##      [,1] [,2] [,3] [,4]
## [1,]    0    1    0    0
## [2,]    1    0    0    1
## [3,]    0    0    0    0
## [4,]    0    1    0    0
```

Comparing the adjacency matrices, we find that maximum likelihood with the standard cutoff recovers the graph correctly.

```
REPLACE  # draw the graph
```

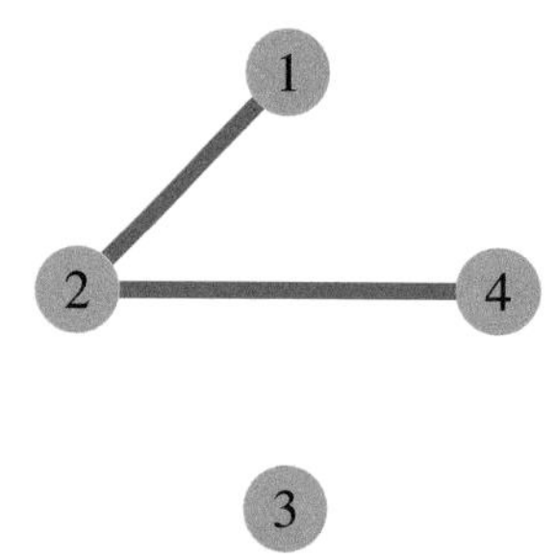

3.6.1.3 Parameter Estimation via Neighborhood Selection

We now implement and apply a neighborhood selection scheme. We do this in four steps.

3.6.1.3.1 Linear Regressions

Implement first a least-squares estimator (without intercept) for usual regression data of the form $y \in \mathbb{R}^n, X \in \mathbb{R}^{n\times(d-1)}$. The output of this function is a $(d-1)$-dimensional vector. Then, study the function `RegressionVectors`: what does it do?

```
LsEstimator <- function(y, X)
{
  return(REPLACE)
}
RegressionVectors <- function(Z, FUN=LsEstimator)
{
  regression.vectors <- NULL
  for (j in 1:dim(Z)[2])  # passing through all nodes
  {
    regression.vectors <- cbind(regression.vectors, FUN(Z[, j], Z[, -j]))
  }
  return(regression.vectors)
}
RegressionVectors(Z)
```

```
##             [,1]         [,2]        [,3]        [,4]
## [1,]  0.23457412  0.182970704 -0.02155855  0.02778872
## [2,] -0.01643790  0.006395282  0.01075305 -0.54409004
## [3,]  0.01118512 -0.170822214  0.04347084  0.08234791
```

3.6.1.3.2 Calculating the Individual Parts of the Estimator in Display (3.6)

Implement a function that augments the $(d-1)$-dimensional columns of the above matrix as described in ▶ Sect. 3.4. Then, implement a function that calculates the estimated diagonal entries $\widehat{\Theta}_{jj}$ as described in ▶ Sect. 3.4.

```
AugmentMatrix <- function(regression.vectors)
{
  REPLACE
}
AugmentMatrix(RegressionVectors(Z))
```

```
##             [,1]         [,2]        [,3]        [,4]
## [1,] -1.00000000  0.182970704 -0.02155855  0.02778872
## [2,]  0.23457412 -1.000000000  0.01075305 -0.54409004
## [3,] -0.01643790  0.006395282 -1.00000000  0.08234791
## [4,]  0.01118512 -0.170822214  0.04347084 -1.00000000
```

```
DiagonalEntries <- function(Z, regression.vectors)
{
  REPLACE
}
DiagonalEntries(Z, RegressionVectors(Z))
```

```
## [1] 1.2398163 1.5894830 0.9453313 0.4990332
```

3.6.1.3.3 Estimating the Inverse Covariance Matrix

We now put the pieces together to estimate the inverse covariance matrix.

```
NeighborhoodSelection <- function(Z, FUN=LsEstimator)
{
  regression.vectors <- RegressionVectors(Z, FUN)
  regression.vectors.augmented <- AugmentMatrix(regression.vectors)
  diagonal.entries <- DiagonalEntries(Z, regression.vectors)
  invcovariance.ns <- matrix(data=0, nrow=dim(Z)[2], ncol=dim(Z)[2])
  for (i in 1:dim(Z)[2])
  {
    for (j in 1:dim(Z)[2])
    {
      invcovariance.ns[i,j] <- REPLACE
    }
  }
  return(invcovariance.ns)
}
invcovariance.ns <- NeighborhoodSelection(Z)
invcovariance.ns
```

```
##             [,1]        [,2]        [,3]        [,4]
## [1,]  1.23981631 -0.29082882  0.02037997 -0.01386750
## [2,] -0.29082882  1.58948298 -0.01016519  0.27151900
## [3,]  0.02037997 -0.01016519  0.94533132 -0.04109434
## [4,] -0.01386750  0.27151900 -0.04109434  0.49903322
```

We find that neighborhood selection yields the same estimate for the inverse covariance matrix as maximum likelihood—which is commensurate with the theoretical finding in Exercise 3.4.

3.6.1.3.4 Estimating the Graph

Calculate the graph estimate (3.5) with cutoff $c = \sqrt{\log[d]/n}$ in terms of an adjacency matrix.

```
adjacencymatrix.ns <- REPLACE
adjacencymatrix.ns
```

```
##      [,1] [,2] [,3] [,4]
## [1,]    0    1    0    0
## [2,]    1    0    0    1
## [3,]    0    0    0    0
## [4,]    0    1    0    0
```

In line with the preceding result, we find that the neighborhood selection scheme provides perfect graph recovery in the test case.

3.6.2 A Low-Dimensional Gene Network

We first estimate a network of only a small number of genes. Throughout the real data analysis, we use neighborhood selection rather than maximum likelihood. A major advantage of neighborhood selection is that once having set up the above pipeline, it is extremely easy to account for high-dimensional data: it suffices to replace the least-squares with a high-dimensional regression method.

3.6.2.1 Loading and Pre-processing the Data

Download the file `GraphicalModels_Lab_Data.rda` from the book's homepage to your `R` working directory. Loading this file into `R` populates a matrix-valued variable `data` with the measurements. The ith row of this matrix corresponds to the ith sample; the jth column corresponds to the jth gene.

Store normalized versions of the first $d = 5$ genes' expressions in a matrix $Z \in \mathbb{R}^{n \times d}$, where n is the number of samples and d the number of genes under consideration. Use the standardization (3.2); the `scale()` function could be helpful for this.

```
# make sure that the file is in the current working directory
load("GraphicalModels_Lab_Data.rda")
Z <- REPLACE
head(Z)
```

```
##          AADK_at    AAPA_at     ABFA_at      ABH_at     ABNA_at
## [1,]   3.2073238  1.2129856  1.40342384  1.71624643  1.30339129
## [2,]   1.5050796 -0.8779609 -1.25524465  1.21686070  0.04949853
## [3,]   2.4009976  0.5989092  0.04432425  0.99872497 -0.21917314
## [4,]   1.9988562  0.8004567  0.57047877  1.00324127  0.18695672
## [5,] -0.1584393 -0.1232478 -0.42849152 -0.32344908  0.58482838
## [6,]   0.5861270  0.6713774 -0.04695200 -0.09209239  0.52639650
```

Verify that the number of samples in `Z` is $n = 71$ and the number of nodes $d = 5$. This means in particular that the number of samples is much larger than the number of model parameters ($n = 71 \gg d(d-1)/2 = 10$), so that we can apply unregularized estimators.

3.6.2.2 Estimating the Inverse Covariance Matrix

Estimate the inverse covariance matrix with the above neighborhood selection scheme. Visualize the result.

```
invcovariance.ls <- REPLACE
# adding back row and column names
colnames(invcovariance.ls) <- rownames(invcovariance.ls) <- colnames(Z)
invcovariance.ls[1:4, 1:4]
```

```
##             AADK_at    AAPA_at    ABFA_at     ABH_at
## AADK_at  2.1664326 -0.4445829  0.4284758 -1.2510060
## AAPA_at -0.4445829  2.1534580 -1.2807526  0.5186785
## ABFA_at  0.4284758 -1.2807526  2.8653192 -0.9264210
## ABH_at  -1.2510060  0.5186785 -0.9264210  2.1110669
```

```
REPLACE  # draw the graph
```

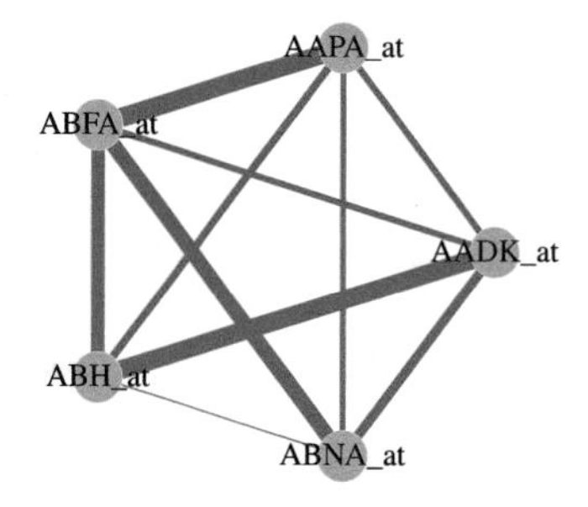

3.6.2.3 Estimating the Graph

Estimate the graph according to Display (3.5) with the standard cutoff $c = \sqrt{\log[d]/n}$ and visualize the result.

```
REPLACE  # draw the graph
```

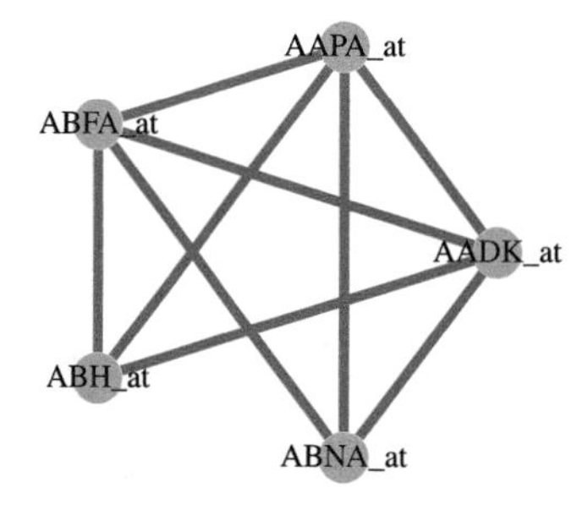

Once more, explain how the meanings of this plot and the preceding one differ.

3.6.3 A High-Dimensional Gene Network

We now increase the number of genes.

3.6.3.1 Loading and Pre-processing the Data

Proceed as before except for increasing the number of genes to $d = 50$.

```
Z <- REPLACE
Z[1:4, 1:4]
```

```
##        AADK_at    AAPA_at     ABFA_at   ABH_at
## [1,] 3.207324  1.2129856  1.40342384 1.716246
## [2,] 1.505080 -0.8779609 -1.25524465 1.216861
## [3,] 2.400998  0.5989092  0.04432425 0.998725
## [4,] 1.998856  0.8004567  0.57047877 1.003241
```

The number of samples is still $n = 71$, but the number of model parameters is now $d(d - 1)/2 = 1225$. This means in particular that we should replace the least-squares estimator in the above neighborhood selection pipeline with a high-dimensional estimator such as the lasso.

3.6.3.2 Estimating the Inverse Covariance Matrix

Implement a lasso estimator for usual regression data of the form $y \in \mathbb{R}^n, X \in \mathbb{R}^{n\times(d-1)}$. For this, use the `cv.glmnet()` function from the `glmnet` package. Because the data is centered, intercepts can be disregarded: set the flag `intercept=FALSE`, and make sure that the outputted regression vector has the correct dimensions.

We then estimate the inverse covariance matrix as in the neighborhood selection pipeline above except for replacing the least-squares estimator with the lasso estimator.

```
library(glmnet)
set.seed(84)   # the glmnet cross-validation routine is randomized
LassoEstimator <- function(y, Z)
{
  return(REPLACE)
}
invcovariance.lasso <- NeighborhoodSelection(Z, FUN=LassoEstimator)
colnames(invcovariance.lasso) <- rownames(invcovariance.lasso) <- colnames(Z)
invcovariance.lasso[1:4, 1:4]
```

```
##            AADK_at   AAPA_at   ABFA_at    ABH_at
## AADK_at   4.939445 -2.365969  0.000000 -1.414621
## AAPA_at  -2.365969 16.519048 -5.725105 -1.988555
## ABFA_at   0.000000 -5.725105  8.764455  0.000000
## ABH_at   -1.414621 -1.988555  0.000000  7.555719
```

3.6.3.3 Visualizing the Inverse Covariance Matrix

We finally visualize the absolute values of the off-diagonals in the estimated inverse covariance matrix. In view of the large number of genes under consideration, we use a heatmap instead of an adjacency matrix or graph.

```
invcovariance.lasso.vis <- invcovariance.lasso - diag(diag(invcovariance.lasso))
invcovariance.lasso.vis <- abs(invcovariance.lasso.vis) /
                               max(abs(invcovariance.lasso.vis))  # mapping into [0,1]
diag(invcovariance.lasso.vis) <- -1 # to make the diagonal stand out visually
heatmap(x         = invcovariance.lasso.vis,
        scale     = "none",
        Rowv      = NA,
        Colv      = "Rowv",
        margins   = c(10, 10),
        cexRow    = 0.45,
        cexCol    = 0.45,
        col = colorRampPalette(c("blue", "white", "red"))(n = 1000))
```

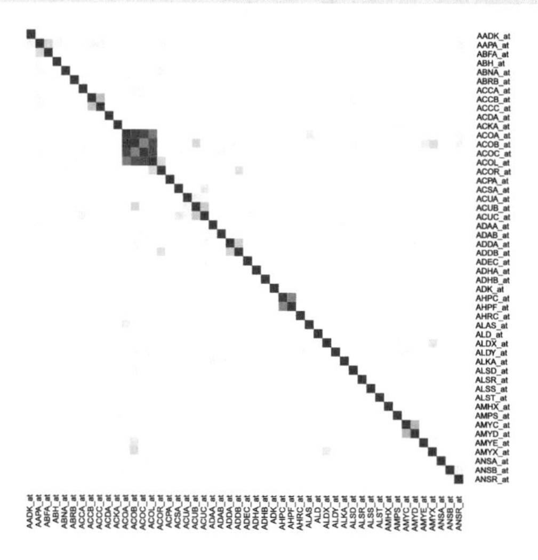

Which genes appear to have the largest pairwise dependence?

3.7 Notes and References

1. Books specialized on (low-dimensional) graphical modeling include Borgelt and Kruse (2002), Edwards (2012), Lauritzen (1996).
2. Applications of graphical models include Statistical Mechanics (Gallavotti, 2013), Quantum Field Theory (Zuber & Itzykson, 1977), Sociology (Diesner & Carley, 2005), and Biology (Kurtz et al., 2015).
3. Mathematical background on conditional independence can be found in Durrett (2010, Chapter 5.1 on pp. 221ff). The same book also introduces the basic notions of probability theory.

4 More precisely, we speak of *undirected, probabilistic graphical models*, also called *Markov random fields*. The word *probabilistic* indicates that the mathematical basis is probability theory. The word *undirected* indicates that the relationships among the nodes are symmetric: for example, `bike` $\not\perp$ `sun` | `dog` if and only if `sun` $\not\perp$ `bike` | `dog`. Hence, the graph on the right-hand side of ◘ Fig. 3.1 describes that the events `bike` and `sun` are related, but it does not specify a hierarchy.

Directed graphical models, on the other hand, go one step further: for example, sunshine makes us take the bike more likely and also increases the chance that the neighbor walks his dog; on the contrary, as much as we might like that, neither taking the bike nor walking the dog influences the weather. Such relationships among the events `bike`, `dog`, and `sun` is, therefore, unsymmetric. Hence, the corresponding graph describes not only that `bike` and `sun` are related, but it also specifies a hierarchy between the two: the chance for `bike` is increased by `sun`. We call such relationships *causal*. In general, however, causal relationships are much less obvious, and they are associated with a number of statistical and philosophical challenges (Spirtes et al., 2000); therefore, we limit ourselves to undirected graphical models.

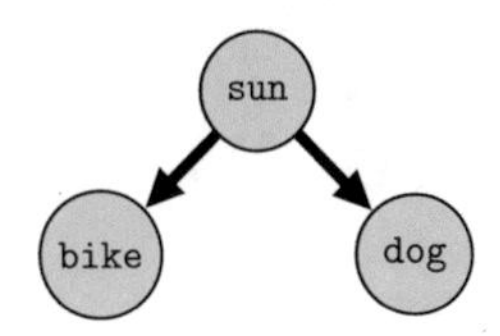

5 A standard approach for count data is the *Anscombe transformation* (Anscombe, 1948). A standard approach for compositional data is the *centered log-ratio transformation* (Aitchison, 1982), which is particularly interesting for microbiome data (Kurtz et al., 2015).

6 See Besag (1974), Grimmett (1973), Preston (1973), Sherman (1973).

7 A more comprehensive version of the Hammersley–Clifford Theorem and a proof can be found in Lauritzen (1996, Theorem 3.9 on p. 36).

8 Yuan and Lin (2007) introduce ℓ_1-regularized maximum likelihood estimation for Gauss-distributed data and discuss its connections to neighborhood selection with the lasso. Further algorithms for the maximum likelihood approach in the Gauss case followed quickly in Banerjee et al. (2008), Friedman et al. (2008). The latter paper also coined the term graphical lasso.

9 If the tuning parameter is calibrated via adaptive validation, one can also select the cutoff along the lines of Example 7.4.1. We refer to Laszkiewicz et al. (2020) for details.

10 Neighborhood selection with the lasso was introduced in Meinshausen and Bühlmann (2006).

11 For the computation of the graphical lasso, for example, see Mazumder and Hastie (2012), Oztoprak et al. (2012).

Tuning-Parameter Calibration

Contents

J. Lederer, *Fundamentals of High-Dimensional Statistics*, Springer Texts in Statistics,
https://doi.org/10.1007/978-3-030-73792-4_4

Regularized estimators consist of two terms, one for comparing model parameters to data and one for including prior information. The tuning parameters define the weighting: small tuning parameters emphasize the data, while large tuning parameters emphasize the prior information. An optimal tuning parameter balances the data and the prior information such that an estimator's error for a given task is minimized. Data-driven calibration schemes try to find such optimal tuning parameters in practice.

In this chapter, we introduce two such calibration schemes: cross-validation and adaptive validation. Cross-validation is recommended for prediction (minimizing $\|X\boldsymbol{\beta} - X\widehat{\boldsymbol{\beta}}\|_2^2$), while adaptive validation is recommended for ℓ_∞-estimation (minimizing $\|\boldsymbol{\beta} - \widehat{\boldsymbol{\beta}}\|_\infty$) and support recovery (minimizing $|\{j : \beta_j \neq 0, \widehat{\beta}_j = 0\}|$ and $|\{j : \beta_j = 0, \widehat{\beta}_j \neq 0\}|$).

4.1 Overview

We spend about one-third of our lives sleeping. It is, therefore, not surprising that good sleep is indispensable for our health; for example, recent research suggests that deep sleep clears the brain from Alzheimer's toxins.[1] Sleep research is based on data that describes brain activities, levels of blood markers, body movements, and other variables of sleeping subjects. These data can be used to fit complex models that reproduce the intricacy of the biology of sleep or, instead, simple models that identify the most important agents in the process under investigation. Regularized estimators such as the lasso can produce both types of models: small tuning parameters generate estimators with many non-zero entries (for example, toxin removal is explained as a concert of many biological factors), and large tuning parameters generate estimates with only a small number of non-zero entries (only the most relevant factors are retained).

However, the margins for adjusting the complexity of a model through the tuning parameter are limited. Data is subject to random noise, which introduces the risk of overfitting—see ◘ Fig. 2.1, for example. Regularized estimators can avoid this overfitting only if the tuning parameters are sufficiently large. In the following, we establish a corresponding lower bound for the tuning parameter.

We again consider a linear regression model

$$y = X\beta + u$$

with outcome $y \in \mathbb{R}^n$, design matrix $X \in \mathbb{R}^{n\times p}$, regression vector $\beta \in \mathbb{R}^p$, and noise $u \in \mathbb{R}^n$. For example, y could summarize the rates of toxin removal in the n subjects, X the recorded variables of those sleepers, β the linear associations between the toxin removal and the variables, and u measurement errors, non-linear associations, and so forth. Our goal is to estimate a sparse surrogate of (the not necessarily sparse) β by using the lasso estimator. If there is no noise $u = \mathbf{0}_n$ (perfect measurements, only linear associations, ...), then $y = X\beta$, and the lasso estimator (2.2) becomes

$$\beta^*_{\text{lasso}} \in \operatorname*{arg\,min}_{\alpha\in\mathbb{R}^p} \left\{ \|X\beta - X\alpha\|_2^2 + r\|\alpha\|_1 \right\}.$$

The first term in the objective function ensures a good fit to the data, and the second term induces sparsity. The tuning parameter r can be chosen at will; in particular, since $X\beta$ is not obscured by any noise, one can balance good fit (r small) and low model complexity (r large) without worries about overfitting.

But in practice, the noise is not zero (for example, toxin removal is hard to measure), which gives tuning-parameter calibration an additional facet. The lasso estimator for linear regression with noise is

$$\widehat{\beta}_{\text{lasso}} \in \operatorname*{arg\,min}_{\alpha\in\mathbb{R}^p} \left\{ \|y - X\alpha\|_2^2 + r\|\alpha\|_1 \right\}.$$

The objective function can be rewritten as

$$\begin{aligned}
&\|y - X\alpha\|_2^2 + r\|\alpha\|_1 \\
&= \|y - X\beta + X\beta - X\alpha\|_2^2 + r\|\alpha\|_1 \qquad \text{adding a zero-valued term} \\
&= \|y - X\beta\|_2^2 + 2\langle y - X\beta,\, X\beta - X\alpha\rangle + \|X\beta - X\alpha\|_2^2 + r\|\alpha\|_1 \\
&\qquad\qquad \text{expanding the data-fitting term} \\
&= \|y - X\beta\|_2^2 + 2\langle X^\top(y - X\beta),\, \beta\rangle - 2\langle X^\top(y - X\beta),\, \alpha\rangle \\
&\qquad + \|X\beta - X\alpha\|_2^2 + r\|\alpha\|_1 \qquad \text{properties of inner products} \\
&= \|u\|_2^2 + 2\langle X^\top u,\, \beta\rangle - 2\langle X^\top u,\, \alpha\rangle + \|X\beta - X\alpha\|_2^2 + r\|\alpha\|_1 . \\
&\qquad\qquad \text{invoking the model}
\end{aligned}$$

4

Since the first two terms are independent of the parameter $\boldsymbol{\alpha}$ over which we optimize, the lasso estimator becomes

$$\widehat{\boldsymbol{\beta}} \in \underset{\boldsymbol{\alpha}\in\mathbb{R}^p}{\arg\min}\left\{\|X\boldsymbol{\beta}-X\boldsymbol{\alpha}\|_2^2+r\|\boldsymbol{\alpha}\|_1-2\langle X^\top\boldsymbol{u},\,\boldsymbol{\alpha}\rangle\right\}.$$

This formulation is not useful in practice (because $\boldsymbol{\beta}$ is unknown), but it allows us to identify the term $2\langle X^\top\boldsymbol{u},\,\boldsymbol{\alpha}\rangle$ as the difference between the lasso estimator with noise and the lasso estimator without noise.

To avoid overfitting, we have to limit the influence of that noise term on the objective function. By the Hölder inequality (2.6), the noise term is bounded by $-2\langle X^\top\boldsymbol{u},\,\boldsymbol{\alpha}\rangle \leq 2\|X^\top\boldsymbol{u}\|_\infty\|\boldsymbol{\alpha}\|_1$. If we write design matrix as $X=(\boldsymbol{x}_1,\ldots,\boldsymbol{x}_p)$ with predictors $\boldsymbol{x}_1,\ldots,\boldsymbol{x}_p\in\mathbb{R}^n$, the part that comprises the noise becomes (cf. Page 40)

$$2\|X^\top\boldsymbol{u}\|_\infty = 2\|\boldsymbol{u}\|_2 \max_{j\in\{1,\ldots,p\}}\left\{|\mathrm{cor}[\boldsymbol{u},\,\boldsymbol{x}_j]|\cdot\|\boldsymbol{x}_j\|_2\right\}.$$

The factor $\|\boldsymbol{u}\|_2$ measures the overall strength of the noise; for example, $\|\boldsymbol{u}\|_2\approx\sqrt{n}\sigma$ if $\boldsymbol{u}\sim\mathcal{N}_n[\mathbf{0}_n,\sigma^2\mathrm{I}_{n\times n}]$—see Exercise 5.4. The factor $|\mathrm{cor}[\boldsymbol{x}_j,\,\boldsymbol{u}]|$ measures the similarities between the noise and the jth predictor. The factor $\|\boldsymbol{x}_j\|_2$ is just the predictor's normalization. The larger the noise and the more similar the noise and the predictor, the more the noise obscures that predictor and, therefore, the less accuracy we can expect from the estimation of the corresponding parameter. Hence, we can think of $2\|X^\top\boldsymbol{u}\|_\infty$ as the maximal effect of the noise on the estimation of a parameter. In line with this, we call $2\|X^\top\boldsymbol{u}\|_\infty$ the *effective noise* of the lasso estimator.

effective noise of the lasso estimator

For tuning parameters larger than the effective noise, the prior term dominates the noise term:

$$r\geq 2\|X^\top\boldsymbol{u}\|_\infty \quad\Rightarrow\quad r\|\boldsymbol{\alpha}\|_1\geq -2\langle X^\top\boldsymbol{u},\,\boldsymbol{\alpha}\rangle.$$

This illustrates that $r\geq 2\|X^\top\boldsymbol{u}\|_\infty$ is a sufficient[2] condition for avoiding overfitting. We will substantiate the mathematics behind this argument later in the theory chapters. In particular, we will show that $r\geq 2\|X^\top\boldsymbol{u}\|_\infty$ is a sufficient condition for prediction guarantees (see Theorem 6.3.1 and Example 6.3.2) and that $r>2\|X^\top\boldsymbol{u}\|_\infty$ can additionally lead to estimation guarantees (see Theorems 7.2.1 and 7.3.2 and Examples 7.2.1 and 7.3.1 and also the below Example 4.4.1).

In practice, the effective noise is unknown. Hence, the goal of this chapter is to transform the above insights into practical calibration schemes.

The outline is as follows: In ▶ Sect. 4.2, we equip the effective noise $2\|X^\top \boldsymbol{u}\|_\infty$ and with a tail bound that shows what to expect from calibration schemes. In ▶ Sect. 4.3, we then introduce cross-validation, a calibration scheme based on data splitting. In ▶ Sect. 4.4, we introduce adaptive validation, a calibration scheme based on error bounds.

4.2 Bounds on the Lasso's Effective Noise

Having identified the effective noise as a lower bound for the tuning parameter, we now quantify this lower bound for noise that is Gauss-distributed. This quantification illustrates what tuning parameters to expect from a successful calibration, while actual calibration schemes will be introduced in the subsequent parts of this chapter.

Our main result is a tail bound for the effective noise:[3]

Lemma 4.2.1

Gauss-Distributed Noise Consider a fixed design matrix $X \in \mathbb{R}^{n\times p}$ and Gauss-distributed noise $\boldsymbol{u} \sim \mathcal{N}_n[\mathbf{0}_n, \sigma^2 \mathrm{I}_{n\times n}]$. Then, for every $t \in (0, 1]$ and $r_t := \sigma\sqrt{8mn\log[p/t]}$, where $m := \max_{j\in\{1,\ldots,p\}} (X^\top X)_{jj}/n$ is a normalization constant, it holds that

$$\mathbb{P}\big\{r_t \geq 2\|X^\top \boldsymbol{u}\|_\infty\big\} \geq 1 - t.$$

Broadly speaking, using the tuning parameter r_t prevents the lasso estimator from overfitting with probability at least $1 - t$. The constant t resembles the significance level of a hypothesis test: for example, setting $t = 0.05$ ensures that the effective noise is bounded by $r_t = \sigma\sqrt{8mn\log[p/t]}$ with probability at least 95%. Summarizing and neglecting constants, we say that "the effective noise is bounded by $\sigma\sqrt{n\log[p]}$ *with high probability*."

with high probability

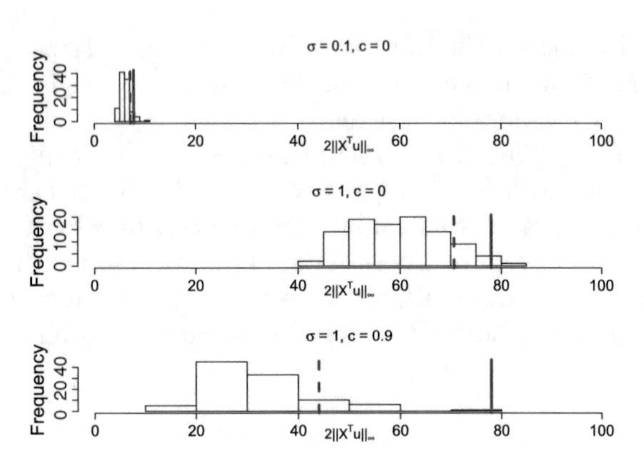

Fig. 4.1 Histograms of the lasso's effective noise $2\|X^\top \boldsymbol{u}\|_\infty$ for repeatedly sampled X and $\boldsymbol{u}$. The rows $\boldsymbol{x}_i$ of the design matrix $X = (\boldsymbol{x}_1, \ldots, \boldsymbol{x}_n)^\top$ are independent samples from $\mathcal{N}_p[0, \Sigma]$ with $\Sigma_{kl} = 1$ if $k = l$ and $\Sigma_{kl} = c$ otherwise; the entries u_i of the noise vector $\boldsymbol{u} = (u_1, \ldots, u_n)^\top$ are independent samples from $\mathcal{N}_1[0, \sigma^2]$. The dashed blue lines are the 90% quantiles; the solid red lines are $\sigma\sqrt{8n\log[p/t]}$ for $t = 1 - 0.9 = 0.1$ ($m \approx 1$ in this example). The plots illustrate that the bound r_t in Lemma 4.2.1 neglects the details of the design matrix but is usually still of the right order

An illustration of the lemma is in Fig. 4.1.

The tail bound looks like a manual for calibrating the lasso's tuning parameter, but r_t cannot be implemented: first, it involves the standard deviation σ, which is usually unknown; second, it requires the coordinates of the noise to be independent and identically Gauss-distributed, which is usually unrealistic; and third, it neglects the correlations among the predictors.[4] Rather than practical advice, the tail bound exemplifies what to expect from a calibration scheme.

We conclude this section by proving the lemma.

Proof of Lemma 4.2.1 The key tool in the proof is the union bound; the rest is simple algebra.

By definition of the sup-norm, it holds that $2\|X^\top \boldsymbol{u}\|_\infty = \max_{j\in\{1,\ldots,p\}} 2|(X^\top \boldsymbol{u})_j|$. We can, therefore, write the complement of the event in question as

$$\begin{aligned}\{r_t \geq 2\|X^\top \boldsymbol{u}\|_\infty\}^{\mathsf{C}} &= \{2\|X^\top \boldsymbol{u}\|_\infty > r_t\}\\ &= \bigcup_{j=1}^{p}\{2|(X^\top \boldsymbol{u})_j| > r_t\}.\end{aligned}$$

Applying the union bound (see Exercise 4.2) to the events on the right-hand side then yields

$$\mathbb{P}\{2\|X^\top \boldsymbol{u}\|_\infty > r_t\} \le \sum_{j=1}^{p} \mathbb{P}\{2|(X^\top \boldsymbol{u})_j| > r_t\}.$$

We can now use the basic fact $\sum_{j=1}^{k} a_j \le k \max_{j\in\{1,\dots,k\}} a_j$ for all numbers $a_1, \dots, a_k \in \mathbb{R}$, $k \in \{1, 2, \dots\}$, to deduce

$$\mathbb{P}\{2\|X^\top \boldsymbol{u}\|_\infty > r_t\} \le p \max_{j\in\{1,\dots,p\}} \mathbb{P}\{2|(X^\top \boldsymbol{u})_j| > r_t\}.$$

With some elementary calculations, we can rewrite this further as follows (verify that we can assume without loss of generality $(X^\top X)_{jj} > 0$ for all $j \in \{1, \dots, p\}$):

$$\mathbb{P}\{2\|X^\top \boldsymbol{u}\|_\infty > r_t\}$$

$$\le p \max_{j\in\{1,\dots,p\}} \mathbb{P}\left\{\frac{|(X^\top \boldsymbol{u})_j|}{\sigma\sqrt{mn}} > \frac{r_t}{2\sigma\sqrt{mn}}\right\}$$

dividing inside the probability in the previous display by $2\sigma\sqrt{mn} > 0$

$$\le p \max_{j\in\{1,\dots,p\}} \mathbb{P}\left\{\frac{|(X^\top \boldsymbol{u})_j|}{\sigma\sqrt{(X^\top X)_{jj}}} > \frac{r_t}{2\sigma\sqrt{mn}}\right\}.$$

definition of m in the above Lemma 4.2.1; $\mathbb{P}\{\mathcal{A}\} \le \mathbb{P}\{\mathcal{B}\}$ for $\mathcal{A} \subset \mathcal{B}$

Recalling that $\boldsymbol{u} \sim \mathcal{N}_n[0, \sigma^2 \mathrm{I}_{n\times n}]$ by assumption, we observe that the random variables $(X^\top \boldsymbol{u})_j/(\sigma\sqrt{(X^\top X)_{jj}}) = \langle \boldsymbol{x}_j, \boldsymbol{u}\rangle/(\|\boldsymbol{x}_j\|_2\sqrt{\sigma^2})$ for $j \in \{1, \dots, p\}$, $X = (\boldsymbol{x}_1, \dots, \boldsymbol{x}_p)$, follow a standard Gauss distribution, and every standard Gauss variable $z \sim \mathcal{N}_1[0, 1]$ fulfills the tail bound (see Exercise 4.3)

$$\mathbb{P}\{|z| \ge a\} \le e^{-\frac{a^2}{2}} \qquad \text{for all } a \ge 0.$$

Combining this tail bound evaluated at $a = r_t/(2\sigma\sqrt{mn})$ and the above display and using that $\mathbb{P}\{\mathcal{A}\} \le \mathbb{P}\{\mathcal{B}\}$ for $\mathcal{A} \subset \mathcal{B}$ yield

$$\mathbb{P}\{2\|X^\top \boldsymbol{u}\|_\infty > r_t\} \le p e^{-\left(\frac{r_t}{2\sigma\sqrt{mn}}\right)^2/2}.$$

We finally use the results to deduce

$$\begin{aligned}
&\mathbb{P}\big\{r_t \geq 2\|X^\top \boldsymbol{u}\|_\infty\big\} \\
&= 1 - \mathbb{P}\big\{2\|X^\top \boldsymbol{u}\|_\infty > r_t\big\} && \mathbb{P}\{\mathscr{A}\} = 1 - \mathbb{P}\{\mathscr{A}^\complement\} \\
&\geq 1 - pe^{-\left(\frac{\sigma\sqrt{8mn\log[p/t]}}{2\sigma\sqrt{mn}}\right)^2/2} && \text{preceding inequality and definition of } r_t \\
&= 1 - t\,, && \text{consolidating}
\end{aligned}$$

as desired. □

4.3 Cross-Validation

Cross-validation calibrates tuning parameters for prediction. It repeatedly partitions the data into two parts: training data for fitting model parameters and validation data for estimating the prediction errors of those fitted parameters. It then selects a tuning parameter that minimizes the average of those estimated errors, trusting that (i) the fitted model parameters resemble the original estimators and (ii) the estimated errors resemble the true ones.[5]

Given a family of linear regression estimators $\{\widehat{\boldsymbol{\beta}}[r] : r \in \mathscr{R}\} \subset \mathbb{R}^p$ indexed by a non-empty but otherwise an arbitrary set of tuning parameters $\mathscr{R}$, an optimal tuning parameter for prediction is

$$r^* \in \operatorname*{arg\,min}_{r\in\mathscr{R}} \ell^*[r] \qquad \text{with } \ell^*[r] := \frac{1}{n}\|X\boldsymbol{\beta} - X\widehat{\boldsymbol{\beta}}[r]\|_2^2\,. \tag{4.1}$$

The scaling $1/n$ has no effect on r^* but makes the below derivations easier. In practice, the regression vector $\boldsymbol{\beta}$ is unknown, which means that the optimal tuning parameter r^* is also unknown. The target of this section is, therefore, a data-driven surrogate of r^*.

The general strategy is to replace the average prediction error ℓ^* by an estimate $\widehat{\ell}$:

$$\widehat{r} \in \operatorname*{arg\,min}_{r\in\mathscr{R}} \widehat{\ell}[r]\,, \tag{4.2}$$

where $\widehat{\ell} : \mathscr{R} \to \mathbb{R}$ involves the data $(\boldsymbol{y}, X)$ but not the unknown regression parameter. If $\widehat{\ell}[r] \approx \ell^*[r]$ for all $r \in$

$\mathscr{R}$, we can expect that $\widehat{r} \approx r^*$ and thus $\|X\boldsymbol{\beta} - X\widehat{\boldsymbol{\beta}}[\widehat{r}]\|_2^2/n \approx \|X\boldsymbol{\beta} - X\widehat{\boldsymbol{\beta}}[r^*]\|_2^2/n$ (cf. Exercise 4.5).

The seemingly most natural estimate of the average prediction error is the least-squares data fit

$$\widehat{\ell}[r] := \frac{1}{n}\|\boldsymbol{y} - X\widehat{\boldsymbol{\beta}}[r]\|_2^2 .$$

But since regularized least-squares estimators already include $\|\boldsymbol{y} - X\boldsymbol{\alpha}\|_2^2$ in their objective functions, this estimate induces overfitting. For example, if $\mathscr{R} = [0, \infty)$ and

$$\widehat{\boldsymbol{\beta}}[r] = \widehat{\boldsymbol{\beta}}_{\text{lasso}}[r] \in \underset{\boldsymbol{\alpha}\in\mathbb{R}^p}{\arg\min}\left\{ \|\boldsymbol{y} - X\boldsymbol{\alpha}\|_2^2 + r\|\boldsymbol{\alpha}\|_1 \right\},$$

it holds that $\widehat{\ell}[0] = \min_{r\in\mathscr{R}} \widehat{\ell}[r]$ and, therefore, that (4.2) has the solution $\widehat{r} = 0$; in other words, the calibration based on the least-squares data fit always selects the plain least-squares estimator.

One approach to amend the estimate of the prediction error is to add a function that measures the models' complexity:

$$\widehat{\ell}[r] := \frac{1}{n}\|\boldsymbol{y} - X\widehat{\boldsymbol{\beta}}[r]\|_2^2 + t \cdot \text{complexity}\left[\widehat{\boldsymbol{\beta}}[r]\right].$$

The complexity function resembles the prior function in (1.6): it favors simple models, thereby attempting a trade-off between a good data fit (typically achieved with small r) and low model complexity (typically achieved with large r). But the complexity and prior functions can differ: for example, the complexity function has fewer computational constraints than the prior function because the optimization for $\widehat{r}$ is typically over a subset of $\mathbb{R}$, while the optimization for $\widehat{\boldsymbol{\beta}}$ is over $\mathbb{R}^p$. Examples for calibration schemes based on least-squares and a complexity function include *AIC* and *BIC*. By specifying $t \in [0, \infty)$ as a function of n and p, they avoid calibrating that parameter.

But in the following, we focus on a different approach to amend the naive estimate of the prediction error: the *holdout method*. The holdout method addresses the problem at source, which is that data are used both for fitting regression vectors and for estimating the prediction errors, by using each sample only for either one of the two tasks. The index set of the samples is split into a *training set*

holdout method

training and validation sets

$\mathcal{T} \subset \{1, \ldots, n\}$ with size $n_{\mathcal{T}} := |\mathcal{T}|$ and a *validation set* (or *holdout set*) $\mathcal{V} := \{1, \ldots, n\} \setminus \mathcal{T}$ with size $n_{\mathcal{V}} := |\mathcal{V}| = n - n_{\mathcal{T}}$. The samples that correspond to the training set are assigned to fitting the regression vectors, and the samples that correspond to the validation set are assigned to estimating the prediction errors:

$$\widehat{r}_{\text{holdout}} \in \underset{r \in \mathcal{R}}{\arg\min}\, \widehat{\ell}[r]$$

with

$$\widehat{\ell}[r] := \frac{1}{n_{\mathcal{V}}} \|\boldsymbol{y}_{\mathcal{V}} - X_{\mathcal{V}} \widehat{\boldsymbol{\beta}}[r, \boldsymbol{y}_{\mathcal{T}}, X_{\mathcal{T}}]\|_2^2 ,$$

where $\boldsymbol{y}_{\mathcal{T}} \in \mathbb{R}^{n_{\mathcal{T}}}$ and $X_{\mathcal{T}} \in \mathbb{R}^{n_{\mathcal{T}} \times p}$ are the vector/matrix-valued training data, $\boldsymbol{y}_{\mathcal{V}} \in \mathbb{R}^{n_{\mathcal{V}}}$ and $X_{\mathcal{V}} \in \mathbb{R}^{n_{\mathcal{V}} \times p}$ are the vector/matrix-valued validation data, and $\widehat{\boldsymbol{\beta}}[r, \boldsymbol{y}_{\mathcal{T}}, X_{\mathcal{T}}] \in \mathbb{R}^p$ is the estimator evaluated on the training data.

The holdout method is expected to work well if: (i) the fitted parameters $\widehat{\boldsymbol{\beta}}[r, \boldsymbol{y}_{\mathcal{T}}, X_{\mathcal{T}}]$ are close to the original estimators $\widehat{\boldsymbol{\beta}}[r] = \widehat{\boldsymbol{\beta}}[r, \boldsymbol{y}, X]$ and (ii) the estimated errors $\|\boldsymbol{y}_{\mathcal{V}} - X_{\mathcal{V}} \widehat{\boldsymbol{\beta}}[r, \boldsymbol{y}_{\mathcal{T}}, X_{\mathcal{T}}]\|_2^2 / n_{\mathcal{V}}$ are close to the true errors $\|X\boldsymbol{\beta} - X\widehat{\boldsymbol{\beta}}[r]\|_2^2/n$. Large training sets and large validation sets benefit (i) and (ii), respectively, but the sizes of the sets are subject to a trade-off: $n_{\mathcal{T}} + n_{\mathcal{V}} = n$. Cross-validation attempts to circumvent this trade-off by averaging multiple splits. In linear regression, this amounts to

$$\widehat{r}_{\text{cv}} \in \underset{r \in \mathcal{R}}{\arg\min}\, \widehat{\ell}[r]$$

with

$$\widehat{\ell}[r] := \frac{1}{k} \sum_{j=1}^{k} \frac{1}{n_{\mathcal{V}_j}} \|\boldsymbol{y}_{\mathcal{V}_j} - X_{\mathcal{V}_j} \widehat{\boldsymbol{\beta}}[r, \boldsymbol{y}_{\mathcal{T}_j}, X_{\mathcal{T}_j}]\|_2^2 ,$$

where $k \in \{1, 2, \ldots\}$ is the number of splits, $\mathcal{T}_1, \ldots, \mathcal{T}_k$ training sets of size $n_{\mathcal{T}_1} := |\mathcal{T}_1|, \ldots, n_{\mathcal{T}_k} := |\mathcal{T}_k| \in \{1, \ldots, n-1\}$, and $\mathcal{V}_1 := \{1, \ldots, n\} \setminus \mathcal{T}_1, \ldots, \mathcal{V}_k := \{1, \ldots, n\} \setminus \mathcal{T}_k$ validation sets of size $n_{\mathcal{V}_1} := |\mathcal{V}_1| = n - n_{\mathcal{T}_1}, \ldots, n_{\mathcal{V}_k} := |\mathcal{V}_k| = n - n_{\mathcal{T}_k} \in \{1, \ldots, n-1\}$. In this way, cross-validation can use each sample both for training and for validation.

Monte Carlo cross-validation

The simplest cross-validation scheme is *Monte Carlo cross-validation* (also called repeated random subsampling

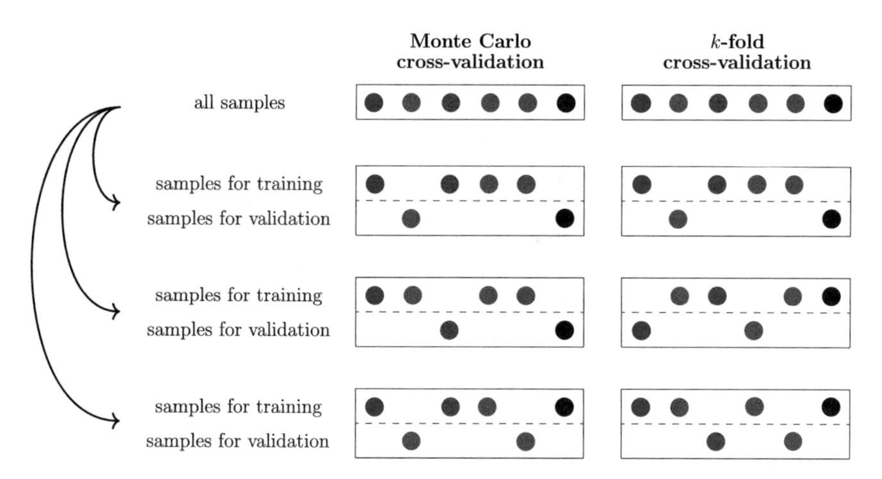

Fig. 4.2 Cross-validation schemes partition the data into training and validation sets multiple times. Monte Carlo cross-validation has two free parameters: the number of folds (here $k = 3$) and the size of the training sets (here $n_{\mathcal{T}} = 4$); k-fold cross-validation has only one free parameter: the number of folds (here $k = 3$). Another difference between the two schemes is that Monte Carlo cross-validation partitions the data each time completely at random, which means that a sample can be used for validation repeatedly (orange and black circles) or not at all (blue and green circles), while k-fold cross-validation uses each sample for validation exactly once

validation). Given $k \in \{1, 2, \dots\}$ and $n_{\mathcal{T}} \in \{1, \dots n-1\}$, it splits the data k times uniformly at random such that the training sets have common size $n_{\mathcal{T}} = n_{\mathcal{T}_1} = \cdots = n_{\mathcal{T}_k}$.

k-fold cross-validation

A slightly more intricate scheme is *k-fold cross-validation*. Given $k \in \{2, 3, \dots\}$, it first partitions the data at random or not at random into k sets $\mathcal{A}_1, \dots, \mathcal{A}_k$ of common size n/k (or approximately of that size if n is not divisible by k) and then defines the training and validation sets by $\mathcal{T}_j := \{1, \dots, n\} \setminus \mathcal{A}_j$ and $\mathcal{V}_j := \mathcal{A}_j, j \in \{1, \dots, k\}$. Two differences to Monte Carlo cross-validation are that the size of the training and validation sets are fixed for a given number of folds k and that each point is used for validation exactly once (see Fig. 4.2). The special case $k = n$, which leads to n-validations that each use one different sample, is called *leave-one-out cross-validation*.

leave-one-out cross-validation

While cross-validation routinely outmatches other approaches in terms of prediction, it produces models that are comparably complex. This tendency to overfit needs to be taken into account when interpreting the results, and more generally, bear in mind that cross-validation is not designed for anything else than prediction.[6]

Cross-validation is also subject to other limitations. First, the holdout approach implicitly assumes that the training and validation data are independent. In practice, this assumption is often violated: for example, time series data are highly dependent by design.

Next, cross-validation uses data and computing resources inefficiently. By design of the holdout scheme, the training and validation steps use only subsets of the data—which means that the effective sample sizes are much smaller than the actual sample size n. Also, each application of one of the discussed cross-validation schemes requires k trainings and validations in addition to the computation of the actual estimator.

Then, cross-validation lacks theoretical support. For example, there is no finite sample theory for how cross-validated tuning parameters $\widehat{r}_{\text{cv}}$ compare to the gold standard r^* for lasso-type estimators.[7]

Moreover, the splitting procedures often comprise random elements: in k-fold cross-validation, for example, the partitioning of the data is typically performed uniformly at random. Unless the randomness is "fixed" (by using the same random seed in all users' programs, for example), different users can then get different outputs $\widehat{\boldsymbol{\beta}}[r]$ on the exact same data.

Finally, cross-validation methods trade the original tuning parameters for new tuning parameters. For example, Monte Carlo cross-validation contains two free parameters, the number of data splits, and the size of the training set; k-fold cross-validation contains one free parameter and the number of folds/data splits. Just as the original tuning parameters, these parameters are subject to trade-offs. Heuristically, the larger the number of data splits, the more stable but computationally demanding the methods are (because the specific compositions of the training and validation sets are averaged out but the training and validation results have to be computed for each split). The larger the training set, the smaller the bias but the larger the variance (because the approximation of $\widehat{\boldsymbol{\beta}}[r]$ is more accurate but the estimation of the error more volatile). For k-fold cross-validation, $k \in \{5, 10\}$ have become standard parameters in this trade-off, but there are few theoretical justifications for any specific choice.

Despite all those limitations, cross-validation schemes are hard to beat in practice. Hence, if data and computational resources are sufficient and the samples fairly independent, cross-validation is the standard calibration approach for prediction.

4.4 Adaptive Validation

The calibration schemes discussed so far estimate prediction errors through least-squares data-fitting errors that are adjusted by using the holdout method (included in the various cross-validation schemes) or complexity measures (included in AIC, BIC, and Mallow's C_p). The selected tuning parameters are then the minimizers of these estimated prediction errors. Adaptive validation, in contrast, evaluates pairwise differences of estimators. The selected tuning parameter is then the stopping point of an algorithm that compares these differences with given error bounds. The two main features of adaptive validation are its optimal guarantees and its computational efficiency.

Our statistical framework for adaptive validation consists of three parts: a family of estimators, a loss function to measure the estimators' errors, and bounds for the estimators in that error measure. The family of estimators $\{\widehat{\boldsymbol{\beta}}[r] : r \in \mathcal{R}\} \subset \mathbb{R}^p$ is indexed by a compact,[8] nonempty set of tuning parameters $\mathcal{R} \subset [0, \infty)$. This setup generalizes the one of ▶ Sect. 4.3 in that the estimators can now correspond to arbitrary model classes, such as logistic regression[9] and graphical modeling,[10] while it restricts that setup in that the tuning parameters must now be real-valued.[11]

The *loss function* $\ell : \mathbb{R}^p \to [0, \infty)$ is assumed to be symmetric ($\ell[-\boldsymbol{a}] = \ell[\boldsymbol{a}]$ for all $\boldsymbol{a} \in \mathbb{R}^p$), to obey the triangle inequality ($\ell[\boldsymbol{a}+\boldsymbol{b}] \leq \ell[\boldsymbol{a}]+\ell[\boldsymbol{b}]$ for all $\boldsymbol{a}, \boldsymbol{b} \in \mathbb{R}^p$), and, without loss of generality, to be definite ($\ell[\mathbf{0}_p] = 0$). A loss function, together with a target vector $\boldsymbol{\alpha} \in \mathbb{R}^p$, induces a measure $\ell[\boldsymbol{\alpha} - \widehat{\boldsymbol{\beta}}[r]]$ for the error of the estimator $\widehat{\boldsymbol{\beta}}[r]$. In linear regression, for example, the loss function $\ell : \boldsymbol{a} \mapsto \|\boldsymbol{a}\|_\infty$, together with the regression vector $\boldsymbol{\beta}$, induces the ℓ_∞-error $\|\boldsymbol{\beta} - \widehat{\boldsymbol{\beta}}[r]\|_\infty$ (cf. Example 7.3.1).

The bounds finally control the estimators' errors in the measure that is induced by the loss function.

▪▪ Assumption 4.4.1

Error Bounds We assume that for a target vector $\boldsymbol{\alpha} \in \mathbb{R}^p$, a (potentially random) factor $f \in [0, \infty)$ that is known in practice or can be approximated, and a (potentially random) tuning parameter $r^* \in \mathcal{R}$, all estimators $\widehat{\boldsymbol{\beta}}[r]$ with $r \in \mathcal{R} \cap [r^*, \infty)$ satisfy

$$\ell\big[\boldsymbol{\alpha} - \widehat{\boldsymbol{\beta}}[r]\big] \leq fr\,.$$

► Chapters 6 and 7 discuss a variety of error bounds, but not all of those bounds fit here: to make the below algorithm feasible, the factor f—or an approximation of it—needs to be known. For example, the prior function bounds in Theorem 7.2.1 do not fit because they involve a measure of the design correlations (namely, the compatibility constant) that can depend crucially on the typically unknown sparsity level (see Example 6.4.2); in contrast, the dual function bounds in Theorem 7.3.2 fit because all necessary parts can be approximated—at least for weakly correlated designs. We illustrate the case of dual function bounds in Example 4.4.1 below.

The tuning parameter r^* is, in the sense of Assumption 4.4.1, the optimal tuning parameter: among all tuning parameters for which there is control, namely all $r \in \mathcal{R} \cap [r^*, \infty)$, it leads to the smallest bound. In contrast to the factor f, the tuning parameter r^* does *not* need to be known. We instead think of r^* with its bound

$$\ell\big[\boldsymbol{\alpha} - \widehat{\boldsymbol{\beta}}[r^*]\big] \leq f r^* \tag{4.3}$$

as the inaccessible gold standard for estimation in terms of the ℓ-loss, and our goal is to have similar guarantees in practice.

adaptive validation

Adaptive validation tries to reach this goal by contrasting the above error bounds with pairwise differences of estimators:[12]

$$\widehat{r}_{\text{av}} := \min\Big\{r \in \mathcal{R} : \ell\big[\widehat{\boldsymbol{\beta}}[r'] - \widehat{\boldsymbol{\beta}}[r'']\big] \leq \tilde{f} r' + \tilde{f} r'' \quad \forall r', r'' \in \mathcal{R} \cap [r, \infty)\Big\}, \tag{4.4}$$

where $\tilde{f}$ is either equal to f or to an approximation of it. Adaptive validation essentially selects the smallest tuning parameter that is commensurate with the error bounds in Assumption 4.4.1 to recover a maximum of relevant signal while avoiding overfitting: see ◘ Fig. 4.3.

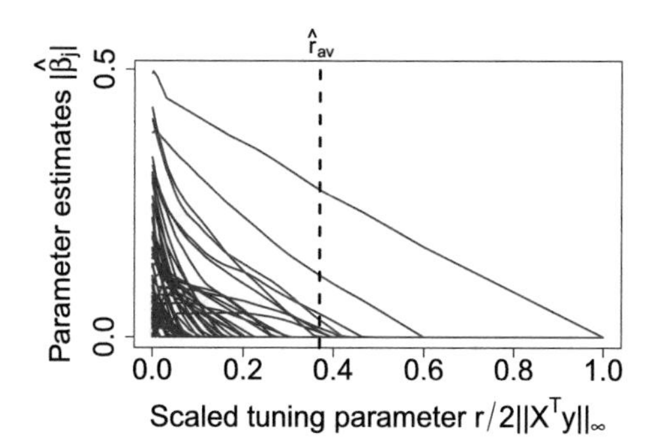

Fig. 4.3 Relative magnitudes of the estimated parameters in a generic lasso analysis as a function of the tuning parameter. For large tuning parameters, most of the non-zero estimates $(\widehat{\beta}_{\text{lasso}})_j \neq 0$ are relevant ($\beta_j \neq 0$; red lines), while for small tuning parameters, many of the non-zero estimates are irrelevant ($\beta_j = 0$; blue lines). Broadly speaking, adaptive validation scans such plots to evaluate when the irrelevant parameters get out of hand. The exact stopping point depends on the loss ℓ

The following theorem shows that this strategy is indeed successful.

Theorem 4.4.1

Optimality of Adaptive Validation If $\tilde{f} \geq f$, it holds that

$$\widehat{r}_{\text{av}} \leq r^* \tag{4.5}$$

and

$$\ell[\boldsymbol{\alpha} - \widehat{\boldsymbol{\beta}}[\widehat{r}_{\text{av}}]] \leq 3\tilde{f}r^* . \tag{4.6}$$

The first bound ensures that the tuning parameter $\widehat{r}_{\text{av}}$ selected by adaptive validation is always smaller or equal to the optimal tuning parameter r^*. This result is very useful for support recovery because it provides a safe cutoff for thresholding (see ► Sect. 7.4, especially Example 7.4.1). The second bound ensures that if $\tilde{f} = f$, the tuning parameter $\widehat{r}_{\text{av}}$ satisfies the optimal bound (4.3) up to a constant factor 3; and it ensures more generally that if $\tilde{f}$ is sufficiently large but still close enough to f, the tuning parameter $\widehat{r}_{\text{av}}$ has similar guarantees as the inaccessible gold standard.

Proof of Theorem 4.4.1 Both claims have short and elementary proofs. The only ingredients needed are the definition of adaptive validation, the symmetry and triangle inequality of the loss function, and the error bounds. In particular, we do not rely on any specific estimators or models.

Claim (4.5) We prove this claim by contradiction: Assume that $\widehat{r}_{\text{av}} > r^*$. Then, by definition of the adaptive validation scheme in (4.4), there must be $r', r'' \in \mathcal{R} \cap [r^*, \infty)$ such that

$$\ell\big[\widehat{\boldsymbol{\beta}}[r'] - \widehat{\boldsymbol{\beta}}[r'']\big] > \tilde{f}r' + \tilde{f}r'' .$$

However,

$$\begin{aligned}
&\ell\big[\widehat{\boldsymbol{\beta}}[r'] - \widehat{\boldsymbol{\beta}}[r'']\big] \\
&= \ell\big[\widehat{\boldsymbol{\beta}}[r'] - \boldsymbol{\alpha} + \boldsymbol{\alpha} - \widehat{\boldsymbol{\beta}}[r'']\big] && \text{adding a zero-valued term} \\
&\le \ell\big[\widehat{\boldsymbol{\beta}}[r'] - \boldsymbol{\alpha}\big] + \ell\big[\boldsymbol{\alpha} - \widehat{\boldsymbol{\beta}}[r'']\big] && \text{triangle inequality for } \ell \\
&= \ell\big[\boldsymbol{\alpha} - \widehat{\boldsymbol{\beta}}[r']\big] + \ell\big[\boldsymbol{\alpha} - \widehat{\boldsymbol{\beta}}[r'']\big] && \text{symmetry of } \ell \\
&\le fr' + fr'' \\
& && \text{error bounds in Assumption 4.4.1 ; } r', r'' \in \mathcal{R} \cap [r^*, \infty) \\
&\le \tilde{f}r' + \tilde{f}r'' , && \tilde{f} \ge f \text{ by assumption}
\end{aligned}$$

which contradicts the preceding inequality and, therefore, shows that $\widehat{r}_{\text{av}} \le r^*$.

Claim (4.6) We prove this claim by using the previous one:

$$\begin{aligned}
&\ell\big[\boldsymbol{\alpha} - \widehat{\boldsymbol{\beta}}[\widehat{r}_{\text{av}}]\big] \\
&= \ell\big[\boldsymbol{\alpha} - \widehat{\boldsymbol{\beta}}[r^*] + \widehat{\boldsymbol{\beta}}[r^*] - \widehat{\boldsymbol{\beta}}[\widehat{r}_{\text{av}}]\big] \\
& && \text{adding a zero-valued term} \\
&\le \ell\big[\boldsymbol{\alpha} - \widehat{\boldsymbol{\beta}}[r^*]\big] + \ell\big[\widehat{\boldsymbol{\beta}}[r^*] - \widehat{\boldsymbol{\beta}}[\widehat{r}_{\text{av}}]\big] \\
& && \text{triangle inequality for } \ell \\
&\le fr^* + \tilde{f}r^* + \tilde{f}\widehat{r}_{\text{av}}]
\end{aligned}$$

$\ell[\boldsymbol{\alpha} - \widehat{\boldsymbol{\beta}}[r^*]] \le fr^*$ by Assumption 4.4.1; $\ell[\widehat{\boldsymbol{\beta}}[r^*] - \widehat{\boldsymbol{\beta}}[\widehat{r}_{\text{av}}]] \le \tilde{f}r^* + \tilde{f}\widehat{r}_{\text{av}}$ *by Definition* (4.4) *and Claim* (4.5)

$$\le 3\tilde{f}r^* , \qquad \widehat{r}_{\text{av}} \le r^* \text{ by Claim (4.5); } \tilde{f} \ge f \text{ by assumption}$$

as desired. □

```
Data: data, candidate set 𝓡 (finite), loss function ℓ, factor f̃
Result: r̂_av ∈ 𝓡
r ← max 𝓡
while r ≠ min 𝓡 do
    compute β̂[r] for the given data
    r' ← max 𝓡
    // r" not needed due to loop structure
    while r' > r do
        if ℓ[β̂[r'] − β̂[r]] > f̃r' + f̃r then
            r ← min{𝓡 ∩ (r, ∞)}
            exit from both loops
        r' ← max{𝓡 ∩ [0, r')}
    end
    r ← max{𝓡 ∩ [0, r)}
end
r̂_av ← r
```

Algorithm 4.1: Pseudocode for adaptive validation (4.4)

Additionally to its guarantees in Theorem 4.4.1, adaptive validation is practical: Algorithm 4.1 shows that adaptive validation is easy to implement and needs to compute each estimator $\widehat{\boldsymbol{\beta}}[r]$ at most once (see Exercise 4.8). In comparison, k-fold cross-validation is also easy to implement but needs to compute each estimator or surrogates of it $k+1$ times (see ▶ Sect. 4.3).

A limitation of adaptive validation is that the tuning parameters need to be real-valued. In contrast, cross-validation and AIC–BIC-type schemes allow—in principle—for vector-valued tuning parameters of any dimension. But calibrating vector-valued tuning parameters typically involves large candidate sets $\mathcal{R}$ (recall ◘ Fig. 1.2, which illustrates that covering spaces of increasing dimensions requires exponentially growing numbers of points) and, therefore, the computation of many estimators $\widehat{\boldsymbol{\beta}}[r]$. In effect, the calibration of vector-valued tuning parameters is very challenging.[13]

But the crucial requirement for adaptive validation is a set of suitable error bounds. Since such bounds typically concern parameter estimation and support recovery rather than prediction[14] (see the example below), adaptive validation and cross-validation complement each other.

▶ Example 4.4.1

Adaptive Validation for the Lasso In this example, we use adaptive validation to calibrate the lasso estimator (2.2). As always in adaptive validation, our starting point is a set of error bounds. For the lasso in orthogonal design $X^\top X =$

$n\mathrm{I}_{n\times n}$, we find such bounds similarly as in Example 7.3.1: for all $r \geq 4\|X^\top \boldsymbol{u}\|_\infty$ (which ensures that $r > 2\|X^\top \boldsymbol{u}\|_\infty$), it holds that

$$\|\boldsymbol{\beta} - \widehat{\boldsymbol{\beta}}_{\text{lasso}}[r]\|_\infty \leq \frac{3}{4n} r.$$

This means that Assumption 4.4.1 is satisfied with loss function $\ell : \boldsymbol{a} \mapsto \|\boldsymbol{a}\|_\infty$, target vector $\boldsymbol{\alpha} = \boldsymbol{\beta}$, factor $f = 3/(4n)$, and optimal tuning parameter[15] $r^* = 4\|X^\top \boldsymbol{u}\|_\infty$.

Since the factor $f = 3/(4n)$ is known, the calibration scheme (4.4) becomes

$$\widehat{r}_{\text{av}} = \min\Big\{ r \in \mathscr{R} : \|\widehat{\boldsymbol{\beta}}_{\text{lasso}}[r'] - \widehat{\boldsymbol{\beta}}_{\text{lasso}}[r'']\|_\infty \leq 3r'/(4n) + 3r''/(4n) \;\forall r', r'' \in \mathscr{R} \cap [r, \infty) \Big\},$$

and Theorem 4.4.1 entails the guarantees $\widehat{r}_{\text{av}} \leq 4\|X^\top \boldsymbol{u}\|_\infty$ and

$$\|\boldsymbol{\beta} - \widehat{\boldsymbol{\beta}}_{\text{lasso}}[\widehat{r}_{\text{av}}]\|_\infty \leq \frac{9}{n}\|X^\top \boldsymbol{u}\|_\infty .$$

For Gauss-distributed noise $\boldsymbol{u} \sim \mathcal{N}_n[\mathbf{0}_n, \sigma^2 \mathrm{I}_{n\times n}]$, this inequality yields together with Lemma 4.2.1

$$\begin{aligned}
&\mathbb{P}\Big\{ \|\boldsymbol{\beta} - \widehat{\boldsymbol{\beta}}_{\text{lasso}}[\widehat{r}_{\text{av}}]\|_\infty \leq 9\sigma\sqrt{\frac{2\log[p/t]}{n}} \Big\} \\
&\geq \mathbb{P}\Big\{ \frac{9}{n}\|X^\top \boldsymbol{u}\|_\infty \leq 9\sigma\sqrt{\frac{2\log[p/t]}{n}} \Big\} && \text{preceding inequality} \\
&\geq \mathbb{P}\big\{ 2\|X^\top \boldsymbol{u}\|_\infty \leq \sigma\sqrt{8mn\log[p/t]} \big\} \\
& && \text{consolidating; } m = \max_{j\in\{1,\dots,p\}} (X^\top X)_{jj}/n = 1 \text{ by assumption} \\
&\geq 1 - t && \text{Lemma 4.2.1 (Gauss-distributed noise)}
\end{aligned}$$

for all $t \in (0, 1]$. In other words, the sup-norm error of the lasso estimator calibrated with adaptive validation is bounded by $\sigma\sqrt{\log[p]/n}$ with high probability. This bound is optimal in the discussed sense: compare to the end of Example 7.3.1.

For designs that are not orthogonal $X^\top X \neq n\mathrm{I}_{n\times n}$, it is more difficult to quantify the factor f. But one can expect—at least for weakly correlated designs—that $3/(4n)$ still approximates f and, therefore, that adaptive validation with $\tilde{f} = 3/(4n)$ still works well.[16]

Example 7.4.1 demonstrates that adaptive validation together with thresholding can also yield accurate support recovery. Hence, adaptive validation is recommended when calibrating the lasso for support recovery and parameter estimation in terms of the ℓ_∞-loss, while cross-validation is the method of choice for prediction. ◀

4.5 Exercises

4.5.1 Exercises for ▶ Sect. 4.2

Exercise 4.1 ◇ In this exercise, we verify the identity that underpins our interpretation of the lasso's effective noise. Show that

$$2\|X^\top \boldsymbol{u}\|_\infty = 2\|\boldsymbol{u}\|_2 \max_{j\in\{1,\dots,p\}} \bigl\{|\mathrm{cor}[\boldsymbol{u}, \boldsymbol{x}_j]| \cdot \|\boldsymbol{x}_j\|_2\bigr\}.$$

Use the definition of the correlation on Page 40 and $X = (\boldsymbol{x}_1, \dots, \boldsymbol{x}_p)$.

Exercise 4.2 ◆◆ In this exercise, we establish the union bound (also called Boole's inequality), which we have used in the proof of Lemma 4.2.1.

Show that for all events $\mathscr{A}_1, \dots, \mathscr{A}_k$, $k \in \{1, 2, \dots\}$, it holds that

$$\mathbb{P}\Bigl\{\bigcup_{j=1}^{k} \mathscr{A}_j\Bigr\} \le \sum_{j=1}^{k} \mathbb{P}\{\mathscr{A}_j\}.$$

Use only the following two properties of probability measures: (i) finite additivity, that is, $\mathbb{P}\{\mathscr{A} \cup \mathscr{B}\} = \mathbb{P}\{\mathscr{A}\} + \mathbb{P}\{\mathscr{B}\}$ for all disjoint events $\mathscr{A}, \mathscr{B}$; (ii) positivity, that is, $\mathbb{P}\{\mathscr{A}\} \ge 0$ for every event $\mathscr{A}$. (That these two properties suffice indicates that the union bound also holds for functions other than probability measures.)

Exercise 4.3 ◆◆ In this exercise, we derive the tail bound for Gauss-distributed random variables that we have used in the proof of Lemma 4.2.1.

Show that any standard Gauss random variable $z \sim \mathscr{N}_1[0, 1]$ fulfills

$$\mathbb{P}\bigl\{|z| \ge a\bigr\} \le e^{-\frac{a^2}{2}}$$

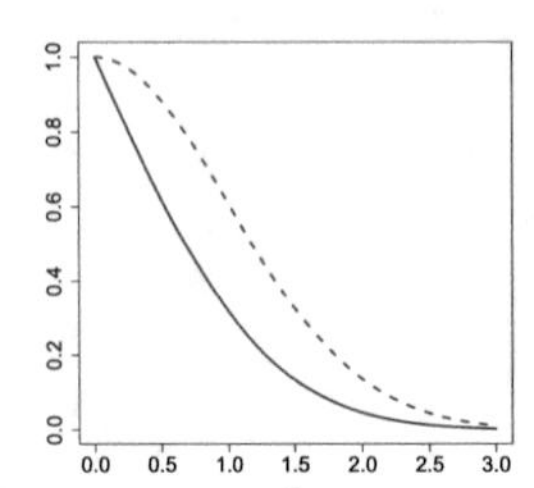

for every $a \in [0, \infty)$. The plot on the left depicts $\mathbb{P}\{|z| \geq a\}$ (red, solid line) and $e^{-\frac{a^2}{2}}$ (blue, dashed line) as functions of a.

Exercise 4.4 ◊ In this exercise, we generalize the tail bound for the effective noise in Lemma 4.2.1.

1. Prove a tail bound as in Lemma 4.2.1 for general $2v\|X^\top \boldsymbol{u}\|_\infty$, $v \in (0, \infty)$.
2. Prove a tail bound as in Lemma 4.2.1 for $2\|X^\top \boldsymbol{u}\|_\infty$ with noise $\boldsymbol{u}$ distributed according to a Laplace distribution (also called double-exponential distribution).

4.5.2 Exercises for ▶ Sect. 4.3

Exercise 4.5 ♦ In this exercise, we study the optimal tuning parameter defined in the minimization (4.1) and its estimation via the minimization (4.2). For this, we consider some general settings in plots A–D:

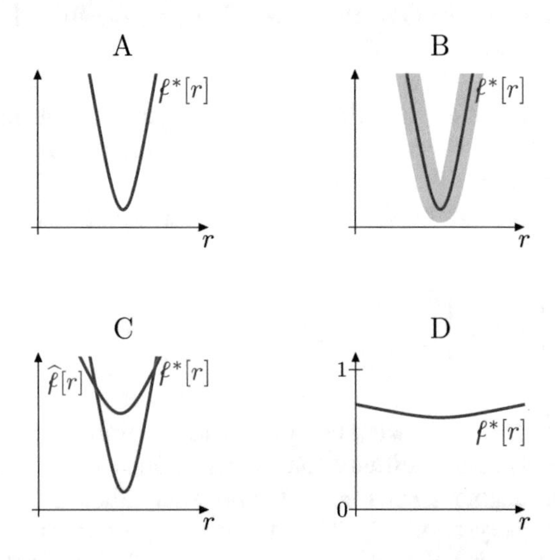

1. Consider Plot A: Mark the optimal tuning parameter r^*. Motivate that in the depicted case, $\widehat{r} \approx r^*$ yields $f^*[\widehat{r}] \approx f^*[r^*]$.
2. Consider Plot B: Assume that the estimated prediction error $\widehat{f}$ is close to the true error f^* in the sense that the values $\widehat{f}[r]$ are in the red shaded area around $f^*[r]$ for all $r \in \mathscr{R}$. Can you restrict the possible values of $\widehat{r}$? Conclude that typically $\widehat{f}$ being close to the true

error ℓ^* across all tuning parameters $r \in \mathcal{R}$ yields $\hat{r} \approx r^*$.

3. Consider Plot C: Mark r^* and $\hat{r}$. Conclude that $\hat{\ell}$ being close to the true error ℓ^* is not a necessary condition for $\hat{r}$ being close to r^*.
4. Consider Plot D: Assume that the x-axis covers the entire set of possible tuning parameters $\mathcal{R}$. Argue that then in the depicted setting, any calibration scheme would do fine in the sense that $\ell^*[\hat{r}] \approx \ell^*[r^*]$. Does this require $\hat{r} \approx r^*$?

Cross-validation aims at finding a tuning parameter $\hat{r}$ such that $\ell^*[\hat{r}] \approx \ell^*[r^*]$, where ℓ^* is the (scaled) prediction error: $\ell^*[r] := \|X\boldsymbol{\beta} - X\widehat{\boldsymbol{\beta}}[r]\|_2^2/n$, $r \in \mathcal{R}$. Question 1 indicates that a typical case where this holds is $\hat{r} \approx r^*$, and Question 2 indicates that a typical case where the latter holds is $\hat{\ell}[r] \approx \ell^*[r]$ for all $r \in \mathcal{R}$.

On the other hand, Question 3 shows that $\hat{\ell} \approx \ell^*$ is *not a necessary* condition for $\hat{r} \approx r^*$, and Question 4 shows that $\hat{r} \approx r^*$ is *not a necessary* condition for $\ell^*[\hat{r}] \approx \ell^*[r^*]$ either. Hence, the only measure of success is how well $\ell^*[\hat{r}]$ approximates $\ell^*[r^*]$.

Exercise 4.6 ♦ In this exercise, we highlight the limitations of cross-validation outside of prediction.

Assume that we want to find a data-driven version of

$$r^* \in \arg\min_{r \in \mathcal{R}} \ell^*[r], \quad \text{where } \ell^*[r] := \|\boldsymbol{\beta} - \widehat{\boldsymbol{\beta}}[r]\|_2^2 .$$

Is cross-validation suited for this?

4.5.3 Exercises for ▶ Sect. 4.4

Exercise 4.7 ◊◊ In this exercise, we verify that $\hat{r}_{\text{av}}$ in the adaptive validation scheme (4.4) is well-defined. Indeed: show that the minimum in the formulation of adaptive validation is always attained in $\mathcal{R}$ and unique. Hint: use the fact that by assumption, $\mathcal{R}$ is compact and non-empty and $\ell[\mathbf{0}_p] = 0$.

Exercise 4.8 ◊◊ In this exercise, we confirm the computational properties of the adaptive validation scheme (4.4).

1. Show that Algorithm 4.1 involves less than $|\mathcal{R}|^2$ contrasts of the form $\ell[\widehat{\boldsymbol{\beta}}[r'] - \widehat{\boldsymbol{\beta}}[r]] > \bar{f}r' + \bar{f}r$. Evaluating

such a contrast is typically cheap in comparison to evaluating an estimator $\widehat{\boldsymbol{\beta}}[r]$, which can require elaborate descent algorithms, for example. This means that for reasonably small $\mathcal{R}$, the computational effort for evaluating the contrasts is negligible.

2. Show that for all r, s such that $r \geq s$, it holds that

$$\exists r', r'' \in \mathcal{R} \cap [r, \infty) \;:\; \ell\big[\widehat{\boldsymbol{\beta}}[r'] - \widehat{\boldsymbol{\beta}}[r'']\big] > \tilde{f}r' + \tilde{f}r''$$
$$\Downarrow$$
$$\exists r', r'' \in \mathcal{R} \cap [s, \infty) \;:\; \ell\big[\widehat{\boldsymbol{\beta}}[r'] - \widehat{\boldsymbol{\beta}}[r'']\big] > \tilde{f}r' + \tilde{f}r''\,.$$

This inclusion implies that if r is an infeasible tuning parameter, that is, $\max\{\ell[\widehat{\boldsymbol{\beta}}[r'] - \widehat{\boldsymbol{\beta}}[r]] - \tilde{f}r' - \tilde{f}r \;:\; r' \in \mathcal{R} \cap (r, \infty)\} > 0$, then also s is an infeasible tuning parameter, that is, $\max\{\ell[\widehat{\boldsymbol{\beta}}[r'] - \widehat{\boldsymbol{\beta}}[s]] - \tilde{f}r' - \tilde{f}s \;:\; r' \in \mathcal{R} \cap (s, \infty)\} > 0$. This property allows Algorithm 4.1 to compute adaptive validation with *early stopping*: as soon the downward search reaches an infeasible tuning parameter, the computations can be stopped. Hence, some estimators $\widehat{\boldsymbol{\beta}}[r]$ do not need to be evaluated altogether.

This exercise demonstrates that adaptive validation can be computationally more efficient than AIC–BIC-type methods (which require exactly one evaluation of each estimator) and cross-validation methods (which require more than one evaluation of each estimator).[17]

Exercise 4.9 $\Diamond\Diamond$ In this exercise, we generalize adaptive validation to incorporate a slightly broader range of error bounds. We assume that for a target vector $\boldsymbol{\alpha} \in \mathbb{R}^p$, a (potentially random) non-decreasing function $\not{f} : \mathbb{R} \to \mathbb{R}$ that is known in practice or can be approximated, and a (potentially random) tuning parameter $r^* \in \mathcal{R}$, all estimators $\widehat{\boldsymbol{\beta}}[r]$ with $r \in \mathcal{R} \cap [r^*, \infty)$ satisfy

$$\ell\big[\boldsymbol{\alpha} - \widehat{\boldsymbol{\beta}}[r]\big] \leq \not{f}[r]\,.$$

You now have two tasks:

1. Show that the above set of assumptions generalizes Assumption 4.4.1.
2. Modify the adaptive validation scheme (4.4) to accommodate the above assumptions and prove a corresponding version of Theorem 4.4.1.

This generalization suggests that the concept of adaptive validation could be useful also outside the scope of high-dimensional statistics.[18]

4.6 R Lab: Cross-Validation

In this lab, we study cross-validation. As always, replace the keyword REPLACE with suitable code and answer the questions in the text.

4.6.1 Data Generation

Generate data from a linear regression model $\boldsymbol{y} = X\boldsymbol{\beta} + \boldsymbol{u}$, where the entries of the design $X \in \mathbb{R}^{100\times 500}$ are sampled independently according to $X_{ij} \sim \mathcal{N}[0, 1]$, the regression vector is $\boldsymbol{\beta} = (1, 1, 1, 0, 0, \ldots, 0)^\top \in \mathbb{R}^{500}$, and the noise is sampled independently from the design according to $\boldsymbol{u} \sim \mathcal{N}_{100}[\boldsymbol{0}_{100}, \mathrm{I}_{100,100}]$.

```
set.seed(1)
n <- 100; p <- 500
design <- REPLACE
regression.vector <- REPLACE
outcome <- REPLACE
cbind(outcome[1:4], design[1:4, 1:4])
```

```
##            [,1]       [,2]        [,3]       [,4]       [,5]
## [1,] -0.3115278 -0.6264538 -0.62036668  0.4094018  0.8936737
## [2,]  1.4270881  0.1836433  0.04211587  1.6888733 -1.0472981
## [3,]  0.9782890 -0.8356286 -0.91092165  1.5865884  1.9713374
## [4,]  2.6375362  1.5952808  0.15802877 -0.3309078 -0.3836321
```

4.6.2 Computing a Set of Estimators

Compute lasso estimates via the `glmnet` package. Let the `glmnet` function generate 50 tuning parameters and store these tuning parameters for later use. Set the flag `intercept=FALSE` throughout. Use `glmnet`'s standard options otherwise. Plot the average prediction error $\|X\boldsymbol{\beta} - X\widehat{\boldsymbol{\beta}}\|_2^2/n$ as a function of the tuning parameter.

```
set.seed(2)
library(glmnet)
AvgPredictionError <- function(estimator, design, regression.vector)
{
```

```
  return(REPLACE)
}
lasso.fit <- REPLACE
estimators <- lasso.fit$beta
tuning.parameters <- lasso.fit$lambda
estimators.prediction.error <- apply(estimators, 2, AvgPredictionError, design, regression.vector)
plot(x    = tuning.parameters,
     y    = estimators.prediction.error,
     xlim = c(0, 1.1),
     ylim = c(0, 4),
     xaxp = c(0, 1, 4),
     yaxp = c(0, 4, 4),
     las  = 1,
     xlab = "Tuning parameter",
     ylab = "True prediction error")
```

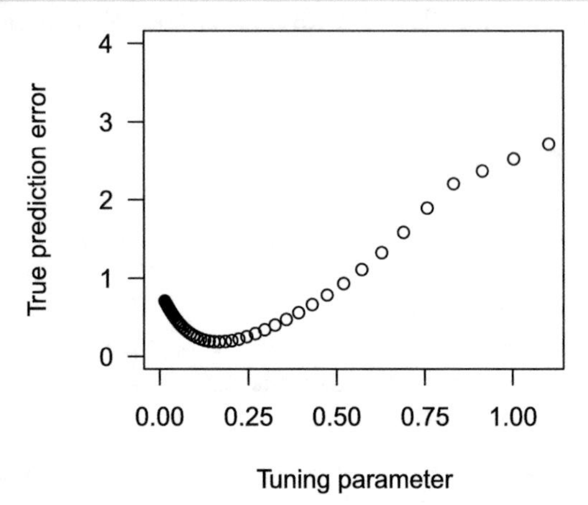

Which tuning parameters are the most favorable ones according to this plot?

4.6.3 Implementing a Monte Carlo Cross-Validation

Implement a Monte Carlo cross-validation scheme for selecting among the tuning parameters stored above. Set the training sample size to half the sample size and the number of splits to 3. Plot the estimated errors $\widehat{f}[r]$ as a function of the tuning parameter. The function `setdiff()` could be convenient in determining the validation set.

```
set.seed(3)
IndividualValidationError <- function(estimator, outcome, design)
{
  return(REPLACE)
}
AvgPredictionErrorEstimated <- function(outcome, design, tuning.parameters, size.training,
                                        number.splits)
{
  estimators.error <- rep(0, length(tuning.parameters))
  for (j in 1:number.splits)
  {
    indexes.training <- sample(c(1:dim(design)[1]), size.training)
    estimators <- REPLACE
    indexes.validation <- REPLACE
```

```
        estimators.error <- estimators.error + apply(estimators, 2, IndividualValidationError,
                                                       outcome[indexes.validation],
                                                       design[indexes.validation, ])
    }
    return(REPLACE)
}
plot(x    = tuning.parameters,
     y    = AvgPredictionErrorEstimated(outcome, design, tuning.parameters,
                                         dim(design)[1] / 2, 3),
     xlim = c(0, 1.1),
     ylim = c(0, 4),
     xaxp = c(0, 1, 4),
     yaxp = c(0, 4, 4),
     las  = 1,
     xlab = "Tuning parameter",
     ylab = "Estimated prediction error")
```

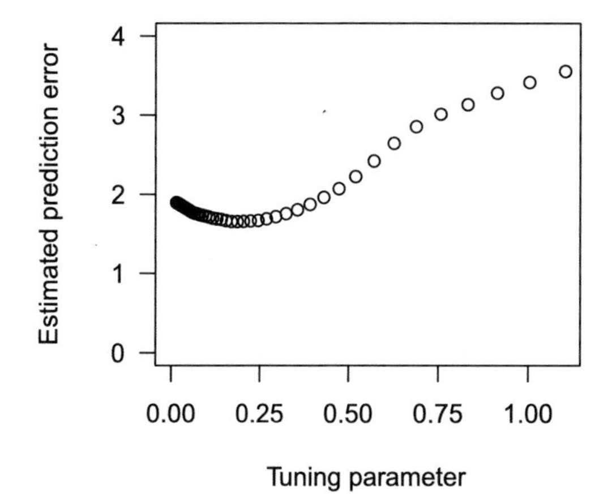

The curve looks a bit like an upward-shifted version of the earlier one, which means especially that cross-validation overestimates the true errors in our example. Can you find a reason for this? Can you corroborate your reasoning by running the code with one of the model specifications changed? For the selection of tuning parameters, is an over- or underestimation of the true errors necessarily a problem?

4.6.4 The Double Role of the Training Sample Size

Complement the first plot with lines that indicate tuning parameters selected by Monte Carlo cross-validation for different training sample sizes.

```
set.seed(4)
plot(x    = tuning.parameters,
     y    = estimators.prediction.error,
     xlim = c(0, 1.1),
     ylim = c(0, 4),
     xaxp = c(0, 1, 4),
     yaxp = c(0, 4, 4),
     las  = 1,
```

```
     xlab = "Tuning parameter",
     ylab = "True prediction error")
nbr.lines <- 19
tuning.parameter.selected <- rep(0, nbr.lines)
colors <- terrain.colors(nbr.lines)
n.values <- seq(1:19) * n / (nbr.lines + 1)
for (i in 1:nbr.lines)
{
  tuning.parameter.selected[i] <- tuning.parameters[which.min(AvgPredictionErrorEstimated(
                              outcome, design, tuning.parameters, n.values[i], 3))]
  abline(v=tuning.parameter.selected[i], col=colors[i], lty=2, lwd=1.5)
}
```

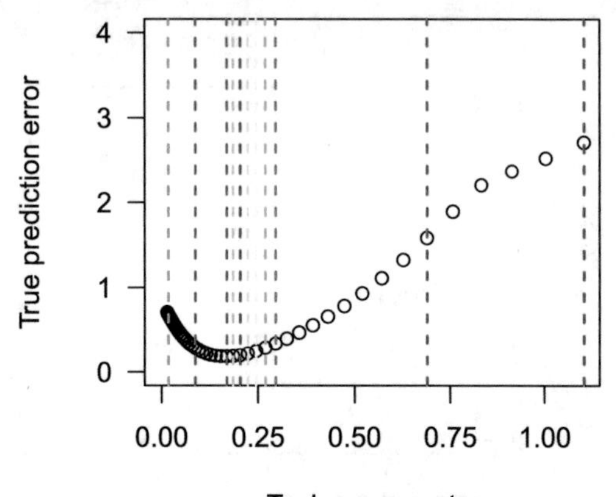


```
plot(x    = n.values,
     y    = tuning.parameter.selected,
     xlim = c(0, 100),
     ylim = c(0, 1.5),
     xaxp = c(0, 100, 5),
     yaxp = c(0, 1.5, 3),
     las  = 1,
     xlab = "Training sample size",
     ylab = "Tuning parameter")
```

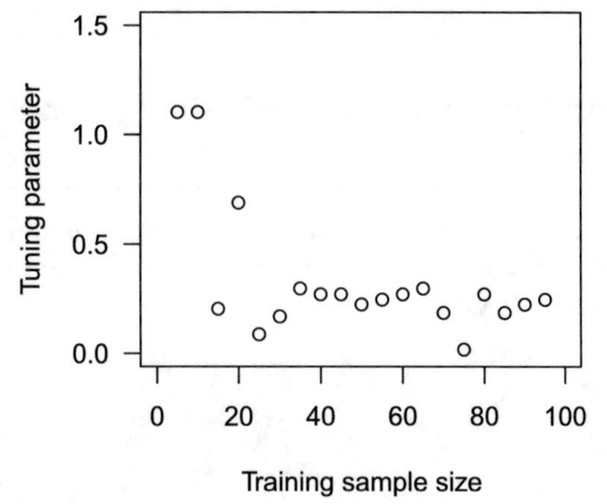

Can you identify a *clear* trend in the number of training samples? Which two effects are competing?

4.6.5 The Role of the Number of Splits

Complement the first plot with lines that indicate tuning parameters selected by (i) Monte Carlo cross-validation with 50 splits and (ii) a simple holdout method. Set the training sample size to 50 for both methods.

```
set.seed(1)
plot(x     = tuning.parameters,
     y     = estimators.prediction.error,
     xlim  = c(0, 1.1),
     ylim  = c(0, 4),
     xaxp  = c(0, 1, 4),
     yaxp  = c(0, 4, 4),
     las   = 1,
     xlab  = "Tuning parameter",
     ylab  = "True prediction error")
for (i in 1:10)
{
  abline(v=tuning.parameters[which.min(AvgPredictionErrorEstimated(outcome, design,
                                                                   tuning.parameters,
                                                                   REPLACE, REPLACE))],
         col="blue", lty=1, lwd=1.5)  # MC with 50 splits
  abline(v=tuning.parameters[which.min(AvgPredictionErrorEstimated(outcome, design,
                                                                   tuning.parameters,
                                                                   REPLACE, REPLACE))],
         col="red", lty=2, lwd=1.5)  # holdout
}
```

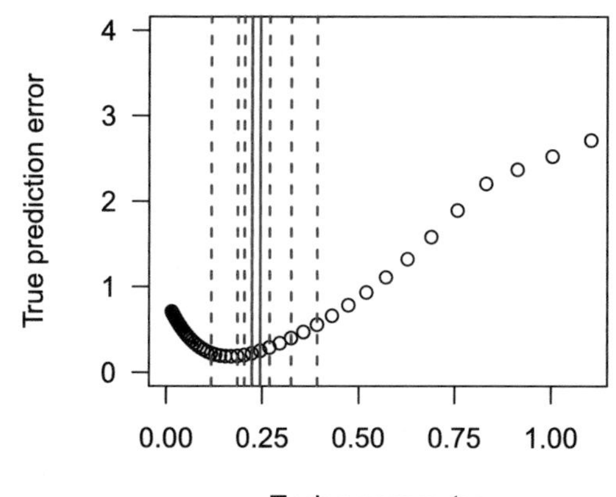

Which method has smaller variance in the selection of the tuning parameter? Why is this expected?

4.7 Notes and References

1 See Fultz et al. (2019).
2 That $r \geq 2v\|X^\top \boldsymbol{u}\|_\infty$ is not a sufficient *and necessary* condition for the lasso to perform well has been shown first in van de Geer and Lederer (2013). They suggest in particular that in correlated settings, tuning parameters should be smaller than what is

suggested by the mentioned condition—see their Corollary 4.2 on p. 308, for example. Further results in this direction have derived in Dalalyan et al. (2017). Hence, although the effective noise $2\|X^\top \boldsymbol{u}\|_\infty$ is intimately connected with the lasso's tuning parameter and with the lasso more generally, it does not account for the entire intricacy of tuning-parameter calibration.

3 See Hebiri and Lederer (2013, Proof of Theorem 3.2 on pp. 16–18), for example.

4 This has been noted in Hebiri and Lederer (2013); in particular, their Theorem 3.2 on pp. 16–18 is a refinement of Lemma 4.2.1 for correlated designs—but see the second note above.

5 Two classical references for cross-validation are Geisser (1975); Stone (1974).

6 For more details on incommensurable goals in estimating $\boldsymbol{\beta}$, including the so-called *AIC–BIC dilemma*, see Arlot and Celisse (2010, Section 2.4 on p. 48).

7 An overview about the existing theory for cross-validation and about the corresponding literature is provided in Arlot and Celisse (2010). Nonasymptotic expressions for the variance of the (again out-of-sample) risk of projection estimators in regression can be found in Celisse (2008, Proposition 3.4.3 on p. 66). Some theoretical bounds for cross-validated lasso can be found in Chatterjee and Jafarov (2015) and Homrighausen and McDonald (2013a,b, 2014). Much more is known about cross-validated ridge regression, see Golub et al. (1979) for example.

8 A set $\mathcal{A} \subset \mathbb{R}$ is *compact* if it is bounded and closed: $\mathcal{A} \subset [b, c]$ for some $b, c \in \mathbb{R}$, and $\lim_{i=1}^{\infty} a_i \in \mathcal{A}$ for every sequence $a_1, a_2, \ldots \in \mathcal{A}$ that converges in $\mathbb{R}$. In particular, finite sets are compact, and since all known implementations of both cross-validation and adaptive validation are limited to finite candidate sets $\mathcal{R}$, compactness does not impose any practical restrictions.

9 Adaptive validation for estimation and support recovery in ℓ_1-regularized logistic regression is discussed in Li and Lederer (2019). The cross-validation schemes described in ▶ Sect. 4.3 can also be adapted to logistic regression—see the general treatment in the classical paper Geisser (1975, Section 2 on pp. 321–322), for example.

10 Adaptive validation for estimation and support recovery in ℓ_1-regularized graphical modeling is discussed in Laszkiewicz et al. (2020). In graphical modeling, the coordinates of the estimators $\widehat{\boldsymbol{\beta}}[r] \in \mathbb{R}^p$ are identified with the entries of the precision matrix or the edges of the corresponding graph; in particular, $p = d \times d$ or $p = d \times (d-1)/2$, respectively, where d the number of nodes—see ▶ Chap. 3. Because graphical models do not generate an immediate prediction task, they are also not amenable to cross-validation directly.

11 The property of real values needed for the treatment here is that they are ordered, which allows a well-defined downward search from large to small tuning parameters.

12 Adaptive validation was introduced by Chichignoud et al. (2016). Our definition in (4.4) generalizes their Definition 2 on p. 4 beyond the lasso and beyond sup-norm bounds, and our Theorem 4.4.1 generalizes their Theorem 3 on p. 5 accordingly. The original paper defines the optimal tuning parameter via tail bounds (Chichignoud et al., 2016, Definition 1 on p. 4), while we

generalize this to potentially random $r^* \in \mathcal{R}$, which allows us to establish a general, purely algebraic description of the concept.

13 A potential approach is to replace the exhaustive search over the set of tuning parameters through black box algorithms (Perrone et al., 2018).

14 For example, the prediction error $\boldsymbol{a} \mapsto \|X\boldsymbol{\beta} - X\boldsymbol{a}\|_2^2$ in linear regression cannot be used in adaptive validation because the corresponding loss function $\boldsymbol{a} \mapsto \|X\boldsymbol{a}\|_2^2$ does not satisfy the triangle inequality. In principle, one can fix this problem by using the square-root of that loss function $\boldsymbol{a} \mapsto \|X\boldsymbol{a}\|_2$ or by relaxing the triangle inequality to $\ell[\boldsymbol{a} + \boldsymbol{b}] \leq 2(\ell[\boldsymbol{a}] + \ell[\boldsymbol{b}])$ and including an additional factor of two in the appropriate places (cf.Lemma B.1.1). But the prediction bounds for lasso-type estimators in ▶ Chap. 6 are still not suitable because they involve factors, such as $\hbar[\boldsymbol{\beta}]$, that are unknown in practice. There are, however, suitable bounds for some estimators: the least-squares refitted lasso estimator is one example (Chételat et al., 2017), which is not surprising in view of the first step of this estimator being support recovery.

15 For simplicity, we assume that $4\|X^\top \boldsymbol{u}\|_\infty \in \mathcal{R}$. More generally, one can set $r^* := \min\{r \in \mathcal{R} : r \geq 4\|X^\top \boldsymbol{u}\|_\infty\}$; in practice, the candidate set $\mathcal{R}$ then needs to (i) contain sufficiently large values—such as $2\|X^\top \boldsymbol{y}\|_\infty$, see Exercise 2.11—to ensure the existence of that minimum and to (ii) contain a sufficiently fine grid to ensure that $r^* \approx 4\|X^\top \boldsymbol{u}\|_\infty$.

16 A way to quantify f beyond orthogonal design is the *ℓ_∞-restricted eigenvalue condition* (Chichignoud et al., 2016, Display (7) on p. 6).

17 For nonparametric regression, a selection scheme for bandwidths that has some commonalities with adaptive validation has already been known much earlier (Lepskii, 1991; Lepski et al., 1997).

18 Theory and algorithms for increasing the computational efficiency of adaptive validation further have been formulated in Taheri et al. (2020).

Inference

Contents

J. Lederer, *Fundamentals of High-Dimensional Statistics*, Springer Texts in Statistics,
https://doi.org/10.1007/978-3-030-73792-4_5

In the preceding sections, we have discussed the estimation of target parameters, such as the elements of the regression vector $\boldsymbol{\beta}$ in linear regression. In this section, our task is to complement these estimates with measures of uncertainty. We call this task *inference*. Our first step is to introduce an algorithm for computing estimators that are defined through systems of equations. However, rather than the actual computations of these estimators, we are interested in modifying other estimators by applying only a single update step of the algorithm. We call estimators that are generated this way *one-step estimators* (see ▶ Sect. 5.1). Our second step is to show that some one-step estimators can be interpreted as intermediate points between a classical estimator and a high-dimensional estimator and can be separated into three parts: (1) the regression vector of the underlying regression model, which ensures unbiasedness, (2) a distributional term that is inherited from the classical estimator and that is, therefore, amenable to classical distribution theory, and (3) a remainder that depends only on the high-dimensional estimator and that is, therefore, amenable to high-dimensional estimation bounds. These observations finally allow us to derive confidence intervals for individual coordinates of regression vectors (see ▶ Sect. 5.2).

5.1 One-Step Estimators

Many classical estimators are Z-estimators, which means that they are solutions of systems of equations. Such estimators can be computed via an iterative scheme called the Newton–Raphson algorithm. In fact, if the initial guess in this algorithm is sufficiently good, a *single* iteration of the algorithm can already yield an estimator that has the desired properties. Estimators that are based on such a single iteration are called one-step estimators.

A *Z-estimator*[1,2] is a solution of a system of equations:

$$\widehat{\boldsymbol{\beta}} \in \mathcal{B} \quad \text{is such that} \quad \mathfrak{z}_Z[\widehat{\boldsymbol{\beta}}] = \mathbf{0}_d \tag{5.1}$$

with a given vector-valued function

$$\begin{aligned} \mathfrak{z}_Z \,:\, \mathcal{B} &\to \mathbb{R}^d \\ \boldsymbol{\alpha} &\mapsto \mathfrak{z}_Z[\boldsymbol{\alpha}] \end{aligned}$$

on a space $\mathscr{B}$ that parametrizes the models. We restrict our analysis to $\mathscr{B} = \mathbb{R}^p$ for ease of presentation. The data enter the definition of the estimators through the specification of $\mathfrak{z}_Z$, that is, different data points Z correspond to different functions $\mathfrak{z}_Z$. Common examples of Z-estimators are maximum likelihood estimators, including the least-squares estimator as one of the most classical representatives:

▶ Example 5.1.1

Maximum Likelihood Estimators In this example, we write maximum likelihood estimators as Z-estimators. The logarithm of the density of the data as a function of the model parameters is called the *likelihood function*, and the maximizers of this likelihood function are called the *maximum likelihood estimators*. If the likelihood function is sufficiently regular (especially differentiable), the maximum likelihood estimators are the parameters that set the derivatives of the likelihood function, called the *score function*, to zero. Consequently, maximum likelihood estimators that are based on regular likelihood functions are Z-estimators with the systems of equations determined by the score functions. In mathematical terms, the maximum likelihood estimators

$$\widehat{\boldsymbol{\beta}} \in \underset{\boldsymbol{\alpha}\in\mathbb{R}^p}{\arg\max}\, \ell[\boldsymbol{\alpha}]$$

for a sufficiently regular likelihood function $\ell : \mathscr{B} \to \mathbb{R}$ are Z-estimators characterized through

$$\widehat{\boldsymbol{\beta}} \in \mathbb{R}^p \quad \text{is such that} \quad \mathfrak{z}_Z[\widehat{\boldsymbol{\beta}}] = \mathbf{0}_d$$

with $\mathfrak{z}_Z$ the score function

$$\mathfrak{z}_Z \,:\, \boldsymbol{\alpha} \mapsto \frac{\partial \ell[\boldsymbol{\alpha}]}{\partial \boldsymbol{\alpha}}\,.$$

As a specific example, we show that the least-squares estimator can be written both as a maximum likelihood estimator and as a Z-estimator. Consider a linear regression with observations $(y_1, \boldsymbol{x}_1), \ldots, (y_n, \boldsymbol{x}_n) \in \mathbb{R} \times \mathbb{R}^p$ that are summarized in $Z = (\boldsymbol{y}, X)$ as usual. Under the assumption that X is non-random and $\boldsymbol{u} \sim \mathcal{N}_n[\mathbf{0}_n, \sigma^2 \mathrm{I}_{n\times n}]$, the likelihood function for the regression vector $\boldsymbol{\beta}$ is $\ell[\boldsymbol{\alpha}] = \log[\prod_{i=1}^n (e^{-(y_i - \boldsymbol{x}_i{}^\top \boldsymbol{\alpha})^2/(2\sigma^2)}/\sqrt{2\pi\sigma^2})] = -\sum_{i=1}^n (y_i - \boldsymbol{x}_i{}^\top \boldsymbol{\alpha})^2/(2\sigma^2) - n\log[2\pi\sigma^2]/2$. The maximizers of this likelihood function are (use the definition of the ℓ_2-norm and that $\max_{a}(b\mathscr{f}[a]+c) = \min_{a} -\mathscr{f}[a]$ for every positive constant b, real-valued constant c, and real-valued function $\mathscr{f}$)

$$\underset{\boldsymbol{\alpha}\in\mathbb{R}^p}{\arg\max}\, \ell[\boldsymbol{\alpha}] \;=\; \underset{\boldsymbol{\alpha}\in\mathbb{R}^p}{\arg\min}\, \|\boldsymbol{y} - X\boldsymbol{\alpha}\|_2^2 \,.$$

Hence, the maximum likelihood estimator in this case is the least-squares estimator. Taking derivatives of the objective function, we find that $\widehat{\boldsymbol{\beta}}_{\text{ls}}$ is a least-squares estimator if and only if $-2X^\top(\boldsymbol{y} - X\widehat{\boldsymbol{\beta}}_{\text{ls}}) = \mathbf{0}_p$ (cf. ▶ Sect. 1.2), which means that the least-squares estimator is the following Z-estimator:

5

$$\widehat{\boldsymbol{\beta}}_{\text{ls}} \in \mathbb{R}^p \quad \text{is such that} \quad \mathfrak{z}_Z[\widehat{\boldsymbol{\beta}}_{\text{ls}}] \;=\; \mathbf{0}_d$$

with $\mathfrak{z}_Z$ the score function

$$\mathfrak{z}_Z \;:\; \boldsymbol{\alpha} \mapsto \; -2X^\top(\boldsymbol{y} - X\boldsymbol{\alpha})\,.$$

It is clearly visible that the specification of the score function $\mathfrak{z}_Z$ depends on the data $Z = (\boldsymbol{y}, X)$.◀

The system of Eqs. (5.1) is typically solved for $\widehat{\boldsymbol{\beta}}$ iteratively. Each iteration is an update step $\widehat{\boldsymbol{\beta}}^i \mapsto \widehat{\boldsymbol{\beta}}^{i+1} := \widehat{\boldsymbol{\beta}}^i + \boldsymbol{\delta}[\widehat{\boldsymbol{\beta}}^i]$, where $\widehat{\boldsymbol{\beta}}^i \in \mathbb{R}^p$ is the current state of the algorithm, and $\boldsymbol{\delta} : \mathbb{R}^p \to \mathbb{R}^p$ is a vector-valued function that is supposed to point from its argument to a solution $\widehat{\boldsymbol{\beta}}$. An ideal function $\boldsymbol{\delta}^*[\widehat{\boldsymbol{\beta}}^i]$ would generate a solution within one iteration:

$$\mathfrak{z}_Z\big[\widehat{\boldsymbol{\beta}}^i + \boldsymbol{\delta}^*[\widehat{\boldsymbol{\beta}}^i]\big] \;=\; \mathbf{0}_d\,.$$

Finding such ideal update vectors is as difficult as finding solutions to the systems of equations in the first place, but the display motivates a practical iteration: We first Taylor expand the function $\mathfrak{z}_Z$ around the current state $\widehat{\boldsymbol{\beta}}^i$ (assuming that $\mathfrak{z}_Z$ is smooth):

$$\mathfrak{z}_Z\big[\widehat{\boldsymbol{\beta}}^i + \boldsymbol{\delta}^*[\widehat{\boldsymbol{\beta}}^i]\big] \;\approx\; \mathfrak{z}_Z[\widehat{\boldsymbol{\beta}}^i] + \Big(\frac{\partial \mathfrak{z}_Z[\boldsymbol{\alpha}]}{\partial \boldsymbol{\alpha}}\Big|_{\boldsymbol{\alpha}=\widehat{\boldsymbol{\beta}}^i}\Big)\boldsymbol{\delta}^*[\widehat{\boldsymbol{\beta}}^i]$$

with the *Jacobi matrix*

$$\Big(\frac{\partial \mathfrak{z}_Z[\boldsymbol{\alpha}]}{\partial \boldsymbol{\alpha}}\Big|_{\boldsymbol{\alpha}=\widehat{\boldsymbol{\beta}}^i}\Big)_{kl} := \frac{\partial \mathfrak{z}_k[\boldsymbol{\alpha}]}{\partial \alpha_l}\Big|_{\boldsymbol{\alpha}=\widehat{\boldsymbol{\beta}}^i}$$

$$\text{for all } k \in \{1, \ldots, d\},\, l \in \{1, \ldots, p\}\,.$$

Plugging this expansion into the previous display yields

$$\mathfrak{z}_Z[\widehat{\boldsymbol{\beta}}^i] + \Bigl(\frac{\partial \mathfrak{z}_Z[\boldsymbol{\alpha}]}{\partial \boldsymbol{\alpha}}\Big|_{\boldsymbol{\alpha}=\widehat{\boldsymbol{\beta}}^i}\Bigr)\boldsymbol{\delta}^*[\widehat{\boldsymbol{\beta}}^i] \approx \mathbf{0}_d\,.$$

Assuming that the Jacobi is a square matrix ($d = p$) and invertible, we can then solve for $\boldsymbol{\delta}^*[\widehat{\boldsymbol{\beta}}^i]$:

$$\boldsymbol{\delta}^*[\widehat{\boldsymbol{\beta}}^i] \approx -\Bigl(\frac{\partial \mathfrak{z}_Z[\boldsymbol{\alpha}]}{\partial \boldsymbol{\alpha}}\Big|_{\boldsymbol{\alpha}=\widehat{\boldsymbol{\beta}}^i}\Bigr)^{-1} \mathfrak{z}_Z[\widehat{\boldsymbol{\beta}}^i]\,.$$

This insight is finally formulated in the update rule

$$\widehat{\boldsymbol{\beta}}^i \mapsto \widehat{\boldsymbol{\beta}}^{i+1} := \widehat{\boldsymbol{\beta}}^i - \Bigl(\frac{\partial \mathfrak{z}_Z[\boldsymbol{\alpha}]}{\partial \boldsymbol{\alpha}}\Big|_{\boldsymbol{\alpha}=\widehat{\boldsymbol{\beta}}^i}\Bigr)^{-1} \mathfrak{z}_Z[\widehat{\boldsymbol{\beta}}^i]\,, \qquad (5.2)$$

which is called the *Newton–Raphson algorithm*.

Newton–Raphson algorithm

▶ Example 5.1.2

Least-Squares Estimator Revisited I In the previous example, we have demonstrated that the least-squares estimator is a Z-estimator of the form

$$\widehat{\boldsymbol{\beta}}_{\mathrm{ls}} \in \mathbb{R}^p \quad \text{is such that} \quad \mathfrak{z}_Z[\widehat{\boldsymbol{\beta}}_{\mathrm{ls}}] = \mathbf{0}_d$$

with

$$\mathfrak{z}_Z : \boldsymbol{\alpha} \mapsto -2X^\top(\boldsymbol{y} - X\boldsymbol{\alpha})\,.$$

Assuming that the Gram matrix $X^\top X$ is invertible, we can solve for $\widehat{\boldsymbol{\beta}}_{\mathrm{ls}}$ directly to recover the well-known formula (cf. ▶ Sect. 1.2)

$$\widehat{\boldsymbol{\beta}}_{\mathrm{ls}} = (X^\top X)^{-1}X^\top \boldsymbol{y}\,.$$

But we can also compute $\widehat{\boldsymbol{\beta}}_{\mathrm{ls}}$ via the Newton–Raphson scheme. The Jacobi matrix is a multiple of the Gram matrix:

$$\frac{\partial \mathfrak{z}_Z[\boldsymbol{\alpha}]}{\partial \boldsymbol{\alpha}} = 2X^\top X \qquad \text{for all } \boldsymbol{\alpha} \in \mathbb{R}^p\,,$$

hence,

$$\Bigl(\frac{\partial \mathfrak{z}_Z[\boldsymbol{\alpha}]}{\partial \boldsymbol{\alpha}}\Big|_{\boldsymbol{\alpha}=\widehat{\boldsymbol{\beta}}^i}\Bigr)^{-1} = \frac{(X^\top X)^{-1}}{2}$$

irrespective of $\widehat{\boldsymbol{\beta}}^i$. The first Newton–Raphson update is, consequently,

$$
\begin{aligned}
\widehat{\boldsymbol{\beta}}^1 &= \widehat{\boldsymbol{\beta}}^0 - \Bigl(\frac{\partial \mathfrak{s}_Z[\boldsymbol{\alpha}]}{\partial \boldsymbol{\alpha}}\Big|_{\boldsymbol{\alpha}=\widehat{\boldsymbol{\beta}}^0}\Bigr)^{-1} \mathfrak{s}_Z[\widehat{\boldsymbol{\beta}}^0] && \text{Newton–Raphson update (5.2)}\\
&= \widehat{\boldsymbol{\beta}}^0 - \frac{(X^\top X)^{-1}}{2}\bigl(-2X^\top(\boldsymbol{y} - X\widehat{\boldsymbol{\beta}}^0)\bigr) && \text{using the previous display and the definition of } \mathfrak{s}_Z \text{ directly}\\
&= \widehat{\boldsymbol{\beta}}^0 + (X^\top X)^{-1}X^\top \boldsymbol{y} - (X^\top X)^{-1}X^\top X\widehat{\boldsymbol{\beta}}^0 && \text{linearity of matrix multiplications}\\
&= (X^\top X)^{-1}X^\top \boldsymbol{y}\,, && \text{consolidating}
\end{aligned}
$$

which, according to (1.4), is the least-squares estimator. Further iterations of the Newton–Raphson scheme have no effect:

$$
\begin{aligned}
\widehat{\boldsymbol{\beta}}^2 &= \widehat{\boldsymbol{\beta}}^1 + (X^\top X)^{-1}X^\top \boldsymbol{y} - (X^\top X)^{-1}X^\top X\widehat{\boldsymbol{\beta}}^1 && \text{as above}\\
&= \widehat{\boldsymbol{\beta}}^1 + (X^\top X)^{-1}X^\top \boldsymbol{y} - (X^\top X)^{-1}X^\top X(X^\top X)^{-1}X^\top \boldsymbol{y} && \widehat{\boldsymbol{\beta}}^1 = (X^\top X)^{-1}X^\top \boldsymbol{y} \text{ according to the previous display}\\
&= \widehat{\boldsymbol{\beta}}^1\,. && \text{consolidating}
\end{aligned}
$$

This means that the Newton–Raphson algorithm converges to a solution in a *single* iteration—irrespective of the starting point. ◀

The Newton–Raphson algorithm can be generalized to avoid computationally challenging inversions of Jacobi matrices or to account for singular or non-square ($d \neq p$) Jacobi matrices, which cannot be inverted altogether. The generalization consists of replacing the inverse of the Jacobi matrix by an approximation, which can be the actual inverse if it exists, a Moore–Penrose inverse, or some other approximate inverse. Given such an approximate inverse $M_{\mathfrak{s}_Z} \in \mathbb{R}^{p\times d}$, the update rule (5.2) generalizes to

$$
\widehat{\boldsymbol{\beta}}^i \mapsto \widehat{\boldsymbol{\beta}}^{i+1} := \widehat{\boldsymbol{\beta}}^i - M_{\mathfrak{s}_Z}\mathfrak{s}_Z[\widehat{\boldsymbol{\beta}}^i]\,, \tag{5.3}
$$

generalized Newton–Raphson algorithm

which is called a *generalized Newton–Raphson algorithm*.

▶ Example 5.1.3

Least-Squares Estimator Revisited II We now generalize Example 5.1.2 to non-invertible Gram matrices. Given a starting vector $\widehat{\boldsymbol{\beta}}^0 \in \mathbb{R}^p$ and an approximate inverse $M_{\mathfrak{z}_Z} \in \mathbb{R}^{p\times p}$ of the Jacobi matrix $2X^\top X$, the first update of the generalized Newton–Raphson algorithm is

$$\begin{aligned}
\widehat{\boldsymbol{\beta}}^1 &= \widehat{\boldsymbol{\beta}}^0 - M_{\mathfrak{z}_Z}\mathfrak{z}_Z[\widehat{\boldsymbol{\beta}}^0] && \text{generalized Newton–Raphson update (5.3)}\\
&= \widehat{\boldsymbol{\beta}}^0 - M_{\mathfrak{z}_Z}\big(-2X^\top(\boldsymbol{y} - X\widehat{\boldsymbol{\beta}}^0)\big) && \text{definition of } \mathfrak{z}_Z\text{—see Example 5.1.2}\\
&= \widehat{\boldsymbol{\beta}}^0 + 2M_{\mathfrak{z}_Z}X^\top\boldsymbol{y} - 2M_{\mathfrak{z}_Z}X^\top X\widehat{\boldsymbol{\beta}}^0 && \text{linearity of matrix–vector multiplications}\\
&= 2M_{\mathfrak{z}_Z}X^\top\boldsymbol{y} + \big(\mathrm{I}_{p\times p} - 2M_{\mathfrak{z}_Z}X^\top X\big)\widehat{\boldsymbol{\beta}}^0\,. && \text{consolidating}
\end{aligned}$$

Selecting $\widehat{\boldsymbol{\beta}}^0 := \mathbf{0}_p$ and $M_{\mathfrak{z}_Z} := (X^\top X)^+/2$, where $(X^\top X)^+$ is a Moore–Penrose inverse of $X^\top X$ (see the definition of Moore–Penrose inverses on Page 19), yields

$$\widehat{\boldsymbol{\beta}}^1 = (X^\top X)^+X^\top\boldsymbol{y}\,,$$

which, according to Exercise 1.2, is a least-squares estimator. Further iterations of the Newton–Raphson scheme have no effect:

$$\begin{aligned}
\widehat{\boldsymbol{\beta}}^2 &= \widehat{\boldsymbol{\beta}}^1 + 2M_{\mathfrak{z}_Z}X^\top\boldsymbol{y} - 2M_{\mathfrak{z}_Z}X^\top X\widehat{\boldsymbol{\beta}}^1 && \text{as above}\\
&= \widehat{\boldsymbol{\beta}}^1 + (X^\top X)^+X^\top\boldsymbol{y} - (X^\top X)^+X^\top X\widehat{\boldsymbol{\beta}}^1 && 2M_{\mathfrak{z}_Z} = (X^\top X)^+ \text{ by definition}\\
&= \widehat{\boldsymbol{\beta}}^1 + (X^\top X)^+X^\top\boldsymbol{y} - (X^\top X)^+X^\top X(X^\top X)^+X^\top\boldsymbol{y} && \widehat{\boldsymbol{\beta}}^1 = (X^\top X)^+X^\top\boldsymbol{y} \text{ according to the previous display}\\
&= \widehat{\boldsymbol{\beta}}^1 + (X^\top X)^+X^\top\boldsymbol{y} - (X^\top X)^+X^\top\boldsymbol{y} && (X^\top X)^+X^\top X(X^\top X)^+ = (X^\top X)^+ \text{ according to 2. in the definition of Moore–Penrose inverses}\\
&= \widehat{\boldsymbol{\beta}}^1\,. && \text{consolidating}
\end{aligned}$$

This means that if the starting point and the approximate inverse are chosen appropriately, the generalized Newton–Raphson algorithm converges again to a solution in a single iteration. ◀

That the Newton–Raphson algorithm converges in a single iteration is not the rule. But such a single iteration can still be valuable from a statistical perspective: roughly speaking, it can transform an estimator that is consistent but has an intractable distribution into an estimator that is amenable to inference. This feature of Newton–Raphson updates has been long known in classical statistics;[3] we will show in the next section that it also stands in high-dimensional statistics. For further reference, we thus call the output of single (generalized) Newton–Raphson iteration applied to an initial estimator a *one-step estimator*.

one-step estimator

5.2 Confidence Intervals

According to ► Sect. 1.3, the prior terms in high-dimensional estimators include prior information by favoring certain model parameters. But this favoring also generates a bias. The bias is usually small enough in terms of prediction and estimation, but it can render inference such as the construction of confidence intervals infeasible.[4] In this section, we try to remove the bias through single Newton–Raphson iterations in the direction of classical Z-estimators such as the least-squares.[5] This debiasing does *not* usually improve the prediction or estimation accuracy,[6] but the distributions of the resulting one-step estimators are suitable for inference.

To fix ideas, we construct confidence intervals for the jth coordinate of a regression vector $\boldsymbol{\beta}$. Our starting point is a high-dimensional estimator $\widehat{\boldsymbol{\beta}}^0 = \widehat{\boldsymbol{\beta}}$ such as the lasso. We update this initial estimator through a generalized Newton–Raphson step (5.3) in the direction of a least-squares solution (see Example 5.1.3 in the previous section):

$$\widehat{\boldsymbol{\beta}}^0 \mapsto \widehat{\boldsymbol{\beta}}^1 := 2M_{\mathfrak{z}_Z}X^\top \boldsymbol{y} + \left(\mathrm{I}_{p\times p} - 2M_{\mathfrak{z}_Z}X^\top X\right)\widehat{\boldsymbol{\beta}}^0\,, \qquad (5.4)$$

where $M_{\mathfrak{z}_Z} \in \mathbb{R}^{p\times p}$ is an approximate inverse of the Jacobi matrix $2X^\top X$. If the Gram matrix $X^\top X$ is invertible and $M_{\mathfrak{z}_Z} = (X^\top X)^{-1}/2$, the update yields the least-squares estimator (see Example 5.1.2). In general, the output is different, which is reassuring, because the least-squares estimator is not suitable for high-dimensional inference: for example, 2. in Exercise 1.2 illustrates that least-squares estimation is even ambiguous as soon as $p > n$. What the above update returns in general is rather a *mix* of the initial estimator and the least-squares estimator in an attempt to borrow the least-squares' unbiasedness (see ▶ Sect. 1.3) while maintaining the initial estimator's ability to cope with high-dimensionality. We thus call the updating step *debiasing*.[7]

debiasing

Debiased estimators can be separated into three parts, which are the regression vector, the approximate distribution around the regression vector, and the remainder:

$$\begin{aligned}
\widehat{\boldsymbol{\beta}}^1 &= 2M_{\mathfrak{z}_Z}X^\top \boldsymbol{y} + \bigl(\mathrm{I}_{p\times p} - 2M_{\mathfrak{z}_Z}X^\top X\bigr)\widehat{\boldsymbol{\beta}}^0 \\
&\qquad\qquad\text{above update rule}\\
&= 2M_{\mathfrak{z}_Z}X^\top(X\boldsymbol{\beta}+\boldsymbol{u}) + \bigl(\mathrm{I}_{p\times p} - 2M_{\mathfrak{z}_Z}X^\top X\bigr)\widehat{\boldsymbol{\beta}}^0 \\
&\qquad\qquad\text{linear regression: } \boldsymbol{y} = X\boldsymbol{\beta}+\boldsymbol{u}\\
&= \underbrace{\boldsymbol{\beta}}_{\substack{\text{regression}\\ \text{vector}}} + \underbrace{2M_{\mathfrak{z}_Z}X^\top \boldsymbol{u}}_{\substack{\text{distributional}\\ \text{term}}} + \underbrace{(2M_{\mathfrak{z}_Z}X^\top X - \mathrm{I}_{p\times p})(\boldsymbol{\beta}-\widehat{\boldsymbol{\beta}}^0)}_{\text{remainder}}\,.\\
&\qquad\qquad\text{linearity of matrix–vector multiplications}
\end{aligned}$$

The distributional term is, given X and $M_{\mathfrak{z}_Z}$, a linear function of the noise $\boldsymbol{u}$; this term has, therefore, a tractable distribution given X and $M_{\mathfrak{z}_Z}$ as long as the noise has a tractable distribution. The remainder is governed by the estimation accuracy of the initial estimator; this term might not have a tractable distribution but is small in comparison to the distributional term if the initial estimator converges to the regression vector of the underlying model sufficiently fast.

If we can handle the distributional part and bound the remainder, we can construct the desired confidence intervals for β_j with $j \in \{1,\dots,p\}$. Consider $z_{t/2}, m_{t/2} \in [0,\infty)$ such that

$$\begin{aligned}
&\mathbb{P}\bigl\{|(2M_{\mathfrak{z}_Z}X^\top \boldsymbol{u})_j| > z_{t/2}\bigr\} \le \frac{t}{2}\\
&\text{and } \mathbb{P}\Bigl\{\bigl|\bigl((2M_{\mathfrak{z}_Z}X^\top X - \mathrm{I}_{p\times p})(\boldsymbol{\beta}-\widehat{\boldsymbol{\beta}}^0)\bigr)_j\bigr| > m_{t/2}\Bigr\} \le \frac{t}{2}\,.
\end{aligned}$$

Then,

$$\begin{aligned}
&\mathbb{P}\bigl\{\beta_j \in [(\widehat{\beta}^1)_j - z_{t/2} - m_{t/2}, (\widehat{\beta}^1)_j + z_{t/2} + m_{t/2}]\bigr\}\\
&= \mathbb{P}\bigl\{\beta_j - (\widehat{\beta}^1)_j \in [-z_{t/2} - m_{t/2}, z_{t/2} + m_{t/2}]\bigr\}\\
&\qquad\qquad\text{subtracting } (\widehat{\beta}^1)_j \text{ throughout}
\end{aligned}$$

$$= \mathbb{P}\big\{\,|\beta_j - (\widehat{\beta}^1)_j| \;\leq\; z_{t/2} + m_{t/2}\big\}$$
$a \in [-b, b] \Leftrightarrow |a| \leq b$ for all $a \in \mathbb{R}, b \in [0, \infty)$

$$= \mathbb{P}\big\{\,\big|(2M_{\mathfrak{z}Z}X^\top \boldsymbol{u})_j + ((2M_{\mathfrak{z}Z}X^\top X - \mathrm{I}_{p\times p})(\boldsymbol{\beta} - \widehat{\boldsymbol{\beta}}^0))_j\big| \leq z_{t/2} + m_{t/2}\big\}$$
above decomposition of $\widehat{\boldsymbol{\beta}}^1$

$$= 1 - \mathbb{P}\big\{\,|(2M_{\mathfrak{z}Z}X^\top \boldsymbol{u})_j + ((2M_{\mathfrak{z}Z}X^\top X - \mathrm{I}_{p\times p}) \times (\boldsymbol{\beta} - \widehat{\boldsymbol{\beta}}^0))_j| \;>\; z_{t/2} + m_{t/2}\big\}$$
$\mathbb{P}\{\mathscr{A}\} = 1 - \mathbb{P}\{\mathscr{A}^{\mathsf{C}}\}$

$$\geq 1 - \mathbb{P}\big\{\,|(2M_{\mathfrak{z}Z}X^\top \boldsymbol{u})_j| \;>\; z_{t/2}\big\} - \mathbb{P}\big\{\,|((2M_{\mathfrak{z}Z}X^\top X - \mathrm{I}_{p\times p})(\boldsymbol{\beta} - \widehat{\boldsymbol{\beta}}^0))_j| \;>\; m_{t/2}\big\}$$
$\mathbb{P}\{\mathscr{A} \cup \mathscr{B}\} \leq \mathbb{P}\{\mathscr{A}\} + \mathbb{P}\{\mathscr{B}\}$

$$\geq 1 - \frac{t}{2} - \frac{t}{2}$$
by assumption on $z_{t/2}, m_{t/2}$ in the above display

$$= 1 - t\,,$$
consolidating

which means that $[(\widehat{\beta}^1)_j - z_{t/2} - m_{t/2}, (\widehat{\beta}^1)_j + z_{t/2} + m_{t/2}]$ is a level $1 - t$ confidence interval for β_j. We formulate a slight generalization of this result in the following theorem.

Theorem 5.2.1

Confidence Intervals in Linear Regression Given constants $t_1, t_2 \in [0, 1]$ and corresponding bounds $z_{t_1}, m_{t_2} \in [0, \infty)$ that satisfy $\mathbb{P}\{\,|(2M_{\mathfrak{z}Z}X^\top \boldsymbol{u})_j| \;>\; z_{t_1}\} \;\leq\; t_1$ and $\mathbb{P}\{\,|((2M_{\mathfrak{z}Z}X^\top X - \mathrm{I}_{p\times p})(\boldsymbol{\beta} - \widehat{\boldsymbol{\beta}}^0))_j| > m_{t_2}\} \leq t_2$, it holds that

$$\mathbb{P}\big\{\,\beta_j \;\in\; [(\widehat{\beta}^1)_j - z_{t_1} - m_{t_2}, (\widehat{\beta}^1)_j + z_{t_1} + m_{t_2}]\big\} \;\geq\; 1 - t_1 - t_2\,,$$

that is,

$$[(\widehat{\beta}^1)_j - z_{t_1} - m_{t_2}, (\widehat{\beta}^1)_j + z_{t_1} + m_{t_2}]$$

is a confidence interval for β_j at level $1 - t_1 - t_2$.

The value z_{t_1} captures the tail of the distributional term, while m_{t_2} essentially describes the convergence of the initial estimator.

Given a target level $1 - t \in [0, 1]$ in practice, we have to specify concrete values for t_1, t_2, where $t_1 + t_2 = t$, and find the corresponding z_{t_1}, m_{t_2}. If the remainder is negligible (that is, the approximate inverse and/or the initial estimator are accurate), the calibration of t_2 and m_{t_2} is uncomplicated: setting $t_2 := t - t_1 := 0$ and $m_{t_2} := 0$ provides for a good approximation of the stated confidence interval. It then remains to find a corresponding z_t. We illustrate the whole procedure in the following two examples.

▶ Example 5.2.1

Confidence Intervals for Least-Squares Estimator It is educational to apply our scheme for constructing confidence intervals first to the classical case where $n \gg p$ and $X^\top X$ is invertible. We can choose $M_{\mathfrak{z}Z} = (X^\top X)^{-1}/2$, which implies that the debiased lasso coincides with the least-squares estimator ($\widehat{\boldsymbol{\beta}}^1 = \widehat{\boldsymbol{\beta}}_{\text{ls}}$)—see Example 5.1.2—and that $2M_{\mathfrak{z}Z}X^\top X - \mathrm{I}_{p\times p} = \mathbf{0}_{p\times p}$, which allows us to set $t_1 := t$, $t_2 := 0$, and $m_{t_2} := 0$ for a given target level $1-t$. We now assume for the sake of illustration that $\boldsymbol{u} \sim \mathcal{N}_n[\mathbf{0}_n, \sigma^2\mathrm{I}_{n\times n}]$ and that X is a non-random matrix.[8] The distributional term then follows $2M_{\mathfrak{z}Z}X^\top\boldsymbol{u} \sim \mathcal{N}_n[\mathbf{0}_n, \sigma^2(2M_{\mathfrak{z}Z})X^\top X(2M_{\mathfrak{z}Z})^\top]$, and thus, the marginal distributions of its coordinates are $(2M_{\mathfrak{z}Z}X^\top\boldsymbol{u})_j \sim \mathcal{N}[0, \sigma^2((2M_{\mathfrak{z}Z})X^\top X(2M_{\mathfrak{z}Z})^\top)_{jj}]$. Since $M_{\mathfrak{z}Z} = (X^\top X)^{-1}/2$ by assumption, the distributions of the coordinates simplify to $2(M_{\mathfrak{z}Z}X^\top\boldsymbol{u})_j \sim \mathcal{N}[0, \sigma^2((X^\top X)^{-1})_{jj}]$. This allows us to set $z_{t_1} := q_{t/2}\sigma\sqrt{((X^\top X)^{-1})_{jj}}$, where $q_{t/2}$ is such that $\mathbb{P}\{|v| \geq q_{t/2}\} = t$ for $v \sim \mathcal{N}[0,1]$. The factor $\sigma\sqrt{((X^\top X)^{-1})_{jj}}$ captures the "scaling" of $2(M_{\mathfrak{z}Z}X^\top\boldsymbol{u})_j$, and the factor $q_{t/2}$ captures the scaled "shape" of $2(M_{\mathfrak{z}Z}X^\top\boldsymbol{u})_j$. Theorem 5.2.1 then yields the confidence interval at level $1-t$

$$\left[(\widehat{\beta}_{\text{ls}})_j - q_{t/2}\sigma\sqrt{\left((X^\top X)^{-1}\right)_{jj}},\, (\widehat{\beta}_{\text{ls}})_j + q_{t/2}\sigma\sqrt{\left((X^\top X)^{-1}\right)_{jj}}\right]$$

for β_j.

The standard deviation σ is usually unknown in practice, but it can also be estimated by using the least-squares estimator. Note first that

$$\begin{aligned}
&\frac{\|\boldsymbol{y} - X\widehat{\boldsymbol{\beta}}_{\text{ls}}\|_2}{\sqrt{n}} \\
&= \frac{\|X\boldsymbol{\beta} + \boldsymbol{u} - X\widehat{\boldsymbol{\beta}}_{\text{ls}}\|_2}{\sqrt{n}} && \text{linear regression model: } \boldsymbol{y} = X\boldsymbol{\beta} + \boldsymbol{u} \\
&\leq \frac{\|\boldsymbol{u}\|_2}{\sqrt{n}} + \frac{\|X\boldsymbol{\beta} - X\widehat{\boldsymbol{\beta}}_{\text{ls}}\|_2}{\sqrt{n}}, && \text{triangle inequality for norms}
\end{aligned}$$

and similarly

$$\frac{\|\boldsymbol{y} - X\widehat{\boldsymbol{\beta}}_{\text{ls}}\|_2}{\sqrt{n}} \geq \frac{\|\boldsymbol{u}\|_2}{\sqrt{n}} - \frac{\|X\boldsymbol{\beta} - X\widehat{\boldsymbol{\beta}}_{\text{ls}}\|_2}{\sqrt{n}}.$$

Since $\|\boldsymbol{u}\|_2/\sqrt{n}$ is sharply concentrated around σ (see Exercise 5.4), and since least-squares estimation provides accurate prediction, that is, $\|X\boldsymbol{\beta} - X\widehat{\boldsymbol{\beta}}_{\text{ls}}\|_2/\sqrt{n} \ll 1$, under mild conditions when $n \gg p$ (see Display (1.5) in ▸ Sect. 1.2), the two displays show that $\|\boldsymbol{y} - X\widehat{\boldsymbol{\beta}}_{\text{ls}}\|_2/\sqrt{n} \approx \sigma$ and, therefore, that

$$\Bigl[(\widehat{\beta}_{\text{ls}})_j - q_{t/2}\|\boldsymbol{y} - X\widehat{\boldsymbol{\beta}}_{\text{ls}}\|_2\sqrt{\bigl((X^\top X)^{-1}\bigr)_{jj}/n},\; (\widehat{\beta}_{\text{ls}})_j + q_{t/2}\|\boldsymbol{y} - X\widehat{\boldsymbol{\beta}}_{\text{ls}}\|_2\sqrt{\bigl((X^\top X)^{-1}\bigr)_{jj}/n}\Bigr] \tag{5.5}$$

is an approximate confidence interval at level $1 - t$ for β_j. ◂

▸ **Example 5.2.2**

Confidence Intervals for Debiased Lasso The lasso estimator satisfies sharp bounds for prediction and estimation (see ▸ Chaps. 6 and 7), but its distribution in terms of the design and the noise is involved. A way to make the distribution more tractable for inference is the one-step update (5.4):

$$\overline{\boldsymbol{\beta}} := 2M_{\mathfrak{z}Z}X^\top\boldsymbol{y} + \bigl(\mathrm{I}_{p\times p} - 2M_{\mathfrak{z}Z}X^\top X\bigr)\widehat{\boldsymbol{\beta}}_{\text{lasso}},$$

where $\widehat{\boldsymbol{\beta}}^0 = \widehat{\boldsymbol{\beta}}_{\text{lasso}}$ is an initial lasso estimator (see Display (2.2)) and $M_{\mathfrak{z}Z}$ an approximate inverse of $2X^\top X$ (see Examples 5.1.2 and 5.1.3). The corresponding one-step estimator $\widehat{\boldsymbol{\beta}}^1 = \overline{\boldsymbol{\beta}}$ is called the *debiased lasso estimator*.

Example 5.2.1 sets the general direction also for the high-dimensional case, but we need to make two adjustments: 1. we have to replace $(X^\top X)^{-1}/2$ by an approximation because the Gram matrix $X^\top X$ is not invertible as soon as $p > n$ (see 2. in Exercise 1.2); 2. we have to estimate the standard deviation through the lasso because the least-squares estimator does not provide reliable prediction as soon as $p \gtrsim n$ (see ▸ Sect. 1.2). We again make the assumptions that $\boldsymbol{u} \sim \mathcal{N}_n[\mathbf{0}_n, \sigma^2\mathrm{I}_{n\times n}]$ and that X is non-random. For Adjustment 1, we construct an approximate inverse through defining its rows as minimizers of convex optimization programs, that is, for each $k \in \{1, \ldots, p\}$, the kth row $\boldsymbol{a}^k$ of $M_{\mathfrak{z}Z}$ is defined as a solution of

minimize $\|\boldsymbol{b}\|_1$ over all $\boldsymbol{b} \in \mathbb{R}^p$

$$\text{that satisfy } \|2X^\top X\boldsymbol{b} - \boldsymbol{e}_k\|_\infty \leq a\sqrt{\frac{\log p}{n}}, \tag{5.6}$$

where $\boldsymbol{e}_k$ is the kth canonical unit vector in $\mathbb{R}^p$ ($(\boldsymbol{e}_k)_l = 1$ for $k = l$ and $(\boldsymbol{e}_k)_l = 0$ for $k \neq l$) and $a \in (0, \infty)$ a tuning parameter.[9] We can then bound the remainder as follows:

$$\begin{aligned}
&\left|\left((2M_{\mathfrak{z}Z}X^\top X - \mathrm{I}_{p\times p})(\boldsymbol{\beta} - \widehat{\boldsymbol{\beta}}^0)\right)_j\right| \\
&= |\langle(2M_{\mathfrak{z}Z}X^\top X - \mathrm{I}_{p\times p})_{j\cdot}, \boldsymbol{\beta} - \widehat{\boldsymbol{\beta}}^0\rangle| \\
&\qquad\qquad \text{indicating the } j\text{th row of a matrix by }_{j\cdot} \\
&= |\langle\left((2M_{\mathfrak{z}Z}X^\top X - \mathrm{I}_{p\times p})^\top\right)_{\cdot j}, \boldsymbol{\beta} - \widehat{\boldsymbol{\beta}}^0\rangle| \\
&\qquad\qquad \text{indicating the } j\text{th column of a matrix by }_{\cdot j} \\
&= |\langle(2X^\top X M_{\mathfrak{z}Z}{}^\top - \mathrm{I}_{p\times p})_{\cdot j}, \boldsymbol{\beta} - \widehat{\boldsymbol{\beta}}^0\rangle| \\
&\qquad\qquad (AB)^\top = B^\top A^\top;\ X^\top X \text{ and } \mathrm{I}_{p\times p} \text{ are symmetric} \\
&= |\langle 2X^\top X\boldsymbol{a}^j - \boldsymbol{e}^j, \boldsymbol{\beta} - \widehat{\boldsymbol{\beta}}^0\rangle| \\
&\qquad\qquad M_{\mathfrak{z}Z} = (\boldsymbol{a}^{1\top}, \ldots, \boldsymbol{a}^{p\top})^\top \text{ and } \mathrm{I}_{p\times p} = (\boldsymbol{e}^1, \ldots, \boldsymbol{e}^p)^\top \\
&\leq \|2X^\top X\boldsymbol{a}^j - \boldsymbol{e}^j\|_\infty \|\boldsymbol{\beta} - \widehat{\boldsymbol{\beta}}^0\|_1 \qquad \text{Hölder inequality (2.6)} \\
&\leq a\sqrt{\frac{\log p}{n}}\|\boldsymbol{\beta} - \widehat{\boldsymbol{\beta}}^0\|_1 . \\
&\qquad\qquad \text{definition of } \boldsymbol{a}^j \text{ through the above program}
\end{aligned}$$

The lasso's estimation accuracy scales like $\sigma\sqrt{\log[p]/n}$ when the noise is Gauss-distributed (see ▶ Chap. 7); it is thus convenient to introduce a function $\tilde{a} : [0, 1] \to [0, \infty)$ (which might be unknown in practice) such that $\|\boldsymbol{\beta} - \widehat{\boldsymbol{\beta}}^0\|_1 \leq \tilde{a}[t_2]\sigma\sqrt{\log[p]/n}$ with probability t_2. Combining this formulation of the lasso's accuracy with the prior display gives

$$\mathbb{P}\left\{\left|\left((2M_{\mathfrak{z}Z}X^\top X - \mathrm{I}_{p\times p})(\boldsymbol{\beta} - \widehat{\boldsymbol{\beta}}^0)\right)_j\right| \leq a\tilde{a}[t_2]\frac{\sigma\log p}{n}\right\} \leq t_2 .$$

Setting $t_1 := t - t_2$, $z_{t_1} := q_{t_1/2}\sigma\sqrt{((2M_{\mathfrak{z}Z})X^\top X(2M_{\mathfrak{z}Z})^\top)_{jj}}$ (recall from the last example that $(2M_{\mathfrak{z}Z}X^\top \boldsymbol{u})_j \sim \mathcal{N}[0, \sigma^2((2M_{\mathfrak{z}Z})X^\top X(2M_{\mathfrak{z}Z})^\top)_{jj}]$ and that $q_{t_1/2}$ is such that $\mathbb{P}\{|v| \geq q_{t/2}\} = t$ for $v \sim \mathcal{N}[0, 1]$), and setting

$m_{t_2} := a\tilde{a}[t_2]\sigma \log[p]/n$, Theorem 5.2.1 provides us with the following confidence interval at level $1 - t$ for β_j:

$$\Big[\overline{\beta}_j - q_{t_1/2}\sigma\sqrt{\big((2M_{\mathfrak{z}Z})X^\top X(2M_{\mathfrak{z}Z})^\top\big)_{jj}} - a\tilde{a}[t_2]\sigma \log[p]/n,$$

$$\overline{\beta}_j + q_{t_1/2}\sigma\sqrt{\big((2M_{\mathfrak{z}Z})X^\top X(2M_{\mathfrak{z}Z})^\top\big)_{jj}} + a\tilde{a}[t_2]\sigma \log[p]/n\Big].$$

The factor $\tilde{a}[t_2]$ is unknown in practice (for example, it can depend on the unknown sparsity level $\|\boldsymbol{\beta}\|_0$), but the remainder term is typically neglected altogether. The rationale is that one hopes that the minimization programs (5.6) have a solution for $a \approx 1$ (see Note 10 at the end of this chapter) and that the lasso is accurate enough to satisfy bounds with $\tilde{a}[t_2] \lesssim 1$ also for small t_2 (see Theorem 7.2.1). Specifically, with the design normalized such that $(X^\top X)_{jj} = n$ for all $j \in \{1, \dots, p\}$, it might make sense to assume that (i) $\sqrt{((2M_{\mathfrak{z}Z})X^\top X(2M_{\mathfrak{z}Z})^\top)_{jj}} \gtrsim 1/\sqrt{n}$ (if $2M_{\mathfrak{z}Z} = (X^\top X)^{-1}$ and the correlations among the predictors are low, that is, $(X^\top X)_{jj} = n \gg (X^\top X)_{ij}$ for all $i \neq j$, then $\sqrt{((2M_{\mathfrak{z}Z})X^\top X(2M_{\mathfrak{z}Z})^\top)_{jj}} = \sqrt{((X^\top X)^{-1})_{jj}} \approx \sqrt{1/(X^\top X)_{jj}} = 1/\sqrt{n}$, for example), (ii) $a \approx 1$ (as commented above), (iii) $\tilde{a}[t_2] \lesssim 1$ for $t_1 \approx t$ and $t_2 \approx 0$ (as commented above), and (iv) $q_{t_1/2} \gtrsim 1$ (which basically means that t_1 is not too close to one). These assumptions taken together yield

$$\frac{a\tilde{a}[t_2]\sigma \log[p]/n}{2q_{t_1/2}\sigma\sqrt{\big((2M_{\mathfrak{z}Z})X^\top X(2M_{\mathfrak{z}Z})^\top\big)_{jj}}}$$

$$= \frac{a\tilde{a}[t_2] \log[p]/n}{2q_{t_1/2}\sqrt{\big((2M_{\mathfrak{z}Z})X^\top X(2M_{\mathfrak{z}Z})^\top\big)_{jj}}} \qquad \text{dividing through by } \sigma$$

$$\ll \frac{\log[p]/n}{1/\sqrt{n}} \qquad \text{Assumptions (i)–(iv)}$$

$$= \frac{\log p}{\sqrt{n}}. \qquad \text{consolidating}$$

Therefore, if $\sqrt{n} \gg \log p$, the above confidence interval can be approximated by

$$\Big[\overline{\beta}_j - q_{t/2}\sigma\sqrt{\big((2M_{\mathfrak{z}Z})X^\top X(2M_{\mathfrak{z}Z})^\top\big)_{jj}},$$

$$\overline{\beta}_j + q_{t/2}\sigma\sqrt{\big((2M_{\mathfrak{z}Z})X^\top X(2M_{\mathfrak{z}Z})^\top\big)_{jj}}\Big].$$

This approximation, and the debiasing scheme in general, requires reasonably large sample sizes but then allows for a comparably large number of model parameters: for example, say, $\sqrt{n} \geq 2\log p$ requires $n \geq 85$ if $p = 100$ but only $n \geq 340$ if $p = 10\,000$.

For Adjustment 2, we simply exchange $\|\boldsymbol{y} - X\widehat{\boldsymbol{\beta}}_{\text{ls}}\|_2/\sqrt{n}$ by $\|\boldsymbol{y} - X\widehat{\boldsymbol{\beta}}_{\text{lasso}}\|_2/\sqrt{n}$ in the estimation of σ, using the fact that the lasso provides accurate prediction, that is, $\|X\boldsymbol{\beta} - X\widehat{\boldsymbol{\beta}}_{\text{lasso}}\|_2/\sqrt{n} \ll 1$, under mild conditions even when $p \gg n$ (see ► Chap. 6). Plugging the lasso estimate of σ into the previous display yields the approximate confidence interval

$$\Bigg[\overline{\beta}_j - q_{t/2}\|\boldsymbol{y} - X\widehat{\boldsymbol{\beta}}_{\text{lasso}}\|_2\sqrt{\big((2M_{\mathfrak{z}_Z})X^\top X(2M_{\mathfrak{z}_Z})^\top\big)_{jj}/n},$$
$$\overline{\beta}_j + q_{t/2}\|\boldsymbol{y} - X\widehat{\boldsymbol{\beta}}_{\text{lasso}}\|_2\sqrt{\big((2M_{\mathfrak{z}_Z})X^\top X(2M_{\mathfrak{z}_Z})^\top\big)_{jj}/n}\Bigg]. \tag{5.7}$$

Two tuning parameters remain to be calibrated: the tuning parameter r of the lasso (2.2) and the tuning parameter a in the minimization programs (5.6) for the approximate inverse. For practical choices of the lasso's tuning parameter, we refer to ► Chap. 4; a suggestion for the programs' tuning parameter is $a = 1.2 \times \inf_{\boldsymbol{b}\in\mathbb{R}^p} \|2X^\top X\boldsymbol{b} - \boldsymbol{e}^j\|_\infty$.[11] Importantly, while we cannot check how accurate the lasso is, we can check how accurate the approximate inverse is by computing $\max_k \|2X^\top X\boldsymbol{a}^k - \boldsymbol{e}^k\|_\infty$. ◄

5.3 Exercises

5.3.1 Exercises for ► Sect. 5.1

Exercise 5.1 ♦ In this exercise, we approach the Z-formulation of the least-squares estimator from another direction. In contrast to Example 5.1.1, where we have established a Z-formulation by taking derivatives of the least-squares' objective function, we start here by assuming that $\mathbb{E}[\boldsymbol{u}^\top X] = \mathbf{0}_p$ (and that all relevant random variables are integrable).[12]

1. Show first that

$$\mathbb{E}\big[X^\top(\boldsymbol{y} - X\boldsymbol{\beta})\big] = \mathbf{0}_p\,.$$

Hint: Background on conditional expectations can be found in Durrett (2010, Chapter 5.1 on pp. 221ff). Two results might be particularly useful: Theorem 5.1.7 on p. 228 and Display (5.1.5); the latter is called the *law of iterated expectations* and the *tower rule*—among many other names.

2. Claim 1 motivates the requirement that an estimator $\widehat{\boldsymbol{\beta}}$ of $\boldsymbol{\beta}$ should satisfy an "empirical version" of that equality:

$$X^\top(\boldsymbol{y} - X\widehat{\boldsymbol{\beta}}) = \mathbf{0}_p\,.$$

In other words, Claim 1 motivates the Z-estimator

$$\widehat{\boldsymbol{\beta}} \in \mathbb{R}^p \quad \text{is such that} \quad \tilde{\mathfrak{z}}_Z[\widehat{\boldsymbol{\beta}}] = \mathbf{0}_p$$

with

$$\tilde{\mathfrak{z}}_Z \,:\, \boldsymbol{\alpha} \mapsto X^\top(\boldsymbol{y} - X\boldsymbol{\alpha})\,.$$

Show that this is again the least-squares estimator.

This exercise illustrates the fact that Z-estimators can have several equivalent yet slightly different formulations that reflect different motivations of the estimator.

Exercise 5.2 ♦ In this exercise, we discuss the convergence of the generalized Newton–Raphson algorithm for the least-squares estimator. We have shown in Example 5.1.2 that the regular Newton–Raphson algorithm converges to a least-squares solution irrespective of the starting point. Does the same hold for the *generalized* Newton–Raphson algorithm as well?

1. Give an $M_{\mathfrak{z}_Z} \in \mathbb{R}^{p\times d}$ such that the generalized Newton–Raphson algorithm converges for all starting points but not necessarily to a least-squares solution.
2. Give an $M_{\mathfrak{z}_Z} \in \mathbb{R}^p$ such that the generalized Newton–Raphson algorithm fails to converge for "almost" all

starting points. You may assume $X^\top X = \mathrm{I}_{p\times p}$ for simplicity.

These results illustrate the fact that the generalized Newton–Raphson algorithm requires carefully chosen approximate inverses.

5.3.2 Exercises for ▶ Sect. 5.2

Exercise 5.3 ♦ In this exercise, we show that the update step in ▶ Sect. 5.2 can indeed be interpreted as debiasing. We consider estimators of the form

$$\widehat{\boldsymbol{\beta}} \in \underset{\boldsymbol{\alpha}\in\mathbb{R}^p}{\arg\min}\left\{\|\boldsymbol{y}-X\boldsymbol{\alpha}\|_2^2+r\hbar[\boldsymbol{\alpha}]\right\},$$

where $r \in [0,\infty)$ is a tuning parameter and $\hbar : \mathbb{R}^p \to \mathbb{R}$ a convex prior function. The KKT conditions for $\widehat{\boldsymbol{\beta}}$ are according to ▶ Sect. 2.5

$$-2X^\top(\boldsymbol{y}-X\widehat{\boldsymbol{\beta}})+r\widehat{\boldsymbol{\kappa}} = \mathbf{0}_p,$$

where $\widehat{\boldsymbol{\kappa}} \in \partial\hbar[\widehat{\boldsymbol{\beta}}]$.

1. Use the KKT conditions to show that

$$\widehat{\boldsymbol{\beta}}+rM_{\mathfrak{z}Z}\widehat{\boldsymbol{\kappa}} = 2M_{\mathfrak{z}Z}X^\top\boldsymbol{y}+\left(\mathrm{I}_{p\times p}-2M_{\mathfrak{z}Z}X^\top X\right)\widehat{\boldsymbol{\beta}}.$$

   This means that the update step $\widehat{\boldsymbol{\beta}}^0 \mapsto \widehat{\boldsymbol{\beta}}^1 = 2M_{\mathfrak{z}Z}X^\top\boldsymbol{y}+(\mathrm{I}_{p\times p}-2M_{\mathfrak{z}Z}X^\top X)\widehat{\boldsymbol{\beta}}^0$ of ▶ Sect. 5.2 applied to the estimator $\widehat{\boldsymbol{\beta}}^0 := \widehat{\boldsymbol{\beta}}$ can be written as $\widehat{\boldsymbol{\beta}} \mapsto \widehat{\boldsymbol{\beta}}+rM_{\mathfrak{z}Z}\widehat{\boldsymbol{\kappa}}$.
2. Use 1. to show that if $M_{\mathfrak{z}Z}X^\top\boldsymbol{u}$ is symmetric and the integrated remainder term $\mathbb{E}[(2M_{\mathfrak{z}Z}X^\top X-\mathrm{I}_{p\times p})(\boldsymbol{\beta}-\widehat{\boldsymbol{\beta}})]$ is negligible, it holds that

$$\mathbb{E}[\widehat{\boldsymbol{\beta}}-\boldsymbol{\beta}] \approx -\mathbb{E}[rM_{\mathfrak{z}Z}\widehat{\boldsymbol{\kappa}}].$$

   This means that $-\mathbb{E}[rM_{\mathfrak{z}Z}\widehat{\boldsymbol{\kappa}}]$ is approximately the bias of the estimator $\widehat{\boldsymbol{\beta}}$, and therefore, adding $rM_{\mathfrak{z}Z}\widehat{\boldsymbol{\kappa}}$ to $\widehat{\boldsymbol{\beta}}$ can be interpreted as a measure for reducing the bias (see also ◘ Fig. 2.3).
3. Discuss the results of 1. and 2. for the special case of the least-squares estimator: $\widehat{\boldsymbol{\beta}} = \widehat{\boldsymbol{\beta}}_{\mathrm{ls}}$.

Exercise 5.4 ♦♦ In this exercise, we show that $\|\boldsymbol{u}\|_2/\sqrt{n}$ is sharply concentrated around σ for $\boldsymbol{u} \sim \mathcal{N}_n[\mathbf{0}_n, \sigma^2 \mathrm{I}_{n\times n}]$. We will use the Properties (i) $\mathbb{E}[z^2] = 1$ and (ii) $\mathbb{E}[z^4] = 3$ for $z \sim \mathcal{N}[0, 1]$.

1. Use Property (i) to show that

$$\mathbb{E}\|\boldsymbol{u}\|_2^2 = n\sigma^2 .$$

If $\sigma = 1$, we call the distribution of $\|\boldsymbol{u}\|_2^2$ a *Chi-squared distribution* with n degrees of freedom. Hence, the equality implies that the mean of a Chi-squared distribution equals its degrees of freedom.

2. Use 1. and both Properties (i) and (ii) to show that

$$\mathbb{E}\Big[\big(\|\boldsymbol{u}\|_2^2 - n\sigma^2\big)^2\Big] = 2n\sigma^4 .$$

This equality implies that the variance of a Chi-squared distribution is equal to two times its degrees of freedom.

3. Use 2. and the Markov inequality to show that for every $t \in (0, 1)$, it holds that

$$\mathbb{P}\left\{\frac{\|\boldsymbol{u}\|_2}{\sqrt{n}} \notin [\sqrt{1-t}\,\sigma, \sqrt{1+t}\,\sigma]\right\} \le \frac{2}{nt^2} .$$

Hint: The Markov inequality (or rather one version of it) states that $\mathbb{P}\{x \ge a\} \le \mathbb{E}[x]/a$ for every non-negative random variable x and every constant $a \in (0, \infty)$. (This inequality is sometimes also called the *Chebyshev inequality* instead.)[13]

4. Conclude from 3. that for every fixed $b \in (0, \infty)$, it holds that

$$\lim_{n\to\infty} \mathbb{P}\left\{\left|\frac{\|\boldsymbol{u}\|_2}{\sqrt{n}} - \sigma\right| \ge b\right\} = 0 ,$$

which means that $\|\boldsymbol{u}\|_2/\sqrt{n}$ converges in probability to σ.

We can thus corroborate the statements in Example 5.2.1 and 5.2.2 that $\|\boldsymbol{y} - X\widehat{\boldsymbol{\beta}}_{\mathrm{ls}}\|_2$ and $\|\boldsymbol{y} - X\widehat{\boldsymbol{\beta}}_{\mathrm{lasso}}\|_2$ can be reasonable estimators of σ.

5.4 R Lab: Confidence Intervals in Low and High Dimensions

In this lab, we establish confidence intervals for coordinates of regression vectors.

Your task is, as always, to replace the keyword `REPLACE` with suitable code and to answer the questions in the text.

5.4.1 Generating Synthetic Data

We first create a generator for synthetic data. Write a function `DataGeneration()` that generates data according to a linear regression model. The entries of the design matrix should be i.i.d. standard Gauss-distributed and then transformed such that the matrix columns are centered and have Euclidean norm equal to $\sqrt{n}$. The entries of the noise should be i.i.d. Gauss-distributed (independent from the design) with mean zero and some `sigma`. The first three entries of the regression vector should be 1, while all other entries should be 0. The outcome vector should also be centered (to avoid dealing with intercepts) but not scaled. Hint: the `scale()` function might be convenient but make sure to adapt its standard scaling according to our description.

```
set.seed(1)
DataGeneration <- function(n, p, sigma)
{
  REPLACE
  return(list("y"=y, "X"=X))
}
data.low <- DataGeneration(n=333, p=9, sigma=1)
cbind(data.low$y[1:5], data.low$X[1:5, 1:4])
```

```
##            [,1]       [,2]        [,3]       [,4]       [,5]
## [1,]  0.9276815 -0.6967259  1.34247973 -1.2322317 -0.6888858
## [2,] -1.7374456  0.1462850 -0.25697206  0.6539392  1.0959945
## [3,] -1.2805843 -0.9143994  0.74770736  0.0799100  1.0735572
## [4,]  5.2386521  1.6152764  0.94904747  2.0512395 -0.8578577
## [5,] -0.4331412  0.2980758  0.06191724 -1.0637167  0.1956718
```

5.4.2 Defining Initial Estimators

We consider two initial estimators: a least-squares and a lasso. Write two functions accordingly. For the lasso, use the `cv.glmnet()` function from the `glmnet` package;

set the intercept flag to `FALSE` (and discard the entry for the intercept from the output), and keep the standard settings otherwise. Hint: the `coef()` function provides easy access to the estimated model parameters in the `cv.glmnet` object.

```
library(glmnet)
LeastSquares <- function(y, X)
{
  return(REPLACE)
}
Lasso <- function(y, X)
{
  return(REPLACE)
}
cbind(LeastSquares(data.low$y, data.low$X), Lasso(data.low$y, data.low$X))[1:5, ]
```



```
##             [,1]      [,2]
## [1,]  1.05028611 0.8909012
## [2,]  0.99201291 0.8283301
## [3,]  1.05737576 0.8972300
## [4,] -0.01262238 0.0000000
## [5,]  0.01558863 0.0000000
```

5.4.3 Constructing Approximate Inverses

We establish a very naive optimization approach to construct approximate inverses according to Display (5.6) in the main text. Describe the two below functions in detail. Do you have any ideas for improvement? (Running the code below can take a bit of time.)

```
library("MASS")  # for the ginv function
ValidateInverse <- function(initial.matrix, test.matrix, tuning.parameter=0, coordinate=0)
{
  maximal.deviation <- 0
  for (index.row in 1:dim(test.matrix)[1])
  {
    unit.vector <- rep(0, dim(initial.matrix)[1]);
    if (coordinate == 0)
      unit.vector[index.row] <- 1
    else
      unit.vector[coordinate] <- 1
    maximal.deviation <- max(maximal.deviation,
                             max(abs(initial.matrix %*% t(test.matrix)[, index.row]
                                     - unit.vector))
                             + tuning.parameter * sum(abs(test.matrix[index.row, ])))
  }
  return(maximal.deviation)
}
ApproximateInverse <- function(matrix.initial, tuning.parameter=0.02, nbr.iter=1000,
                               step.size=0.01)
{
  matrix.inv <- ginv(matrix.initial)
  for (index.row in 1:dim(matrix.initial)[1])
  {
    for (index.rep in 1:nbr.iter)
    {
      proposal.direction <- rnorm(dim(matrix.initial)[1])
      proposal.direction <- proposal.direction / sum((proposal.direction)^2)
      mult.factor <- step.size
      repeat
      {
        proposal.vector <- matrix.inv[index.row, ] + mult.factor * proposal.direction
```

```
        # the rbind is to ensure a row vector
        min.proposal <- ValidateInverse(matrix.initial, rbind(proposal.vector),
                                  tuning.parameter, coordinate=index.row)
        min.current <- ValidateInverse(matrix.initial, rbind(matrix.inv[index.row, ]),
                                 tuning.parameter, coordinate=index.row)
        if (min.proposal >= min.current) break
        matrix.inv[index.row, ] <- proposal.vector
        mult.factor <- mult.factor + step.size
      }
    }
  }
  return(matrix.inv)
}
```

5.4.4 Testing the Inversion Algorithm

We test our inversion scheme in low dimensions and in moderately high dimensions. Run the below code.

```
set.seed(2)
gram.low <- t(data.low$X) %*% data.low$X
gram.low.inv <- ApproximateInverse(gram.low)
ValidateInverse(gram.low, gram.low.inv)
```

```
## [1] 5.846018e-16
```

Interpret this result.

```
set.seed(3)
data.high <- DataGeneration(n=180, p=200, sigma=1)
gram.high <- t(data.high$X) %*% data.high$X
gram.high.inv <- ApproximateInverse(gram.high)
ValidateInverse(gram.high, gram.high.inv) / sqrt(log(dim(data.high$X)[2]) /
                                          dim(data.high$X)[1])
```

```
## [1] 0.722643
```

Interpret also this result. Argue in particular that the approximate inverse satisfies the conditions of all minimization problems (5.6) for the tuning parameter $a = 1$. What does this mean for the remainder in Theorem 5.2.1?

Our naive optimization approach serves us well in this lab but does not necessarily provide a good inverse in a reasonable amount of time in practice; therefore, in practice, it is recommended to implement more scalable alternatives to our optimization such as the one referred to in the following bonus question. In any case, one should always check the quality of the approximate inverse with the `ValidateInverse()` function in practice.

5.4.5 Bonus: A Scalable Optimization Algorithm

Implement a refined inversion scheme along the lines of https://github.com/LedererLab/HDIV.

5.4.6 Debiasing

We now implement a debiasing routine. Define a function `Debiasing()` that takes the data, the initial estimator, and the approximate inverse and returns the one-step estimator in Display (5.4) of the main text. Test the debiasing as indicated. Hint: recall that $2M$ (rather than M) is the approximate inverse of $X^\top X$.

```
set.seed(4)
Debias <- function(y, X, initial.estimator, gram.inv)
{
  return(REPLACE)
}
least.squares <- LeastSquares(data.low$y, data.low$X)
least.squares.deb <- Debias(data.low$y, data.low$X, least.squares, gram.low.inv)
cbind(least.squares, least.squares.deb)[1:5, ]
```

```
##            [,1]        [,2]
## [1,]  1.05028611  1.05028611
## [2,]  0.99201291  0.99201291
## [3,]  1.05737576  1.05737576
## [4,] -0.01262238 -0.01262238
## [5,]  0.01558863  0.01558863
```

```
lasso.low <- Lasso(data.low$y, data.low$X)
lasso.deb.low <- Debias(data.low$y, data.low$X, lasso.low, gram.low.inv)
cbind(lasso.low, lasso.deb.low)[1:5, ]
```

```
##           [,1]        [,2]
## [1,] 0.8909012  1.05028611
## [2,] 0.8283301  0.99201291
## [3,] 0.8972300  1.05737576
## [4,] 0.0000000 -0.01262238
## [5,] 0.0000000  0.01558863
```

```
lasso.high <- Lasso(data.high$y, data.high$X)
lasso.deb.high <- Debias(data.high$y, data.high$X, lasso.high, gram.high.inv)
cbind(lasso.high, lasso.deb.high)[1:5, ]
```

```
##              [,1]       [,2]
## [1,] 0.7790845  0.6886401
## [2,] 0.7859893  0.9681673
## [3,] 0.6282234  1.0068510
## [4,] 0.0000000 -0.1089748
## [5,] 0.0000000  0.4463807
```

Are the results as expected? Explain.

5.4.7 Constructing Confidence Intervals

We now construct confidence intervals. Write a function `ConfidenceIntervals` that corresponds to our results in ▶ Sect. 5.2. Hint: the function `qnorm()` might be helpful.

```
set.seed(5)
ConfidenceInterval <- function(y, X, gram.inv, coordinate, level, FUN=LeastSquares)
{
  REPLACE
}
ConfidenceInterval(data.low$y, data.low$X, gram.low.inv, coordinate=1, level=0.95,
                   FUN=LeastSquares)
```

```
## $left
## [1] 0.9327692
##
## $right
## [1] 1.167803
```

```
ConfidenceInterval(data.low$y, data.low$X, gram.low.inv, coordinate=1, level=0.95,
                   FUN=Lasso)
```

```
## $left
## [1] 0.9291717
##
## $right
## [1] 1.171401
```

```
ConfidenceInterval(data.high$y, data.high$X, gram.high.inv, coordinate=1, level=0.95,
                   FUN=Lasso)
```

```
## $left
## [1] 0.2893542
##
## $right
## [1] 1.08438
```

5.4.8 Validating the Pipeline

We now check the validity of the confidence intervals by comparing nominal levels with their empirical counterparts. Write a function `EmpiricalLevels()` that returns the empirical levels for the confidence intervals of the regression vector's first coordinate. The empirical levels are the fraction of draws leading to confidence intervals that contain the first coordinate of the regression vector. Each draw consists of the generation of fresh data and the computation of confidence intervals on these data. Set `nbr.iter=10` when calling `ApproximateInverse()` to speed up the computations (the computations can take a while nonetheless).

```
set.seed(6)
EmpiricalLevels <- function(n, p, sigma, FUN, nominal.levels, nbr.draws)
{
  REPLACE
}
PlotLevels <- function (n, p, sigma, FUN, nbr.draws=50)
{
  nominal.levels <- seq(from=0.05, to=0.95, by=0.05)
  plot(x     = nominal.levels,
       y     = EmpiricalLevels(n, p, sigma, FUN, nominal.levels, nbr.draws),
       xlim = c(0, 1),
       ylim = c(0, 1),
       xaxp = c(0, 1, 2),
       yaxp = c(0, 1, 2),
       las  = 1,
       xlab = "Nominal level",
       ylab = "Empirical level")
}
PlotLevels(n=333, p=9, sigma=1, FUN=LeastSquares)
```

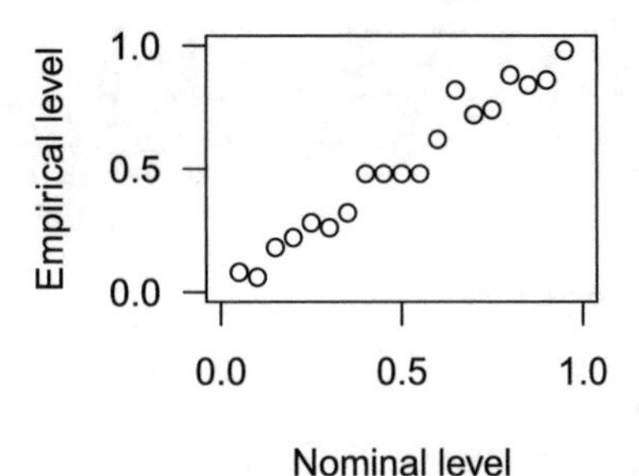


```
PlotLevels(n=333, p=9, sigma=1, FUN=Lasso)
```

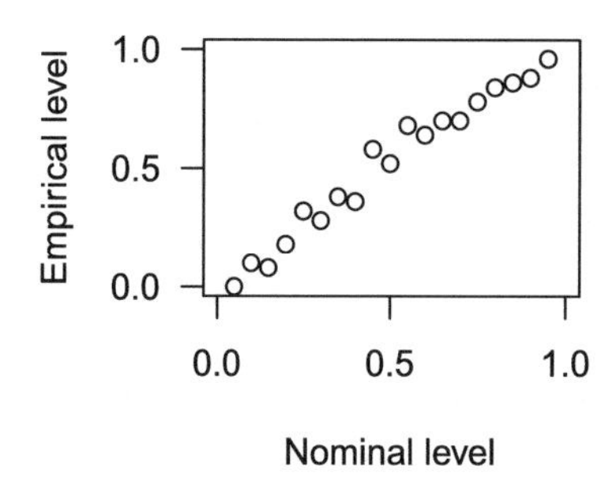


```
PlotLevels(n=180, p=200, sigma=1, FUN=Lasso)
```

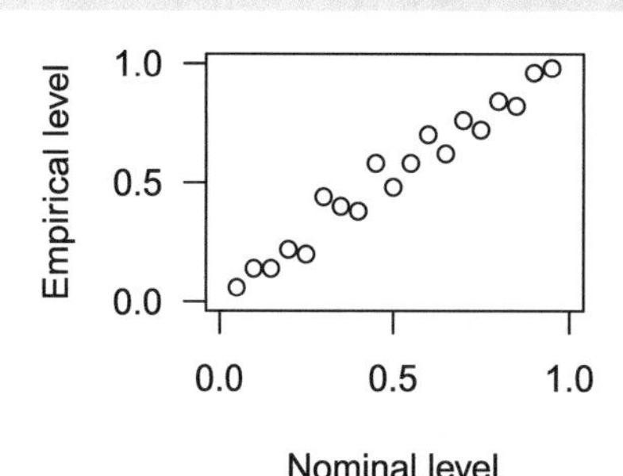

What do these results indicate?

5.4.9 Real Data Analysis

We finally analyze real data. We chose data with many more samples than observations, which allows us to test our pipeline against the standard `lm()` function.

5.4.9.1 Data Loading

We consider the `Fertility` data set from the `Stat2Data` package. Load the data and take the column `Embryos` as the preliminary outcome vector and the remaining data as the preliminary design matrix. Normalize the data such that the final outcome vector $\boldsymbol{y}$ and all columns of the final design matrix X are centered and that the columns of X have Euclidean norm equal to $\sqrt{n}$. Hint: to ease later manipulations, transform the data into matrix format by applying the `as.matrix()` function.

```
library(Stat2Data)
data("Fertility")
y <- REPLACE
X <- REPLACE
cbind(y, X)[1:5, ]
```

```
##      Embryos        Age   LowAFC  MeanAFC        FSH          E2      MaxE2
## 1  6.2732733  0.9948009 4.010100 5.119848 -0.3274049  0.24693263 -0.1527636
## 2 -0.7267267  0.3552860 4.154807 3.704057  0.6004745  0.77319545 -0.9544059
## 3  8.2732733  0.9948009 3.720684 3.704057 -0.5336003 -0.08198163  3.8310776
## 4 -2.7267267  0.9948009 3.431269 3.232127 -1.0490889 -1.00294157  0.3307870
## 5  5.2732733 -1.1369153 3.431269 3.029871 -0.9975400  0.51006404  1.2568441
##    MaxDailyGn    TotalGn    Oocytes
## 1 -0.09320925 -0.0954916  2.2295757
## 2 -0.74201110 -0.7525575 -0.8194950
## 3  1.20439445  1.4741658  2.5683614
## 4 -0.09320925 -0.0954916 -0.4807093
## 5 -1.39081295 -0.9715795  1.2132188
```

The number of samples is $n = 333$ and the number of model parameters is $p = 9$.

5.4.9.2 Estimating Confidence Intervals

We now estimate confidence intervals for all nine model parameters in the above data set. Write a function `ConfidenceIntervalsAll()` accordingly and compute all (individual) 99% confidence intervals. Hint: Keep the standard settings for `ApproximateInverse()`.

```
set.seed(7)
ConfidenceIntervalsAll <- function(y, X, level, FUN)
{
  REPLACE
}
confidence.intervals <- ConfidenceIntervalsAll(y, X, 0.99, LeastSquares)
confidence.intervals
```

```
##          left       right
##    [1,] -0.7129082 0.1922226
##    [2,] -0.3003823 2.222127
##    [3,] -2.000322  0.5117284
##    [4,] -0.3931534 0.4753687
##    [5,] -0.3518565 0.40498
##    [6,] -0.1485149 0.7253007
##    [7,] -0.6854799 1.178465
##    [8,] -0.8809723 0.9158202
##    [9,] 2.480274   3.413196
```

What would you need to change in the above code if p were larger than n?

5.4.9.3 Plotting the Intervals

We plot the intervals. Write a corresponding plotting function `PlotInvervals()`.

```
PlotIntervals <- function(confidence.intervals, estimator)
{
  REPLACE
}
least.squares <- LeastSquares(y, X)
least.squares
```

```
##                  Embryos
## Age          -0.26034283
## LowAFC        0.96087230
## MeanAFC      -0.74429689
## FSH           0.04110764
## E2            0.02656174
## MaxE2         0.28839293
## MaxDailyGn    0.24649258
## TotalGn       0.01742394
## Oocytes       2.94673502
```

```
PlotIntervals(confidence.intervals, least.squares)
```

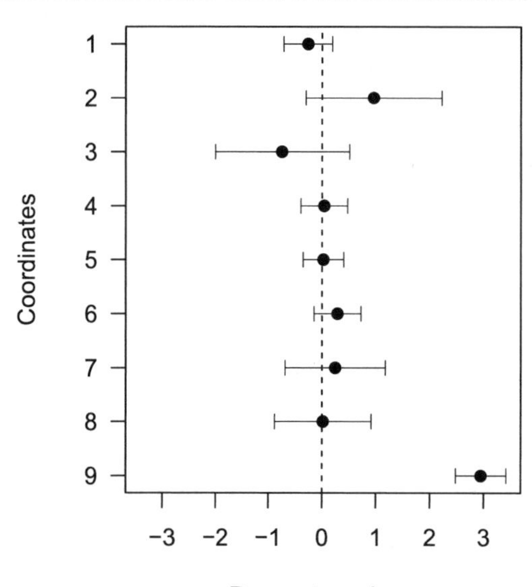

Which model parameters are significant at a 99% level? Explain.

5.4.9.4 Testing Against a Standard Function

We finally test against the `lm()` function.

```
summary(lm(y ~ X - 1))  # the - 1 avoids an intercept
```

```
##
## Call:
## lm(formula = y ~ X - 1)
##
## Residuals:
##     Min      1Q  Median      3Q     Max
## -9.5313 -1.1743  0.0822  1.4170 10.1756
##
## Coefficients:
##              Estimate Std. Error t value Pr(>|t|)
## XAge         -0.26034    0.17812  -1.462   0.1448
## XLowAFC       0.96087    0.49640   1.936   0.0538 .
## XMeanAFC     -0.74430    0.49435  -1.506   0.1331
## XFSH          0.04111    0.17092   0.241   0.8101
## XE2           0.02656    0.14894   0.178   0.8586
## XMaxE2        0.28839    0.17196   1.677   0.0945 .
## XMaxDailyGn   0.24649    0.36681   0.672   0.5021
## XTotalGn      0.01742    0.35359   0.049   0.9607
## XOocytes      2.94674    0.18359  16.051   <2e-16 ***
## ---
## Signif. codes:  0 '***' 0.001 '**' 0.01 '*' 0.05 '.' 0.1 ' ' 1
##
## Residual standard error: 2.656 on 324 degrees of freedom
## Multiple R-squared:  0.5865, Adjusted R-squared:  0.5751
## F-statistic: 51.07 on 9 and 324 DF,  p-value: < 2.2e-16
```

Are these results commensurate with the outputs of our pipeline? Is this expected?

5.5 Notes and References

1. Background on Z-estimators can be found in van der Vaart (2000, Chapter 5 on pp. 41ff).
2. The letter Z in Z-estimators refers to the *zeros* on the right-hand side of the equations.
3. Refer to Bickel et al. (1993, Sections 2.5 and 7.3) and van der Vaart (2000, Chapter 5.7 on pp. 71ff).
4. See, for example, Knight and Fu (2000).
5. The point of view adopted here was introduced in Gold et al. (2020, Section 2).
6. There might not even exist an estimator that is suitable for both prediction/estimation and inference; essentially, the debiasing disentangles these two tasks.
7. Yet another name for this specific updating step is *desparsifying* (van de Geer et al., 2014, Section 2.1 on p. 1169). This name speaks to the fact that updated estimators are typically non-sparse, that is, most or even all of their components are different from zero (as it is the case for the least-squares estimator) even if the initial estimators are sparse, that is, many of their components are equal to zero (as it is the case for the lasso). One can observe this in Part 5.6 of our lab.

8 One could also consider, for example, X random and $\boldsymbol{u} \mid X \sim \mathcal{N}_n[\mathbf{0}_n, \sigma^2 \mathrm{I}_{n\times n}]$. Then, the results would hold conditionally on X.
9 This is Program 3.2 in Gold et al. (2020), which is a modification of the CLIME estimator (Cai et al., 2011, Equation (1) on p. 595). Other programs for finding approximate inverses are formulated by Javanmard and Montanari (2014); van de Geer et al. (2014).
10 See Gold et al. (2020, Lemma 4.9).
11 See Gold et al. (2020, Section 5).
12 If $\mathbb{E}[\boldsymbol{u} \mid X] = \mathbf{0}_p$ (which implies $\mathbb{E}[\boldsymbol{u}^\top X] = \mathbf{0}_p$ in view of the law of iterated expectations), we call the predictors *exogenous*. Exogeneity and its counterpart *endogeneity* are important concepts in econometric models such as instrumental variable regression (Stock and Trebbi, 2003).
13 See Durrett (2010, pp. 28–29), for example.

Theory I: Prediction

Contents

J. Lederer, *Fundamentals of High-Dimensional Statistics*, Springer Texts in Statistics, https://doi.org/10.1007/978-3-030-73792-4_6

In the remainder of this book, we establish mathematical guarantees for high-dimensional estimators. The concepts underpinning our derivations are the basis for high-dimensional theories in general, but for the sake of clarity we focus here on linear regression with regularized least-squares estimators. Specifically, we consider the model $\boldsymbol{y} = X\boldsymbol{\beta} + \boldsymbol{u}$ of (2.1) and the corresponding estimators of the form

$$\widehat{\boldsymbol{\beta}} \in \underset{\boldsymbol{\alpha}\in\mathbb{R}^p}{\arg\min}\left\{\mathscr{g}\left[\|\boldsymbol{y} - X\boldsymbol{\alpha}\|_2^2\right] + r\mathscr{h}[\boldsymbol{\alpha}]\right\} \tag{6.1}$$

for a *link function* $\mathscr{g} : [0, \infty) \to [0, \infty]$, a tuning parameter $r \in [0, \infty)$, and a prior function $\mathscr{h} : \mathbb{R}^p \to [0, \infty]$. Typical link functions are the identity function $\mathscr{g} : a \mapsto a$ (which applies to the lasso (2.2) and the group lasso (2.3), for example) and the square-root function $\mathscr{g} : a \mapsto \sqrt{a}$ (which applies to the square-root lasso (6.2) below and the square-root group lasso (2.9), for example).

We derive two types of guarantees: In this chapter, we state conditions under which estimators $\widehat{\boldsymbol{\beta}}$ can disentangle the signal $X\boldsymbol{\beta}$ from the noise $\boldsymbol{u}$. We formulate this type of guarantees in terms of the *prediction error*[1] $\|X\boldsymbol{\beta} - X\widehat{\boldsymbol{\beta}}\|_2^2$. In the next chapter, we state conditions under which estimators can recover the regression vector $\boldsymbol{\beta}$ itself. We formulate that type of guarantees for estimation and support recovery errors, such as, for example, $\|\boldsymbol{\beta} - \widehat{\boldsymbol{\beta}}\|_\infty$.

prediction error

6.1 Overview

Prediction guarantees are derived in two steps: In the first step, the prediction error is separated from the other terms in the estimator's objective function or its KKT conditions. This separation produces unwieldy inner product terms, which are controlled in the second step. The key assumption in that second step is that the regularization is sufficiently strong: in a sense, the influence of the prior term must outbalance the randomness of the problem.

For an illustration, we consider the lasso estimator

$$\widehat{\boldsymbol{\beta}}_{\text{lasso}} \in \underset{\boldsymbol{\alpha}\in\mathbb{R}^p}{\arg\min}\left\{\|\boldsymbol{y} - X\boldsymbol{\alpha}\|_2^2 + r\|\boldsymbol{\alpha}\|_1\right\}.$$

Since $\widehat{\boldsymbol{\beta}}_{\text{lasso}}$ minimizes the objective function $\boldsymbol{a} \mapsto \|\boldsymbol{y} - X\boldsymbol{a}\|_2^2 + r\|\boldsymbol{a}\|_1$, we obtain for every $\boldsymbol{\alpha} \in \mathbb{R}^p$ the inequality

$$\|\boldsymbol{y} - X\widehat{\boldsymbol{\beta}}_{\text{lasso}}\|_2^2 + r\|\widehat{\boldsymbol{\beta}}_{\text{lasso}}\|_1 \leq \|\boldsymbol{y} - X\boldsymbol{\alpha}\|_2^2 + r\|\boldsymbol{\alpha}\|_1 .$$

Adding a zero-valued term in the ℓ_2-norms on both sides then gives us

$$\|\boldsymbol{y} - X\boldsymbol{\beta} + X\boldsymbol{\beta} - X\widehat{\boldsymbol{\beta}}_{\text{lasso}}\|_2^2 + r\|\widehat{\boldsymbol{\beta}}_{\text{lasso}}\|_1 \leq \|\boldsymbol{y} - X\boldsymbol{\beta} + X\boldsymbol{\beta} - X\boldsymbol{\alpha}\|_2^2 + r\|\boldsymbol{\alpha}\|_1 ,$$

and expanding ($\|\boldsymbol{a}+\boldsymbol{b}\|_2^2 = \|\boldsymbol{a}\|_2^2 + 2\langle\boldsymbol{a}, \boldsymbol{b}\rangle + \|\boldsymbol{b}\|_2^2$ for all $\boldsymbol{a}, \boldsymbol{b} \in \mathbb{R}^p$—see Lemma B.1.2)

$$\|\boldsymbol{y} - X\boldsymbol{\beta}\|_2^2 + 2\langle\boldsymbol{y} - X\boldsymbol{\beta}, X\boldsymbol{\beta} - X\widehat{\boldsymbol{\beta}}_{\text{lasso}}\rangle + \|X\boldsymbol{\beta} - X\widehat{\boldsymbol{\beta}}_{\text{lasso}}\|_2^2 + r\|\widehat{\boldsymbol{\beta}}_{\text{lasso}}\|_1 \leq \|\boldsymbol{y} - X\boldsymbol{\beta}\|_2^2 + 2\langle\boldsymbol{y} - X\boldsymbol{\beta}, X\boldsymbol{\beta} - X\boldsymbol{\alpha}\rangle + \|X\boldsymbol{\beta} - X\boldsymbol{\alpha}\|_2^2 + r\|\boldsymbol{\alpha}\|_1 .$$

Invoking the linear regression model (2.1) and consolidating the display, we can then derive the *basic inequality*

basic inequality

$$\|X\boldsymbol{\beta} - X\widehat{\boldsymbol{\beta}}_{\text{lasso}}\|_2^2 \leq \|X\boldsymbol{\beta} - X\boldsymbol{\alpha}\|_2^2 + 2\langle\boldsymbol{u}, X\widehat{\boldsymbol{\beta}}_{\text{lasso}} - X\boldsymbol{\alpha}\rangle + r\|\boldsymbol{\alpha}\|_1 - r\|\widehat{\boldsymbol{\beta}}_{\text{lasso}}\|_1 .$$

The basic inequality separates the prediction error of the estimator from other parts of the problem.

We now proceed by controlling the inner product term on the right-hand side. There are two ways to do this. On the one hand, the properties of the inner product ($\langle\boldsymbol{u}, X\widehat{\boldsymbol{\beta}}_{\text{lasso}} - X\boldsymbol{\alpha}\rangle = \langle X^\top\boldsymbol{u}, \widehat{\boldsymbol{\beta}}_{\text{lasso}} - \boldsymbol{\alpha}\rangle = \langle X^\top\boldsymbol{u}, \widehat{\boldsymbol{\beta}}_{\text{lasso}}\rangle + \langle X^\top\boldsymbol{u}, -\boldsymbol{\alpha}\rangle$), the Hölder inequality ($\langle X^\top\boldsymbol{u}, \widehat{\boldsymbol{\beta}}_{\text{lasso}}\rangle \leq \|X^\top\boldsymbol{u}\|_\infty\|\widehat{\boldsymbol{\beta}}_{\text{lasso}}\|_1$ and $\langle X^\top\boldsymbol{u}, -\boldsymbol{\alpha}\rangle \leq \|X^\top\boldsymbol{u}\|_\infty\|-\boldsymbol{\alpha}\|_1$), and the symmetry of norms ($\|-\boldsymbol{\alpha}\|_1 = \|\boldsymbol{\alpha}\|_1$) lead to

$$\|X\boldsymbol{\beta} - X\widehat{\boldsymbol{\beta}}_{\text{lasso}}\|_2^2 \leq \|X\boldsymbol{\beta} - X\boldsymbol{\alpha}\|_2^2 + 2\|X^\top\boldsymbol{u}\|_\infty\big(\|\widehat{\boldsymbol{\beta}}_{\text{lasso}}\|_1 + \|\boldsymbol{\alpha}\|_1\big) + r\|\boldsymbol{\alpha}\|_1 - r\|\widehat{\boldsymbol{\beta}}_{\text{lasso}}\|_1 .$$

The crucial assumption is now that the regularization is sufficiently strong in the sense that $r \geq 2\|X^\top\boldsymbol{u}\|_\infty$. Using this assumption, we can control the inner product term further: $2\|X^\top \boldsymbol{u}\|_\infty(\|\widehat{\boldsymbol{\beta}}_{\text{lasso}}\|_1 + \|\boldsymbol{\alpha}\|_1) \le r\|\widehat{\boldsymbol{\beta}}_{\text{lasso}}\|_1 + r\|\boldsymbol{\alpha}\|_1$. This yields

$$\|X\boldsymbol{\beta} - X\widehat{\boldsymbol{\beta}}_{\text{lasso}}\|_2^2 \le \|X\boldsymbol{\beta} - X\boldsymbol{\alpha}\|_2^2 + 2r\|\boldsymbol{\alpha}\|_1 .$$

power-one prediction bound

Since $\boldsymbol{\alpha}$ was arbitrary, we eventually find the *power-one bound*

$$\|X\boldsymbol{\beta} - X\widehat{\boldsymbol{\beta}}_{\text{lasso}}\|_2^2 \le \min_{\boldsymbol{\alpha}\in\mathbb{R}^p} \left\{ \|X\boldsymbol{\beta} - X\boldsymbol{\alpha}\|_2^2 + 2r\|\boldsymbol{\alpha}\|_1 \right\} .$$

This means that up to the complexity term $2r\|\boldsymbol{\alpha}\|_1$, the lasso with sufficiently large tuning parameter minimizes the prediction error.

6

On the other hand, the properties of the inner product ($\langle \boldsymbol{u}, X\widehat{\boldsymbol{\beta}}_{\text{lasso}} - X\boldsymbol{\alpha}\rangle = \langle X^\top\boldsymbol{u}, \widehat{\boldsymbol{\beta}}_{\text{lasso}} - \boldsymbol{\alpha}\rangle$), the Hölder inequality ($\langle X^\top\boldsymbol{u}, \widehat{\boldsymbol{\beta}}_{\text{lasso}} - \boldsymbol{\alpha}\rangle \le \|X^\top\boldsymbol{u}\|_\infty\|\widehat{\boldsymbol{\beta}}_{\text{lasso}} - \boldsymbol{\alpha}\|_1$), and the triangle inequality ($\|\widehat{\boldsymbol{\beta}}_{\text{lasso}}\|_1 - \|\boldsymbol{\alpha}\|_1 \le \|\widehat{\boldsymbol{\beta}}_{\text{lasso}} - \boldsymbol{\alpha}\|_1$) also lead to

$$\begin{aligned}\|X\boldsymbol{\beta} - X\widehat{\boldsymbol{\beta}}_{\text{lasso}}\|_2^2 \le \|X\boldsymbol{\beta} - X\boldsymbol{\alpha}\|_2^2 + 2\|X^\top\boldsymbol{u}\|_\infty\|\boldsymbol{\alpha} - \widehat{\boldsymbol{\beta}}_{\text{lasso}}\|_1 \\ + r\|\boldsymbol{\alpha} - \widehat{\boldsymbol{\beta}}_{\text{lasso}}\|_1 .\end{aligned}$$

We assume again that the regularization is strong enough: $r \ge 2\|X^\top\boldsymbol{u}\|_\infty$. Using this assumption, the inequality yields in a similar way as before

$$\|X\boldsymbol{\beta} - X\widehat{\boldsymbol{\beta}}_{\text{lasso}}\|_2^2 \le \|X\boldsymbol{\beta} - X\boldsymbol{\alpha}\|_2^2 + 2r\|\boldsymbol{\alpha} - \widehat{\boldsymbol{\beta}}_{\text{lasso}}\|_1 .$$

This result ensures that if (i) $\boldsymbol{\alpha}$ is close to the regression vector in terms of the prediction error and (ii) $\boldsymbol{\alpha}$ is close to $\widehat{\boldsymbol{\beta}}_{\text{lasso}}$ in terms of the ℓ_1-error, the estimator is close to the regression vector $\boldsymbol{\beta}$ in terms of prediction.

However, the term $2r\|\boldsymbol{\alpha} - \widehat{\boldsymbol{\beta}}_{\text{lasso}}\|_1$ on the right-hand side of the above inequality still needs more treatment. For this, we relate prediction and ℓ_1-estimation further: we assume that the estimator $\widehat{\boldsymbol{\beta}}_{\text{lasso}}$ is close to the regression vector $\boldsymbol{\alpha}$ in terms of the ℓ_1-error whenever $\widehat{\boldsymbol{\beta}}_{\text{lasso}}$ is close to $\boldsymbol{\alpha}$ in terms of the prediction error, that is, $\boldsymbol{\alpha} \in \widehat{\mathscr{B}}_m$, where

$$\widehat{\mathscr{B}}_m := \left\{\boldsymbol{a} \in \mathbb{R}^p : \|\boldsymbol{a} - \widehat{\boldsymbol{\beta}}_{\text{lasso}}\|_1 \le m\|X\boldsymbol{a} - X\widehat{\boldsymbol{\beta}}_{\text{lasso}}\|_2/\sqrt{n}\right\}$$

structural condition

for a fixed $m \in [0, \infty]$. We say that such $\boldsymbol{\alpha}$ satisfy the *structural condition*. The previous display entails for those $\boldsymbol{\alpha}$

$$\|X\boldsymbol{\beta} - X\widehat{\boldsymbol{\beta}}_{\text{lasso}}\|_2^2 \le \|X\boldsymbol{\beta} - X\boldsymbol{\alpha}\|_2^2 + 2mr\|X\boldsymbol{\alpha} - X\widehat{\boldsymbol{\beta}}_{\text{lasso}}\|_2/\sqrt{n} .$$

Using the inequality $2ab \leq 4a^2 + b^2/4$ for all $a, b \in \mathbb{R}$ (second part of Lemma B.1.3 on Page 311 with $p = 1$, $u = 2$, and $v = 1/4$), we further find

$$\|X\boldsymbol{\beta} - X\widehat{\boldsymbol{\beta}}_{\text{lasso}}\|_2^2 \leq \|X\boldsymbol{\beta} - X\boldsymbol{\alpha}\|_2^2 + 4m^2r^2/n + \|X\boldsymbol{\alpha} - X\widehat{\boldsymbol{\beta}}_{\text{lasso}}\|_2^2/4\,,$$

which becomes with $\|\boldsymbol{a} + \boldsymbol{b}\|_2^2 \leq 2\|\boldsymbol{a}\|_2^2 + 2\|\boldsymbol{b}\|_2^2$ for all $\boldsymbol{a}, \boldsymbol{b} \in \mathbb{R}^p$ (second part of Lemma B.1.1)

$$\|X\boldsymbol{\beta} - X\widehat{\boldsymbol{\beta}}_{\text{lasso}}\|_2^2 \leq \|X\boldsymbol{\beta} - X\boldsymbol{\alpha}\|_2^2 + 4m^2r^2/n + \|X\boldsymbol{\beta} - X\boldsymbol{\alpha}\|_2^2/2 + \|X\boldsymbol{\beta} - X\widehat{\boldsymbol{\beta}}_{\text{lasso}}\|_2^2/2\,.$$

In summary, we find the *power-two prediction bound*

power-two bound

$$\|X\boldsymbol{\beta} - X\widehat{\boldsymbol{\beta}}_{\text{lasso}}\|_2^2 \leq \min_{\boldsymbol{\alpha} \in \widehat{\mathcal{B}}_m} \left\{ 3\|X\boldsymbol{\beta} - X\boldsymbol{\alpha}\|_2^2 + \frac{8m^2r^2}{n} \right\}.$$

This means that up to the complexity term $8m^2r^2/n$ and a factor 3, the lasso with a sufficiently large tuning parameter minimizes the prediction error over $\widehat{\mathcal{B}}_m$.

The power-two bound differs from the power-one bound above in three main aspects: the constant in front of $\|X\boldsymbol{\beta} - X\boldsymbol{\alpha}\|_2^2$ is 3 rather than 1, that is, the bound is not *sharp*; the complexity term involves m rather than $\|\boldsymbol{\alpha}\|_1$, and it is quadratic in the tuning parameter r rather than linear (in other words, it contains the tuning parameter raised to the power of two rather than to the power of one—hence the naming);[2] and the set over which the minimum is taken is $\widehat{\mathcal{B}}_m$ rather than the entire $\mathbb{R}^p$. The two types of bounds cannot be ranked globally: grosso modo, power-two bounds dominate if the regression vector can be approximated well by a sparse vector and the predictors are only weakly correlated, while power-one bounds dominate otherwise—see ▶ Sect. 6.4.

In both bounds, the dependence on the random noise is governed by the term $2\|X^\top \boldsymbol{u}\|_\infty$. We have called this term earlier the effective noise of the lasso estimator. The larger the effective noise, the larger the tuning parameters have to be, and therefore the larger the right-hand sides of the bounds. Thus, the lasso's effective noise plays the same role in the above bounds as the least-squares' effective noise in the risk bound on Page 9. We can compare, say, the power-one bound to that risk bound by invoking the two assumptions of that section: $\boldsymbol{u} \sim \mathcal{N}_n[\mathbf{0}_n, \sigma^2 \mathrm{I}_{n\times n}]$ and $(X^\top X)_{jj} = n$ for all $j \in \{1, \ldots, p\}$. We then find that if $r = 2\|X^\top \boldsymbol{u}\|_\infty$ and $t \in (0, 1]$,[3]

$$
\begin{aligned}
&\mathbb{P}\left\{\frac{\|X\boldsymbol{\beta} - X\widehat{\boldsymbol{\beta}}_{\text{lasso}}\|_2^2}{n} \le \sigma\sqrt{\frac{32\log[p/t]}{n}}\|\boldsymbol{\beta}\|_1\right\}\\
&\ge \mathbb{P}\left\{\frac{\min_{\boldsymbol{\alpha}\in\mathbb{R}^p}\left\{\|X\boldsymbol{\beta} - X\boldsymbol{\alpha}\|_2^2 + 4\|X^\top \boldsymbol{u}\|_\infty\|\boldsymbol{\alpha}\|_1\right\}}{n}\right.\\
&\qquad\left.\le \sigma\sqrt{\frac{32\log[p/t]}{n}}\|\boldsymbol{\beta}\|_1\right\} && \text{power-one bound}\\
&\ge \mathbb{P}\left\{\frac{4\|X^\top \boldsymbol{u}\|_\infty\|\boldsymbol{\beta}\|_1}{n} \le \sigma\sqrt{\frac{32\log[p/t]}{n}}\|\boldsymbol{\beta}\|_1\right\} && \text{bounding the minimum by setting } \boldsymbol{\alpha} = \boldsymbol{\beta}\\
&= \mathbb{P}\left\{2\|X^\top \boldsymbol{u}\|_\infty \le \sigma\sqrt{8mn\log[p/t]}\right\} && \text{consolidating; } m = \max_{j\in\{1,\ldots,p\}}(X^\top X)_{jj}/n = 1 \text{ by assumption}\\
&\ge 1 - t\,. && \text{Lemma 4.2.1}
\end{aligned}
$$

Neglecting constants, we can say that the lasso's average prediction error is bounded by $\sigma\sqrt{\log[p]/n}\|\boldsymbol{\beta}\|_1$ with high probability.

The bound's dependence on the dimensions n and p of the statistical model is captured by the factor $\sqrt{\log[p]/n}$. This factor decreases in the number of samples as $1/\sqrt{n}$ and increases in the number of model parameters p logarithmically; hence, if the prior assumption is satisfied, that is, the regression vector (or a good approximation of it) is not too large in terms of the ℓ_1-norm, and if σ is not too large, the lasso estimator predicts reliably whenever $n \gg \log[p]$—which even allows for models with $p \gg n$. In strong contrast, the risk bound for the least-squares estimator on Page 9 decreases in the number of samples as $1/n$ but increases in the number of model parameters p linearly; hence, the least-squares estimator predicts reliably only if $n \gg p$.

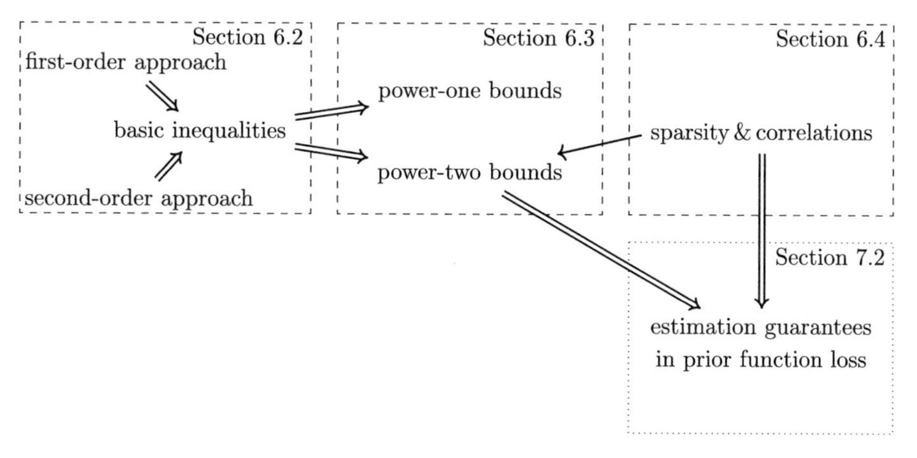

Fig. 6.1 Overview of this chapter. In ▶ Sect. 6.2, we introduce two approaches for deriving basic inequalities. In ▶ Sect. 6.3, we then use these basic inequalities to derive two types of probability bounds, which are the main results of this chapter. In ▶ Sect. 6.4, we provide further background on the assumptions needed for power-two bounds

The goal of this chapter is to generalize the above prediction bounds. The outline is depicted in Fig. 6.1: Mimicking the above derivations, we first establish basic inequalities (▶ Sect. 6.2) and then transform them into power-one and power-two prediction bounds (▶ Sect. 6.3). These bounds generalize the ones above from the lasso to a wide spectrum of regularized least-squares estimators. We then deepen our discussion of power-two bounds in the context of sparsity and correlations (▶ Sect. 6.4). This discussion will also be the basis for estimation bounds later in the book (▶ Sect. 7.2). Our proofs in this chapter and in the following one are purely algebraic, which means that we impose assumptions on the noise distribution only in the examples.

6.2 Basic Inequalities

Basic inequalities are our stepping stone for establishing prediction bounds because they express the prediction error through inner product and prior function terms that are readily amenable to further analysis. We introduce two approaches for deriving such inequalities for regularized least-squares estimators. Our first approach generalizes the strategy outlined in the previous section: it uses that, directly by definition, the objective function evaluated at the estimator itself is smaller or equal to the objective function evaluated at any other vector. Because this is based on the estimators' formulation directly, we speak of the *first-order* approach. Our second approach is different: it uses that, by Theorem 2.5.1, the subdifferential of a *convex* objective function evaluated again at the estimator itself must contain the all-zeros vector. Because this involves (sub)derivatives, we speak of the *second-order* approach. The two approaches differ in the sets of estimators they apply to, but they essentially agree in the inequalities they produce.

Our first basic inequality is valid if the link function is the identity function.

Lemma 6.2.1

First-Order Basic Inequality Assume that the link function $\mathscr{g}$ is the identity: $\mathscr{g}[a] = a$ for all $a \in \mathbb{R}$. Then, it holds for every $\boldsymbol{\alpha} \in \mathbb{R}^p$ that

$$\|X\boldsymbol{\beta} - X\widehat{\boldsymbol{\beta}}\|_2^2 \leq \|X\boldsymbol{\beta} - X\boldsymbol{\alpha}\|_2^2 + 2\langle \boldsymbol{u}, X\widehat{\boldsymbol{\beta}} - X\boldsymbol{\alpha}\rangle + r\hbar[\boldsymbol{\alpha}] - r\hbar[\widehat{\boldsymbol{\beta}}].$$

This result allows for *every* prior function $\hbar$ at the price of restricting the link function $\mathscr{g}$ to the identity function. As a special case, the bound comprises the basic inequality for the lasso in the previous section (set $\hbar$ equal to the ℓ_1-norm).

Proof of Lemma 6.2.1 The proof generalizes the strategy outlined in ▶ Sect. 6.1.

By definition of $\widehat{\boldsymbol{\beta}}$ as a minimizer of the objective function in (6.1), it holds for every $\boldsymbol{\alpha} \in \mathbb{R}^p$ that (recall that here $\mathscr{g} : a \mapsto a$)

$$\|\boldsymbol{y} - X\widehat{\boldsymbol{\beta}}\|_2^2 + r\hbar[\widehat{\boldsymbol{\beta}}] \leq \|\boldsymbol{y} - X\boldsymbol{\alpha}\|_2^2 + r\hbar[\boldsymbol{\alpha}].$$

We add a zero-valued term inside the ℓ_2-norm on the left-hand side and then open up that term by using $\|\boldsymbol{a} + \boldsymbol{b}\|_2^2 = \|\boldsymbol{a}\|_2^2 + 2\langle \boldsymbol{a}, \boldsymbol{b}\rangle + \|\boldsymbol{b}\|_2^2$ for every $\boldsymbol{a}, \boldsymbol{b} \in \mathbb{R}^p$ according to

Lemma B.1.2:

$$\begin{aligned}\|y - X\widehat{\beta}\|_2^2 &= \|\underbrace{y - X\beta}_{a} + \underbrace{X\beta - X\widehat{\beta}}_{b}\|_2^2\\ &= \|\underbrace{y - X\beta}_{a}\|_2^2 + 2\langle\underbrace{y - X\beta}_{a},\, \underbrace{X\beta - X\widehat{\beta}}_{b}\rangle + \|\underbrace{X\beta - X\widehat{\beta}}_{b}\|_2^2 .\end{aligned}$$

We also perform a similar attack on ℓ_2-term on the right-hand side of the initial inequality:

$$\begin{aligned}\|y - X\alpha\|_2^2 &= \|y - X\beta + X\beta - X\alpha\|_2^2\\ &= \|y - X\beta\|_2^2 + 2\langle y - X\beta,\, X\beta - X\alpha\rangle + \|X\beta - X\alpha\|_2^2 .\end{aligned}$$

Plugging these two observations into that initial inequality yields

$$\begin{aligned}&\|y - X\beta\|_2^2 + 2\langle y - X\beta,\, X\beta - X\widehat{\beta}\rangle + \|X\beta - X\widehat{\beta}\|_2^2 + r\hbar[\widehat{\beta}]\\ &\le \|y - X\beta\|_2^2 + 2\langle y - X\beta,\, X\beta - X\alpha\rangle + \|X\beta - X\alpha\|_2^2 + r\hbar[\alpha] ,\end{aligned}$$

which can be consolidated into

$$\begin{aligned}\|X\beta - X\widehat{\beta}\|_2^2 \le \|X\beta - X\alpha\|_2^2 &+ 2\langle y - X\beta,\, X\widehat{\beta} - X\alpha\rangle\\ &+ r\hbar[\alpha] - r\hbar[\widehat{\beta}] .\end{aligned}$$

From this, the result follows by substituting $\boldsymbol{u}$ for $\boldsymbol{y} - X\boldsymbol{\beta}$ by virtue of the linear regression model (2.1). □

If the prior function $\hbar$ is convex (see Definition 2.5.1), we can include link functions g beyond the identity. For this, we introduce an "induced version" of g:

$$\begin{aligned}\tilde{g} &: \mathbb{R}^p \to \mathbb{R} ;\\ &\alpha \mapsto g\big[\|y - X\alpha\|_2^2\big] .\end{aligned}$$

While the arguments of the initial link function g are real-valued, the arguments of the induced function $\tilde{g}$ are vector-valued. We then allow for the following link functions:

Assumption 6.2.1

Link Functions We assume that the link function g is differentiable at $\|\boldsymbol{y} - X\widehat{\boldsymbol{\beta}}\|_2^2$ with strictly positive derivative, that is, $g'\big[\|\boldsymbol{y} - X\widehat{\boldsymbol{\beta}}\|_2^2\big] > 0$, and we assume that the induced link function $\tilde{g}$ is convex.

6

One example that satisfies the assumption is again the identity function $g : a \mapsto a$: it is differentiable with constant derivative equal to 1, and its induced version $\tilde{g} : \boldsymbol{a} \mapsto \|\boldsymbol{y} - X\boldsymbol{a}\|_2^2$ is convex (see 1. in Exercise 1.4). Another example that satisfies the assumption is $g : a \mapsto \sqrt{a}$ (assuming $\|\boldsymbol{y} - X\widehat{\boldsymbol{\beta}}\|_2^2 \neq 0$):[4] it is differentiable (assuming $a \neq 0$) with derivative equal to $1/(2\sqrt{a})$—which is strictly positive for $a > 0$), and its induced version $\tilde{g} : \boldsymbol{a} \mapsto \|\boldsymbol{y} - X\boldsymbol{a}\|_2$ is convex (because every norm is convex). The square-root function can be used to write the *square-root lasso*[5]

$$\widehat{\boldsymbol{\beta}}_{\sqrt{\text{lasso}}} \in \mathop{\arg\min}_{\boldsymbol{\alpha} \in \mathbb{R}^p} \Big\{ \|\boldsymbol{y} - X\boldsymbol{\alpha}\|_2 + r\|\boldsymbol{\alpha}\|_1 \Big\} \tag{6.2}$$

as

$$\widehat{\boldsymbol{\beta}}_{\sqrt{\text{lasso}}} \in \mathop{\arg\min}_{\boldsymbol{\alpha} \in \mathbb{R}^p} \Big\{ g\big[\|\boldsymbol{y} - X\boldsymbol{\alpha}\|_2^2\big] + r\|\boldsymbol{\alpha}\|_1 \Big\},$$

which is of the assumed form (6.1). Thus, in contrast to the lemma derived above, the lemma to follow applies in particular to the lasso *and* the square-root lasso.

Lemma 6.2.2

Second-Order Basic Inequality Assume that the link function g satisfies Assumption 6.2.1 and that the prior function h is convex. Then, it holds for every $\boldsymbol{\alpha} \in \mathbb{R}^p$ that

$$\begin{aligned}\|X\boldsymbol{\beta} - X\widehat{\boldsymbol{\beta}}\|_2^2 &\le \|X\boldsymbol{\beta} - X\boldsymbol{\alpha}\|_2^2 + 2\langle \boldsymbol{u}, X\widehat{\boldsymbol{\beta}} - X\boldsymbol{\alpha}\rangle \\ &\quad + \frac{r}{g'\big[\|\boldsymbol{y} - X\widehat{\boldsymbol{\beta}}\|_2^2\big]} h[\boldsymbol{\alpha}] - \frac{r}{g'\big[\|\boldsymbol{y} - X\widehat{\boldsymbol{\beta}}\|_2^2\big]} h[\widehat{\boldsymbol{\beta}}].\end{aligned}$$

The first-order and second-order basic inequalities differ only in their assumptions (the first-order bound assumes that the link function is the identity, while the second-order bound assumes that the prior function is convex) and sometimes in factors—see Exercise 6.1 and Note [6] at the end of the chapter.

We have introduced the name "first-order basic inequality" for Lemma 6.2.1 to indicate that the proof uses the estimator's defining property directly:

$$\|y - X\widehat{\beta}\|_2^2 + r\mathscr{h}[\widehat{\beta}] \leq \|y - X\alpha\|_2^2 + r\mathscr{h}[\alpha] \qquad \text{for all } \alpha \in \mathbb{R}^p .$$

Similarly, we have introduced the name "second-order basic inequality" for Lemma 6.2.2 to indicate that the proof does not use that property directly but instead the KKT conditions it implies.

Proof of Lemma 6.2.2 The steps in this proof are more involved than those in the proof of the first-order bound, but the overall strategy is still simple: (i) We first establish the estimator's optimality conditions, that is, we set generalized derivatives of the objective function to zero. (ii) We then transform that equality into an inequality and, thereby, replace the potentially ambiguous subgradient by a term that is based on the prior function. (iii) We finally separate the estimator's prediction error from all other quantities in that inequality.

(i) We first show that the KKT conditions for the estimator $\widehat{\beta}$ in (6.1) yield

$$\mathbf{0}_p = -2\mathscr{g}'\big[\|y - X\widehat{\beta}\|_2^2\big]\big(X^\top(y - X\widehat{\beta})\big) + r\widehat{\kappa}$$

for a $\widehat{\kappa} \in \partial\mathscr{h}[\widehat{\beta}]$.

We write (6.1) as

$$\widehat{\beta} \in \mathop{\arg\min}_{\alpha \in \mathbb{R}^p} \mathscr{f}[\alpha]$$

with objective function

$$\begin{aligned} \mathscr{f} : \mathbb{R}^p &\to \mathbb{R} \\ a &\mapsto \mathscr{f}[\alpha] := \tilde{\mathscr{g}}[\alpha] + r\mathscr{h}[a] . \end{aligned}$$

The objective function $\mathscr{f}$ is convex, because by assumption both the induced link function $\tilde{\mathscr{g}} : a \mapsto \mathscr{g}\big[\|y - Xa\|_2^2\big]$ and the prior function $\hbar$ are convex and $r \geq 0$ (see Lemma 2.5.1 about the convexity of non-negative combinations).

The optimality conditions for the estimator $\widehat{\boldsymbol{\beta}}$ are $\mathbf{0}_p \in \partial \mathscr{f}[\widehat{\boldsymbol{\beta}}]$ (see Theorem 2.5.1). Using the differentiability of g (see Lemma 2.5.2) and the additivity of subdifferentials (see Lemma 2.5.3), we find that $\mathbf{0}_p \in \partial \mathscr{f}[\widehat{\boldsymbol{\beta}}]$ is equivalent to

$$\mathbf{0}_p = \nabla \tilde{g}[\widehat{\boldsymbol{\beta}}] + r\widehat{\boldsymbol{\kappa}} \qquad \text{for a } \widehat{\boldsymbol{\kappa}} \in \partial \hbar[\widehat{\boldsymbol{\beta}}].$$

The chain rule for differentials then gives us

$$\nabla \tilde{g}[\widehat{\boldsymbol{\beta}}] = -2g'\big[\|\boldsymbol{y} - X\widehat{\boldsymbol{\beta}}\|_2^2\big]\big(X^\top(\boldsymbol{y} - X\widehat{\boldsymbol{\beta}})\big).$$

Combining the two displays finally yields

$$\mathbf{0}_p = -2g'\big[\|\boldsymbol{y} - X\widehat{\boldsymbol{\beta}}\|_2^2\big]\big(X^\top(\boldsymbol{y} - X\widehat{\boldsymbol{\beta}})\big) + r\widehat{\boldsymbol{\kappa}},$$

as desired.

(ii) We now use (i) to prove that for every $\boldsymbol{\alpha} \in \mathbb{R}^p$

$$-2g'\big[\|\boldsymbol{y} - X\widehat{\boldsymbol{\beta}}\|_2^2\big]\big(X^\top(\boldsymbol{y}-X\widehat{\boldsymbol{\beta}})\big)^\top(\boldsymbol{\alpha}-\widehat{\boldsymbol{\beta}})+r\big(\hbar[\boldsymbol{\alpha}]-\hbar[\widehat{\boldsymbol{\beta}}]\big) \geq 0.$$

We first conclude from (i) that for every $\boldsymbol{\alpha} \in \mathbb{R}^p$,

$$0 = \mathbf{0}_p{}^\top(\boldsymbol{\alpha}-\widehat{\boldsymbol{\beta}}) = \big(-2g'\big[\|\boldsymbol{y} - X\widehat{\boldsymbol{\beta}}\|_2^2\big](X^\top(\boldsymbol{y}-X\widehat{\boldsymbol{\beta}}))+r\widehat{\boldsymbol{\kappa}}\big)^\top(\boldsymbol{\alpha}-\widehat{\boldsymbol{\beta}}).$$

Indeed, the first equality is trivial, and the second equality follows directly from replacing $\mathbf{0}_p$ with $-2g'\big[\|\boldsymbol{y} - X\widehat{\boldsymbol{\beta}}\|_2^2\big](X^\top(\boldsymbol{y} - X\widehat{\boldsymbol{\beta}})) + r\widehat{\boldsymbol{\kappa}}$ as suggested by (i). Since $\widehat{\boldsymbol{\kappa}} \in \partial \hbar[\widehat{\boldsymbol{\beta}}]$, the definition of subgradients (see Definition 2.5.2) implies that for all $\boldsymbol{\alpha} \in \mathbb{R}^p$,

$$\hbar[\boldsymbol{\alpha}] \geq \hbar[\widehat{\boldsymbol{\beta}}] + \langle \widehat{\boldsymbol{\kappa}}, \boldsymbol{\alpha} - \widehat{\boldsymbol{\beta}} \rangle,$$

which (recall again that $r \geq 0$) can be rearranged to

$$r\big(\hbar[\boldsymbol{\alpha}] - \hbar[\widehat{\boldsymbol{\beta}}]\big) \geq r\widehat{\boldsymbol{\kappa}}^\top(\boldsymbol{\alpha} - \widehat{\boldsymbol{\beta}}).$$

Combining this with the first equality yields

$$-2g'\big[\|\boldsymbol{y} - X\widehat{\boldsymbol{\beta}}\|_2^2\big]\big(X^\top(\boldsymbol{y}-X\widehat{\boldsymbol{\beta}})\big)^\top(\boldsymbol{\alpha}-\widehat{\boldsymbol{\beta}})+r\big(\hbar[\boldsymbol{\alpha}]-\hbar[\widehat{\boldsymbol{\beta}}]\big) \geq 0,$$

as desired.

(iii) We finally derive the desired bound

$$\|X\boldsymbol{\beta} - X\widehat{\boldsymbol{\beta}}\|_2^2 \leq \|X\boldsymbol{\beta} - X\boldsymbol{\alpha}\|_2^2 + 2\langle \boldsymbol{u},\, X\widehat{\boldsymbol{\beta}} - X\boldsymbol{\alpha}\rangle + \frac{r}{g'\big[\|\boldsymbol{y} - X\widehat{\boldsymbol{\beta}}\|_2^2\big]}\mathscr{h}[\boldsymbol{\alpha}] - \frac{r}{g'\big[\|\boldsymbol{y} - X\widehat{\boldsymbol{\beta}}\|_2^2\big]}\mathscr{h}[\widehat{\boldsymbol{\beta}}]\,.$$

We first observe that

$$\begin{aligned}
&\big(X^\top(\boldsymbol{y} - X\widehat{\boldsymbol{\beta}})\big)^\top(\boldsymbol{\alpha} - \widehat{\boldsymbol{\beta}})\\
&= \big(X^\top(X\boldsymbol{\beta} - X\widehat{\boldsymbol{\beta}} + \boldsymbol{y} - X\boldsymbol{\beta})\big)^\top(\boldsymbol{\alpha} - \widehat{\boldsymbol{\beta}})\\
&\qquad\qquad \text{adding a zero-valued term and rearranging quantities}\\
&= (X\boldsymbol{\beta} - X\widehat{\boldsymbol{\beta}})^\top(X\boldsymbol{\alpha} - X\widehat{\boldsymbol{\beta}}) + (\boldsymbol{y} - X\boldsymbol{\beta})^\top(X\boldsymbol{\alpha} - X\widehat{\boldsymbol{\beta}})\\
&\qquad\qquad \text{splitting the term into two parts}\\
&= (X\boldsymbol{\beta} - X\widehat{\boldsymbol{\beta}})^\top(X\boldsymbol{\beta} - X\widehat{\boldsymbol{\beta}} + X\boldsymbol{\alpha} - X\boldsymbol{\beta})\\
&\quad + (\boldsymbol{y} - X\boldsymbol{\beta})^\top(X\boldsymbol{\alpha} - X\widehat{\boldsymbol{\beta}})\\
&\qquad\qquad \text{adding another zero-valued term in the first summand}\\
&\qquad\qquad \text{and rearranging quantities}\\
&= \|X\boldsymbol{\beta} - X\widehat{\boldsymbol{\beta}}\|_2^2 + (X\boldsymbol{\beta} - X\widehat{\boldsymbol{\beta}})^\top(X\boldsymbol{\alpha} - X\boldsymbol{\beta})\\
&\quad + (\boldsymbol{y} - X\boldsymbol{\beta})^\top(X\boldsymbol{\alpha} - X\widehat{\boldsymbol{\beta}})\,.\\
&\qquad\qquad \text{splitting the first term into two parts}\\
&\qquad\qquad \text{and invoking the definition of the } \ell_2\text{-norm}
\end{aligned}$$

The second summand in the last line can be bounded from below according to Lemma B.1.3 (decomposition of the inner product): setting in the first part of that lemma $\boldsymbol{a} = X\boldsymbol{\beta} - X\widehat{\boldsymbol{\beta}}$, $\boldsymbol{b} = X\boldsymbol{\alpha} - X\boldsymbol{\beta}$, and $c = 1/a$ for every fixed $a \in (0, 1)$ yields

$$-a\|X\boldsymbol{\beta} - X\widehat{\boldsymbol{\beta}}\|_2^2 - \frac{\|X\boldsymbol{\alpha} - X\boldsymbol{\beta}\|_2^2}{4a} \leq (X\boldsymbol{\beta} - X\widehat{\boldsymbol{\beta}})^\top(X\boldsymbol{\alpha} - X\boldsymbol{\beta})\,.$$

Using this bound in the foregoing display and consolidating gives us

$$\begin{aligned}
&\big(X^\top(\boldsymbol{y} - X\widehat{\boldsymbol{\beta}})\big)^\top(\boldsymbol{\alpha} - \widehat{\boldsymbol{\beta}})\\
&\geq (1-a)\,\|X\boldsymbol{\beta} - X\widehat{\boldsymbol{\beta}}\|_2^2 - \frac{\|X\boldsymbol{\alpha} - X\boldsymbol{\beta}\|_2^2}{4a} + (\boldsymbol{y} - X\boldsymbol{\beta})^\top(X\boldsymbol{\alpha} - X\widehat{\boldsymbol{\beta}})\,.
\end{aligned}$$

Plugging this back into the result of (ii) and noting that $g'\big[\|y - X\widehat{\beta}\|_2^2\big]$ is positive by Assumption 6.2.1 yield

$$-2g'\big[\|y - X\widehat{\beta}\|_2^2\big]\Big((1-a)\|X\beta - X\widehat{\beta}\|_2^2 - \frac{\|X\alpha - X\beta\|_2^2}{4a} + \langle y - X\beta,\, X\alpha - X\widehat{\beta}\rangle\Big) + r\big(h[\alpha] - h[\widehat{\beta}]\big) \geq 0\,.$$

Dividing both sides by $-2(1-a)g'\big[\|y - X\widehat{\beta}\|_2^2\big]$ (recall again that $g'\big[\|y - X\widehat{\beta}\|_2^2\big] > 0$ by Assumption 6.2.1 and $a \in (0, 1)$) gives us

$$\|X\beta - X\widehat{\beta}\|_2^2 - \frac{\|X\alpha - X\beta\|_2^2}{4(1-a)a} + \frac{\langle y - X\beta, X\alpha - X\widehat{\beta}\rangle}{1-a} - \frac{r}{2(1-a)g'\big[\|y - X\widehat{\beta}\|_2^2\big]}\big(h[\alpha] - h[\widehat{\beta}]\big) \leq 0\,.$$

Rearranging yields

$$\|X\beta - X\widehat{\beta}\|_2^2 \leq \frac{\|X\beta - X\alpha\|_2^2}{4(1-a)a} + \frac{\langle y - X\beta,\, X\widehat{\beta} - X\alpha\rangle}{1-a} + \frac{r}{2(1-a)g'\big[\|y - X\widehat{\beta}\|_2^2\big]}h[\alpha] - \frac{r}{2(1-a)g'\big[\|y - X\widehat{\beta}\|_2^2\big]}h[\widehat{\beta}]\,,$$

from which the desired inequality follows by setting $a = 1/2$ and substituting $\boldsymbol{u}$ for $y - X\beta$ according to the linear regression model (2.1). □

6.3 Prediction Guarantees

We now establish prediction guarantees by bounding the basic inequalities' inner product term. Our main tool for this is the Hölder inequality, which allows us to factor the inner product term into effective noise and a prior function quantity. Assuming that the effective noise is smaller than the tuning parameter, we can consolidate the factored expression with the estimators' regularization terms to obtain upper bounds for the prediction errors. These bounds are the main results of this chapter. They provide insights into how the estimators' prediction accuracies depend on the model specifications and into what accuracies to expect in practice.[7]

As outlined in the overview section, the proving scheme laid out above has two distinct implementations. The first implementation compares the estimators' performance to the performance of arbitrary regression vectors, while the second implementation includes only regression vectors that satisfy the structural condition. The resulting bounds, called power-one and power-two prediction bounds, respectively, differ from each other in their conditions and expressions; as a rule of thumb, power-two bounds give better results in approximately sparse, weakly correlated settings and power-one bounds otherwise—see in particular our ▶ Sect. 6.4.

We consider again regularized least-squares estimators of the form (6.1).[8] We make two assumptions: The first assumption essentially stipulates either of the two basic inequalities derived in the previous section; this inequality will be the starting point of our derivations. The second assumption stipulates properties of the prior function; these properties will allow us to manipulate the terms of that basic inequality.

Assumption 6.3.1

Generic Basic Inequality We assume that there is a potentially random quantity $\widehat{w} \in (0, \infty)$ such that the estimator $\widehat{\boldsymbol{\beta}}$ satisfies for all $\boldsymbol{\alpha} \in \mathbb{R}^p$ the basic inequality

$$\|X\boldsymbol{\beta} - X\widehat{\boldsymbol{\beta}}\|_2^2 \leq \|X\boldsymbol{\beta} - X\boldsymbol{\alpha}\|_2^2 + 2\langle \boldsymbol{u},\, X\widehat{\boldsymbol{\beta}} - X\boldsymbol{\alpha}\rangle + \widehat{w}r\hbar[\boldsymbol{\alpha}] - \widehat{w}r\hbar[\widehat{\boldsymbol{\beta}}]\,.$$

The assumption is satisfied with $\widehat{w} = 1$ (which is deterministic) if the estimator meets the conditions of the first-order basic inequality of Lemma 6.2.1; the assumption is satisfied with $\widehat{w} = 1/g'\big[\|\boldsymbol{y} - X\widehat{\boldsymbol{\beta}}\|_2^2\big]$ (which is random) if the estimator meets the conditions of the second-order basic inequality of Lemma 6.2.2.

Assumption 6.3.2

Prior Function We use three assumptions on the prior function $\hbar$:

1. $\hbar$ meets the conditions of Theorem 2.4.1 (Hölder inequality).

2. $\hbar$ is symmetric: $\hbar[\boldsymbol{a}] = \hbar[-\boldsymbol{a}]$ for all $\boldsymbol{a} \in \mathbb{R}^p$.
3. $\hbar$ satisfies the triangle inequality: $\hbar[\boldsymbol{a}+\boldsymbol{b}] \leq \hbar[\boldsymbol{a}]+\hbar[\boldsymbol{b}]$ for all $\boldsymbol{a}, \boldsymbol{b} \in \mathbb{R}^p$.

The first part of this assumption is crucial in proving our power-one bounds, and the first and third parts are crucial in proving our power-two bounds. The second part, on the other hand, is used only for simplifications.

▶ Example 6.3.1

Non-negative Lasso In this example, we introduce the *non-negative lasso*[9]

$$\widehat{\boldsymbol{\beta}}_{\text{nn}} \in \underset{\boldsymbol{\alpha} \in \mathbb{R}^p}{\arg\min} \left\{ \|\boldsymbol{y} - X\boldsymbol{\alpha}\|_2^2 + r\hbar[\boldsymbol{\alpha}] \right\}$$

with prior function

$$\hbar : \boldsymbol{a} \mapsto \sum_{j=1}^{p} \big(a_j \cdot \mathbb{1}\{a_j \geq 0\} + \infty \cdot \mathbb{1}\{\alpha_j < 0\}\big) .$$

The non-negative lasso excludes negative parameter values by setting the objective function at such values to infinity; in other words, the non-negative lasso is the lasso with the additional constraint that all estimated model parameters are non-negative.

The prior function $\hbar$ is not a norm: for example, it is not positive definite and not symmetric. However, the non-negative lasso is still of the form (6.1) and meets the conditions of the first-order basic inequality in Lemma 6.2.1,[10] so that the basic inequality in Assumption 6.3.1 is satisfied with $\widehat{w} = 1$. Also, the prior function of the non-negative lasso meets 1. and 3. of Assumption 6.3.2 (see 1. of Exercise 6.2). Therefore, the techniques introduced in this section also apply to the non-negative lasso (see 2.–4. of Exercise 6.2).◀

We first generalize the power-one bound from the overview section.

Theorem 6.3.1

Power-One Prediction Bounds Assume that the estimator $\widehat{\boldsymbol{\beta}}$ of (6.1) satisfies a basic inequality as specified in Assumption 6.3.1. Now, if the prior function $\hbar$ satisfies 1. of Assumption 6.3.2, it holds that

$$\|X\boldsymbol{\beta} - X\widehat{\boldsymbol{\beta}}\|_2^2 \leq \min_{\boldsymbol{\alpha}\in\mathbb{R}^p}\Big\{\|X\boldsymbol{\beta} - X\boldsymbol{\alpha}\|_2^2 + 2\overline{\hbar}[X^\top\boldsymbol{u}]\hbar[-\boldsymbol{\alpha}] + \widehat{w}r\hbar[\boldsymbol{\alpha}] + \big(2\overline{\hbar}[X^\top\boldsymbol{u}] - \widehat{w}r\big)\hbar[\widehat{\boldsymbol{\beta}}]\Big\}.$$

If additionally $\widehat{w}r \geq 2v\overline{\hbar}[X^\top\boldsymbol{u}]$ for a constant $v \in [1, \infty)$ and $\hbar$ satisfies 2. of Assumption 6.3.2, the bound implies (consolidate the $\hbar$-terms in the above inequality)

$$\|X\boldsymbol{\beta} - X\widehat{\boldsymbol{\beta}}\|_2^2 \leq \min_{\boldsymbol{\alpha}\in\mathbb{R}^p}\Big\{\|X\boldsymbol{\beta} - X\boldsymbol{\alpha}\|_2^2 + \Big(1 + \frac{1}{v}\Big)\widehat{w}r\hbar[\boldsymbol{\alpha}]\Big\},$$

and if further $v > 1$ and $r > 0$, the first bound also implies (set $\boldsymbol{\alpha} = \boldsymbol{\beta}$ in the first inequality, consolidate the $\hbar$-terms, bound the prediction term from below by 0, and note that $0 < \widehat{w} < \infty$ and $r < \infty$ by assumption)

$$\hbar[\widehat{\boldsymbol{\beta}}] \leq \frac{v+1}{v-1}\hbar[\boldsymbol{\beta}].$$

Recall the specification of dual functions in Definition 2.4.1. Dual functions are ubiquitous here and in the following sections because they allow us to bound the inner product term $2\langle\boldsymbol{u}, X\widehat{\boldsymbol{\beta}} - X\boldsymbol{\alpha}\rangle$ from Assumption (6.3.1) via the Hölder inequality.

The first two bounds in the theorem generalize the power-one bound of the overview section. They involve the tuning parameter to the first power, hence the name power-one bounds. The third bound shows that the size of the estimated model in terms of $\hbar$ is small if the tuning parameter is sufficiently large.

The bounds in Theorem 6.3.1 and in Theorem 6.3.2 below guarantee prediction accuracies in terms of X, $\boldsymbol{\beta}$, and $\boldsymbol{u}$. Since $\boldsymbol{\beta}$ and $\boldsymbol{u}$ are unknown in applications, the bounds cannot be computed in practice; in particular, the bounds do not provide any practical confidence intervals. Still, the guarantees can provide a rough idea for what to expect from a given estimator in practice:

6

► Example 6.3.2

Power-One Prediction Bound for the Square-Root Lasso In this example, we establish a specific power-one prediction bound for the square-root lasso estimator (6.2). In view of Lemma 6.2.2 (second-order basic inequality) and the comments preceding it, the generic basic inequality in Assumption 6.3.1 is satisfied for the square-root lasso with $\widehat{w} = 2\|\boldsymbol{y} - X\widehat{\boldsymbol{\beta}}\|_2$ (assuming $\|\boldsymbol{y} - X\widehat{\boldsymbol{\beta}}\|_2^2 \neq 0$—see again Note [4] at the end of the chapter). The ℓ_1-norm is a norm indeed and therefore (see Page IX) meets all conditions imposed on the prior function by Assumption 6.3.2. The ℓ_1-norm's dual function is the ℓ_∞-norm (see 3. in Exercise 2.2). Hence, the second part of Theorem 6.3.1 implies that if the tuning parameters are such that,[11] say, $\widehat{w}r = 2\|X^\top \boldsymbol{u}\|_\infty$ (that is, $v = 1$), then

$$\|X\boldsymbol{\beta} - X\widehat{\boldsymbol{\beta}}_{\sqrt{\text{lasso}}}\|_2^2 \leq \min_{\boldsymbol{\alpha}\in\mathbb{R}^p} \left\{ \|X\boldsymbol{\beta} - X\boldsymbol{\alpha}\|_2^2 + 4\|X^\top \boldsymbol{u}\|_\infty \|\boldsymbol{\alpha}\|_1 \right\}.$$

This bound equals the power-one bound derived in ► Sect. 6.1 applied to the lasso with tuning parameter $r = 2\|X^\top \boldsymbol{u}\|_\infty$.[12]

We now assume Gauss-distributed noise and normalized design: $\boldsymbol{u} \sim \mathcal{N}_n[\mathbf{0}_n, \sigma^2 \mathrm{I}_{n\times n}]$ for some standard deviation $\sigma \in (0, \infty)$, and $(X^\top X)_{jj} = n$ for all $j \in \{1, \ldots, p\}$. Using the tail bound for Gauss-distributed noise in Lemma 4.2.1 in the exact same way as outlined in the overview section, we then find for every $t \in (0, 1]$ that

$$\mathbb{P}\left\{ \frac{\|X\boldsymbol{\beta} - X\widehat{\boldsymbol{\beta}}_{\sqrt{\text{lasso}}}\|_2^2}{n} \leq \sigma\sqrt{\frac{32\log[p/t]}{n}}\|\boldsymbol{\beta}\|_1 \right\} \geq 1 - t,$$

which again equals the corresponding lasso bound of ► Sect. 6.1.

To show why these bounds can support the use of the lasso/square-root lasso estimator instead of the least-squares estimator in high dimensions, we transform the least-squares' risk bound in ► Sect. 1.2 via Markov inequality (see 3. in Exercise 5.4) into a probability bound:

$$\mathbb{P}\left\{ \frac{\|X\boldsymbol{\beta} - X\widehat{\boldsymbol{\beta}}_{\text{ls}}\|_2^2}{n} \geq \frac{\sigma^2 p}{nt} \right\} \leq \frac{\mathbb{E}[\|X\boldsymbol{\beta} - X\widehat{\boldsymbol{\beta}}_{\text{ls}}\|_2^2/n]}{\sigma^2 p/(nt)} \qquad \text{Markov inequality}$$

$$= t. \qquad \text{Eq. (1.5)}$$

Focusing on the sample size n, this bound guarantees the average prediction error of the least-squares estimator to decrease as $1/n$, while the above bound guarantees the average prediction error of the square-root lasso to decrease only as $1/\sqrt{n}$; on the other hand, focusing on the number of model parameters p, the bound for the least-squares estimator increases linearly in p, while the bound for the square-root lasso increases only logarithmically in p. These results corroborate our narrative that the larger the number of model parameters is, as compared to the number of samples, the more essential are high-dimensional estimators. ◀

We now prove our first set of probability bounds.

Proof of Theorem 6.3.1 The proof goes along the same lines as in the lasso case in the overview section.

The inner product term on the right-hand side of the basic inequality in Assumption 6.3.1 can be bounded via the Hölder inequality:

$$
\begin{aligned}
&2\langle \boldsymbol{u},\, X\widehat{\boldsymbol{\beta}} - X\boldsymbol{\alpha}\rangle \\
&= 2\langle \boldsymbol{u},\, X\widehat{\boldsymbol{\beta}}\rangle + 2\langle \boldsymbol{u},\, -X\boldsymbol{\alpha}\rangle && \text{linearity of inner product} \\
&= 2\langle X^\top \boldsymbol{u},\, \widehat{\boldsymbol{\beta}}\rangle + 2\langle X^\top \boldsymbol{u},\, -\boldsymbol{\alpha}\rangle \\
& && \text{property (B.1) of transposition} \\
&\le 2\overline{\hbar}[X^\top \boldsymbol{u}]\hbar[\widehat{\boldsymbol{\beta}}] + 2\overline{\hbar}[X^\top \boldsymbol{u}]\hbar[-\boldsymbol{\alpha}]\,. \\
& && \text{1. in Assumption 6.3.2 on } \hbar \text{ (Hölder inequality)}
\end{aligned}
$$

Plugging this back into the assumed bound yields for every $\boldsymbol{\alpha} \in \mathbb{R}^p$

$$
\begin{aligned}
&\|X\boldsymbol{\beta} - X\widehat{\boldsymbol{\beta}}\|_2^2 \le \|X\boldsymbol{\beta} - X\boldsymbol{\alpha}\|_2^2 \\
&+2\overline{\hbar}[X^\top \boldsymbol{u}]\hbar[\widehat{\boldsymbol{\beta}}]+2\overline{\hbar}[X^\top \boldsymbol{u}]\hbar[-\boldsymbol{\alpha}]+\widehat{r}\hbar[\boldsymbol{\alpha}]-\widehat{r}\hbar[\widehat{\boldsymbol{\beta}}]\,,
\end{aligned}
$$

and therefore, rearranging,

$$
\begin{aligned}
&\|X\boldsymbol{\beta} - X\widehat{\boldsymbol{\beta}}\|_2^2 \le \|X\boldsymbol{\beta} - X\boldsymbol{\alpha}\|_2^2 \\
&+2\overline{\hbar}[X^\top \boldsymbol{u}]\hbar[-\boldsymbol{\alpha}]+\widehat{r}\hbar[\boldsymbol{\alpha}]+\bigl(2\overline{\hbar}[X^\top \boldsymbol{u}]-\widehat{r}\bigr)\hbar[\widehat{\boldsymbol{\beta}}]\,,
\end{aligned}
$$

which concludes the proof of the first claim since $\boldsymbol{\alpha}$ was arbitrary. The other two claims follow as indicated in the theorem. □

We now generalize the power-two bound from the overview section.

Theorem 6.3.2

Power-Two Prediction Bounds Assume that the estimator $\widehat{\boldsymbol{\beta}}$ in (6.1) satisfies a basic inequality as specified in Assumption 6.3.1. Now, if the prior function $\hbar$ satisfies 1. and 3. of Assumption 6.3.2, it holds for all $b \in (1, \infty]$, $m \in (0, \infty)$ that

$$\|X\boldsymbol{\beta} - X\widehat{\boldsymbol{\beta}}\|_2^2 \leq \min_{\boldsymbol{\alpha} \in \widehat{\mathscr{B}}_m} \Big\{ b\|X\boldsymbol{\beta} - X\boldsymbol{\alpha}\|_2^2 + \frac{(b+1)^2 m^2}{4(b-1)n} \big(2\overline{\hbar}[-X^\top \boldsymbol{u}] + \widehat{wr}\big)^2 \Big\},$$

where $\widehat{\mathscr{B}}_m := \{\boldsymbol{a} \in \mathbb{R}^p : \hbar[\boldsymbol{a}-\widehat{\boldsymbol{\beta}}] \leq m\|X\boldsymbol{a} - X\widehat{\boldsymbol{\beta}}\|_2/\sqrt{n}\}$. If additionally 2. of Assumption 6.3.2 holds and $\widehat{wr} \geq 2v\overline{\hbar}[X^\top \boldsymbol{u}]$ for a positive and finite constant $v \in (0, \infty)$, the bound implies directly ($\hbar$ symmetric implies $\overline{\hbar}$ symmetric according to 5. in Exercise 2.3)

$$\|X\boldsymbol{\beta} - X\widehat{\boldsymbol{\beta}}\|_2^2 \leq \min_{\boldsymbol{\alpha} \in \widehat{\mathscr{B}}_m} \Big\{ b\|X\boldsymbol{\beta} - X\boldsymbol{\alpha}\|_2^2 + \frac{(b+1)^2 m^2 (v+1)^2 \widehat{w}^2 r^2}{4(b-1)v^2 n} \Big\}.$$

These bounds differ from the power-one bounds of Theorem 6.3.1 mainly in that they involve the tuning parameter to the power two (hence the naming) and in that they impose restrictions on the design. These restrictions come through $\widehat{\mathscr{B}}_m$: rather than minimizing over arbitrary $\boldsymbol{\alpha}$, the bounds minimize only over $\boldsymbol{\alpha}$ that satisfy the structural condition, that is, over $\boldsymbol{\alpha} \in \widehat{\mathscr{B}}_m$ for

$$\widehat{\mathscr{B}}_m = \{\boldsymbol{a} \in \mathbb{R}^p : \hbar[\boldsymbol{a} - \widehat{\boldsymbol{\beta}}] \leq m\|X\boldsymbol{a} - X\widehat{\boldsymbol{\beta}}\|_2/\sqrt{n}\}. \tag{6.3}$$

This structural condition generalizes the corresponding condition of ▶ Sect. 6.1 from the ℓ_1-norm to arbitrary prior functions $\hbar$. A detailed discussion about when the set $\widehat{\mathscr{B}}_m$ is large enough to allow for favorable bounds follows in the next section; for the moment, we just observe that power-two bounds involve this additional restriction.

▶ Example 6.3.3

Power-Two Prediction Bound for the Square-Root Lasso In this example, we establish a specific power-two bound for the square-root lasso estimator (6.2). Its main advantage over the power-one bound in Example 6.3.2 is the $1/n$-rate in the sample size; its main disadvantage is the involvement of the structural condition.

We make the same assumptions as in Example 6.3.2: $\widehat{wr} = 2\|X^\top \boldsymbol{u}\|_\infty$, $\boldsymbol{u} \sim \mathcal{N}_n[\mathbf{0}_n, \sigma^2 \mathrm{I}_{n\times n}]$ for some standard deviation $\sigma \in (0, \infty)$, and $(X^\top X)_{jj} = n$ for all $j \in \{1, \dots, p\}$. Additionally, we make the assumption that the regression vector $\boldsymbol{\beta}$ satisfies the structural condition, that is, $\boldsymbol{\beta} \in \widehat{\mathcal{B}}_m$ for a "reasonably small" m. Setting $b = 3$ in the second part of Theorem 6.3.2 and invoking the mentioned assumptions, we find that

$$\|X\boldsymbol{\beta} - X\widehat{\boldsymbol{\beta}}_{\sqrt{\text{lasso}}}\|_2^2 \leq \min_{\boldsymbol{\alpha} \in \widehat{\mathcal{B}}_m} \left\{ 3\|X\boldsymbol{\beta} - X\boldsymbol{\alpha}\|_2^2 + \frac{32m^2\|X^\top \boldsymbol{u}\|_\infty^2}{n} \right\}.$$

Now, if $\boldsymbol{\beta} \in \widehat{\mathcal{B}}_m$,

$$\begin{aligned}
&\mathbb{P}\left\{ \frac{\|X\boldsymbol{\beta} - X\widehat{\boldsymbol{\beta}}_{\sqrt{\text{lasso}}}\|_2^2}{n} \leq \frac{128m^2\sigma^2 \log[p/t]}{n} \right\} \\
&\geq \mathbb{P}\left\{ \frac{\min_{\boldsymbol{\alpha} \in \widehat{\mathcal{B}}_m} \left\{ 3\|X\boldsymbol{\beta} - X\boldsymbol{\alpha}\|_2^2 + 32m^2\|X^\top \boldsymbol{u}\|_\infty^2/n \right\}}{n} \leq \frac{128m^2\sigma^2 \log[p/t]}{n} \right\} && \text{power-two bound above} \\
&\geq \mathbb{P}\left\{ \frac{32m^2\|X^\top \boldsymbol{u}\|_\infty^2}{n^2} \leq \frac{128m^2\sigma^2 \log[p/t]}{n} \right\} && \text{bounding the minimum by setting } \boldsymbol{\alpha} = \boldsymbol{\beta} \text{ assuming } \boldsymbol{\beta} \in \widehat{\mathcal{B}}_m \\
&= \mathbb{P}\left\{ 2\|X^\top \boldsymbol{u}\|_\infty \leq \sigma\sqrt{8mn \log[p/t]} \right\} && \text{consolidating and taking square-roots; } m = \max_{j \in \{1,\dots,p\}} (X^\top X)_{jj}/n = 1 \text{ by assumption} \\
&\geq 1 - t. && \text{Lemma 4.2.1 (Gauss-distributed noise)}
\end{aligned}$$

Whether the power-two bound here improves on the power-one bound of Example 6.3.2 depends on the model specifications: the bound here decreases faster[13] in the sample size ($1/n$ as compared to $1/\sqrt{n}$ before), but it also stipulates an obscure condition about the regression vector and the design matrix ($\boldsymbol{\beta} \in \widehat{\mathcal{B}}_m$ for a reasonably small m—see the following section). ◀

effective noise

The quantity $2\overline{\hbar}[X^\top \boldsymbol{u}]$ in the restrictions on the tuning parameter is called the *effective noise* of the regularized least-squares estimator $\widehat{\boldsymbol{\beta}}$. For example, the effective noise for ℓ_1-regularization is $2\overline{\hbar}[X^\top \boldsymbol{u}] = 2\|X^\top \boldsymbol{u}\|_\infty$. If $\boldsymbol{u} \sim \mathcal{N}_n[\mathbf{0}_n, \sigma^2 \mathrm{I}_{n\times n}]$ and $\widehat{wr} = 2\|X^\top \boldsymbol{u}\|_\infty$ (see the two foregoing examples), then $\widehat{wr}$ is proportional to the standard deviation: $2\|X^\top \boldsymbol{u}\|_\infty = \sigma \cdot 2\|X^\top \boldsymbol{u}/\sigma\|_\infty$ and $\boldsymbol{u}/\sigma \sim \mathcal{N}_n[\mathbf{0}_n, \mathrm{I}_{n\times n}]$ is independent of σ. This then also means that the prediction bounds in Theorems 6.3.1 and 6.3.2, which involve $\widehat{wr}$ and $(\widehat{wr})^2$, respectively, increase with σ. More generally, the effective noise embodies the influence of the noise vector $\boldsymbol{u}$ on the prediction guarantees: the larger $2\overline{\hbar}[X^\top \boldsymbol{u}]$, the larger $\widehat{wr}$ needs to satisfy the restriction $\widehat{wr} \geq 2v\overline{\hbar}[X^\top \boldsymbol{u}]$ for given v; and since the right-hand sides of the prediction bounds increase with $\widehat{wr}$, this means that the larger the effective noise, the looser the prediction guarantees. This relationship is commensurate with our naive expectation that prediction accuracies decrease when the noise level increases.

We finally prove our second set of probability bounds.

Proof of Theorem 6.3.2 The proof goes again along the same lines as in the lasso case in the overview section.

The inner product term on the right-hand side of the basic inequality in Assumption 6.3.1 can be bounded via the Hölder inequality:

$$
\begin{aligned}
&2\langle \boldsymbol{u},\, X\widehat{\boldsymbol{\beta}} - X\boldsymbol{\alpha}\rangle \\
&= 2\langle -\boldsymbol{u},\, X\boldsymbol{\alpha} - X\widehat{\boldsymbol{\beta}}\rangle && \text{linearity of inner products} \\
&= 2\langle -X^\top \boldsymbol{u},\, \boldsymbol{\alpha} - \widehat{\boldsymbol{\beta}}\rangle && \text{Property (B.1) of transposition} \\
&\leq 2\overline{\hbar}[-X^\top \boldsymbol{u}]\hbar[\boldsymbol{\alpha} - \widehat{\boldsymbol{\beta}}]\,. && \text{1. in Assumption 6.3.2 on } \hbar \text{ (Hölder inequality)}
\end{aligned}
$$

Plugging this back into the assumed bound yields for every $\boldsymbol{\alpha} \in \mathbb{R}^p$

$$
\begin{aligned}
\|X\boldsymbol{\beta} - X\widehat{\boldsymbol{\beta}}\|_2^2 \leq \|X\boldsymbol{\beta} - X\boldsymbol{\alpha}\|_2^2 + 2\overline{\hbar}[-X^\top \boldsymbol{u}]\hbar[\boldsymbol{\alpha} - \widehat{\boldsymbol{\beta}}] \\
+ \widehat{wr}\hbar[\boldsymbol{\alpha}] - \widehat{wr}\hbar[\widehat{\boldsymbol{\beta}}]\,,
\end{aligned}
$$

and further,

$$
\begin{aligned}
&\|X\boldsymbol{\beta} - X\widehat{\boldsymbol{\beta}}\|_2^2 \\
&\le \|X\boldsymbol{\beta} - X\boldsymbol{\alpha}\|_2^2 + 2\overline{\hbar}[-X^\top \boldsymbol{u}]\hbar[\boldsymbol{\alpha} - \widehat{\boldsymbol{\beta}}] + \widehat{wr}\hbar[\boldsymbol{\alpha} - \widehat{\boldsymbol{\beta}}] \\
&\quad + \widehat{wr}\hbar[\widehat{\boldsymbol{\beta}}] - \widehat{wr}\hbar[\widehat{\boldsymbol{\beta}}]
\end{aligned}
$$

3. in Assumption 6.3.2 on $\hbar$ (triangle inequality): $\hbar[\boldsymbol{\alpha}] = \hbar[(\boldsymbol{\alpha} - \widehat{\boldsymbol{\beta}}) + \widehat{\boldsymbol{\beta}}] \le \hbar[\boldsymbol{\alpha} - \widehat{\boldsymbol{\beta}}] + \hbar[\widehat{\boldsymbol{\beta}}]$

$$
= \|X\boldsymbol{\beta} - X\boldsymbol{\alpha}\|_2^2 + \bigl(2\overline{\hbar}[-X^\top \boldsymbol{u}] + \widehat{wr}\bigr)\hbar[\boldsymbol{\alpha} - \widehat{\boldsymbol{\beta}}]\,.
$$

consolidating terms

Invoking the first part of Lemma B.1.3 (decomposing the inner product) with $\mathbb{R}^p = \mathbb{R}$ and $c = 2(b-1)n/((b+1)m^2)$, where $b \in (1, \infty]$, to bound the last term in the above display yields

$$
\begin{aligned}
&\|X\boldsymbol{\beta} - X\widehat{\boldsymbol{\beta}}\|_2^2 \\
&\quad\le \|X\boldsymbol{\beta} - X\boldsymbol{\alpha}\|_2^2 + \frac{(b+1)m^2}{2(b-1)n}\bigl(2\overline{\hbar}[-X^\top \boldsymbol{u}] + \widehat{wr}\bigr)^2 \\
&\qquad + \frac{(b-1)n}{2(b+1)m^2}\bigl(\hbar[\boldsymbol{\alpha} - \widehat{\boldsymbol{\beta}}]\bigr)^2\,.
\end{aligned}
$$

Next, we have by definition $\widehat{\mathscr{B}}_m$ that $\hbar[\boldsymbol{\alpha} - \widehat{\boldsymbol{\beta}}] \le m\|X\boldsymbol{\alpha} - X\widehat{\boldsymbol{\beta}}\|_2/\sqrt{n}$ for every $\boldsymbol{\alpha} \in \widehat{\mathscr{B}}_m$. Using this to bound the last term of the above display implies for such $\boldsymbol{\alpha}$

$$
\begin{aligned}
&\|X\boldsymbol{\beta} - X\widehat{\boldsymbol{\beta}}\|_2^2 \\
&\quad\le \|X\boldsymbol{\beta} - X\boldsymbol{\alpha}\|_2^2 + \frac{(b+1)m^2}{2(b-1)n}\bigl(2\overline{\hbar}[-X^\top \boldsymbol{u}] + \widehat{wr}\bigr)^2 \\
&\qquad + \frac{b-1}{2(b+1)}\|X\boldsymbol{\alpha} - X\widehat{\boldsymbol{\beta}}\|_2^2\,.
\end{aligned}
$$

Now, adding a zero-valued term and using $\|\boldsymbol{a} + \boldsymbol{b}\|_2^2 \le 2\|\boldsymbol{a}\|_2^2 + 2\|\boldsymbol{b}\|_2^2$ for all $\boldsymbol{a}, \boldsymbol{b} \in \mathbb{R}^n$ (see Lemma B.1.1), we find

$$
\begin{aligned}
\|X\boldsymbol{\alpha} - X\widehat{\boldsymbol{\beta}}\|_2^2 &= \|\underbrace{X\boldsymbol{\alpha} - X\boldsymbol{\beta}}_{\boldsymbol{a}} + \underbrace{X\boldsymbol{\beta} - X\widehat{\boldsymbol{\beta}}}_{\boldsymbol{b}}\|_2^2 \\
&\le 2\|X\boldsymbol{\alpha} - X\boldsymbol{\beta}\|_2^2 + 2\|X\boldsymbol{\beta} - X\widehat{\boldsymbol{\beta}}\|_2^2 \\
&= 2\|X\boldsymbol{\beta} - X\boldsymbol{\alpha}\|_2^2 + 2\|X\boldsymbol{\beta} - X\widehat{\boldsymbol{\beta}}\|_2^2\,.
\end{aligned}
$$

Plugging this into the preceding display yields

$$\begin{aligned}
&\|X\boldsymbol{\beta} - X\widehat{\boldsymbol{\beta}}\|_2^2 \\
&\le \|X\boldsymbol{\beta} - X\boldsymbol{\alpha}\|_2^2 + \frac{(b+1)m^2}{2(b-1)n}\bigl(2\overline{\hbar}[-X^\top \boldsymbol{u}] + \widehat{wr}\bigr)^2 \\
&\quad + \frac{b-1}{b+1}\|X\boldsymbol{\beta} - X\widehat{\boldsymbol{\beta}}\|_2^2 + \frac{b-1}{b+1}\|X\boldsymbol{\beta} - X\boldsymbol{\alpha}\|_2^2 .
\end{aligned}$$

Therefore, by consolidating terms,

$$\begin{aligned}
&\frac{2}{b+1}\|X\boldsymbol{\beta} - X\widehat{\boldsymbol{\beta}}\|_2^2 \\
&\le \frac{2b}{b+1}\|X\boldsymbol{\beta} - X\boldsymbol{\alpha}\|_2^2 + \frac{(b+1)m^2}{2(b-1)n}\bigl(2\overline{\hbar}[-X^\top \boldsymbol{u}] + \widehat{wr}\bigr)^2
\end{aligned}$$

and then

$$\|X\boldsymbol{\beta} - X\widehat{\boldsymbol{\beta}}\|_2^2 \le b\|X\boldsymbol{\beta} - X\boldsymbol{\alpha}\|_2^2 + \frac{(b+1)^2m^2}{4(b-1)n}\bigl(2\overline{\hbar}[-X^\top \boldsymbol{u}] + \widehat{wr}\bigr)^2 .$$

This concludes the proof. □

6.4 Prediction Guarantees for Sparse and Weakly Correlated Models

The minima in power-one bounds are taken over the entire parameter space $\mathbb{R}^p$, while the minima in power-two bounds are taken only over subsets of it. These subsets can well be too small to contain good minimizers, and then power-two bounds are less informative than power-one bounds—or even completely void. On the other hand, there are also cases where power-two bounds do provide very useful guarantees. In this section, we identify such cases. The corresponding criteria are approximate sparsity and weak correlations: the regression vector must allow for a sparse approximation such that the correlations both among the predictors that correspond to the support of that surrogate vector and between those predictors and the remaining ones are low. These criteria essentially ensure correct estimation of the regression vector (see ► Sect. 7.2), which connects this section to the following chapter on estimation and support recovery theory.

The central quantity is the random set $\widehat{\mathscr{B}}_m$ of (6.3), which has been introduced in Theorem 6.3.2 to formalize the structural condition. The following example demonstrates that this set is closely connected with the correlations among the predictors.

▶ Example 6.4.1

Link Between $\widehat{\mathscr{B}}_m$ and the Correlations in the Design In this example, we illustrate that the structural condition is closely linked to the correlations in the design: the larger the correlations, the more restrictive the condition. Assuming that the columns of X have Euclidean lengths of, say, $\sqrt{n}$, a measure for the correlations among the predictors is the square-root of the smallest eigenvalue of the scaled Gram matrix $X^\top X/n$:

$$c := \min_{\boldsymbol{\delta}\in\mathbb{R}^p\setminus\mathbf{0}_p} \sqrt{\frac{\boldsymbol{\delta}^\top X^\top X\boldsymbol{\delta}}{n\|\boldsymbol{\delta}\|_2^2}} \in [0, 1].$$

The smaller c, the stronger the correlations; the extreme cases are $c = 0$ (some predictors are linearly dependent) and $c = 1$ (all predictors are orthogonal; cf. 1. in Exercise 2.10).

Assume now that $c > 0$, which ensures for all $\boldsymbol{\alpha} \in \mathbb{R}^p$ the inclusion $X\boldsymbol{\alpha} = X\widehat{\boldsymbol{\beta}} \Rightarrow \boldsymbol{\alpha} = \widehat{\boldsymbol{\beta}}$, and consider $\hbar : \boldsymbol{\alpha} \mapsto \|\boldsymbol{\alpha}\|_2$. For $\boldsymbol{\alpha} \in \mathbb{R}^p$ such that $X\boldsymbol{\alpha} = X\widehat{\boldsymbol{\beta}}$, we then find

$$\hbar[\boldsymbol{\alpha} - \widehat{\boldsymbol{\beta}}] = \frac{1}{c\sqrt{n}}\|X\boldsymbol{\alpha} - X\widehat{\boldsymbol{\beta}}\|_2 = 0,$$

which means that the inequality in (6.3) is satisfied for every m. For $\boldsymbol{\alpha} \in \mathbb{R}^p$ such that $X\boldsymbol{\alpha} \neq X\widehat{\boldsymbol{\beta}}$, we find

$$\begin{aligned}
&\hbar[\boldsymbol{\alpha} - \widehat{\boldsymbol{\beta}}]\\
&= \|\boldsymbol{\alpha} - \widehat{\boldsymbol{\beta}}\|_2 && \text{choice of } \hbar\\
&= \sqrt{\frac{n\|\boldsymbol{\alpha} - \widehat{\boldsymbol{\beta}}\|_2^2}{(\boldsymbol{\alpha} - \widehat{\boldsymbol{\beta}})^\top X^\top X(\boldsymbol{\alpha} - \widehat{\boldsymbol{\beta}})}}\sqrt{\frac{(\boldsymbol{\alpha} - \widehat{\boldsymbol{\beta}})^\top X^\top X(\boldsymbol{\alpha} - \widehat{\boldsymbol{\beta}})}{n}} && \text{multiplying by a one-valued factor}\\
&\le \max_{\boldsymbol{\delta}\in\mathbb{R}^p\setminus\mathbf{0}_p}\sqrt{\frac{n\|\boldsymbol{\delta}\|_2^2}{\boldsymbol{\delta}^\top X^\top X\boldsymbol{\delta}}}\sqrt{\frac{(\boldsymbol{\alpha} - \widehat{\boldsymbol{\beta}})^\top X^\top X(\boldsymbol{\alpha} - \widehat{\boldsymbol{\beta}})}{n}} && \text{maximizing the first term}\\
&= \frac{1}{c}\sqrt{\frac{(\boldsymbol{\alpha} - \widehat{\boldsymbol{\beta}})^\top X^\top X(\boldsymbol{\alpha} - \widehat{\boldsymbol{\beta}})}{n}} && \text{above definition of } c\\
&= \frac{1}{c\sqrt{n}}\|X\boldsymbol{\alpha} - X\widehat{\boldsymbol{\beta}}\|_2, && \text{definition of the } \ell_2\text{-norm}
\end{aligned}$$

which means that the inequality in (6.3) is satisfied for every $m \geq 1/c$. In addition, for $\boldsymbol{\alpha} = \boldsymbol{\delta} - \widehat{\boldsymbol{\beta}}$ with $\boldsymbol{\delta}$ minimizing the expression in the definition of c, we deduce from that definition that

$$\hbar[\boldsymbol{\alpha} - \widehat{\boldsymbol{\beta}}] = \frac{1}{c\sqrt{n}}\|X\boldsymbol{\alpha} - X\widehat{\boldsymbol{\beta}}\|_2 .$$

Therefore, $\widehat{\mathscr{B}}_m = \mathbb{R}^p$ if and only if $m \geq 1/c$. This illustrates the general fact that the larger the correlations, the larger m needs to be to ensure that the structural condition holds for all possible regression vectors. ◀

6

The power-two bounds of Theorem 6.3.2 are most useful if both $\widehat{\mathscr{B}}_m$ is large (to ensure flexibility in the minimization) and m is small (to keep the terms quadratic in m at bay). The preceding example relates these characteristics of power-two bounds to the correlations among the predictors; in particular, the example shows that $\widehat{\mathscr{B}}_m$ is even the full $\mathbb{R}^p$ for reasonably small m if the eigenvalues of the Gram matrix are sufficiently large, that is, the correlations among all predictors are weak. However, this scenario is unrealistic in high dimensions: the more predictors there are, the more likely there are some strong correlations, maybe even collinearities. If $p > n$, collinearities are unavoidable altogether, and then $c = 0$ (see 1. in Exercise 1.2), which means that $\widehat{\mathscr{B}}_m \neq \mathbb{R}^p$ irrespective of m.

Nevertheless, the remainder of this section identifies cases where power-two bounds are informative even in high dimensions. These cases require certain predictors to be correlated weakly among themselves and with all other predictors, but they allow those other predictors to be correlated among themselves arbitrarily—which relaxes the assumption in the example that *all* predictors are weakly correlated.

To understand why this relaxation is possible, let us think about connections between prediction and estimation. Having power-two bounds providing good prediction guarantees for an estimator $\widehat{\boldsymbol{\beta}}$ obviously means that (i) $\widehat{\boldsymbol{\beta}}$ is a good predictor of the regression vector, that is, $\|X\boldsymbol{\beta} - X\widehat{\boldsymbol{\beta}}\|_2^2$ is small, and also implies by the form of those bounds that (ii) the set in question contains good prediction surrogates of the regression vector, that is, there are $\boldsymbol{\alpha} \in \widehat{\mathscr{B}}_m$ with $\|X\boldsymbol{\beta} - X\boldsymbol{\alpha}\|_2^2$ small. The first one of these two observations ensures that $\|X\boldsymbol{\beta} - X\boldsymbol{\alpha}\|_2^2 \approx \|X\widehat{\boldsymbol{\beta}} - X\boldsymbol{\alpha}\|_2^2$ is small, which in turn by the definition of $\widehat{\mathcal{B}}_m$ and the second observation, means that $\hbar[\boldsymbol{\alpha} - \widehat{\boldsymbol{\beta}}]$ is small, that is, every such $\boldsymbol{\alpha}$ has a small estimation error (in $\hbar$-loss). Hence, power-two bounds, and especially their involvement of $\widehat{\mathcal{B}}_m$, intertwine prediction and estimation.

However, if there are linear dependencies among the predictors (again, this is always the case when $p > n$), the regression vector $\boldsymbol{\beta}$ itself becomes ambiguous: there are then $\boldsymbol{\gamma} \neq \mathbf{0}_p$ such that $X\boldsymbol{\beta} = X(\boldsymbol{\beta} + \boldsymbol{\gamma})$, and no surrogate $\boldsymbol{\alpha}$ can be close (in Euclidean norm, for example) to all such regression vectors $\boldsymbol{\beta} + \boldsymbol{\gamma}$ simultaneously. Hence, the connection between prediction and estimation outlined above cannot hold in general, and consequently, power-two bounds cannot provide good prediction guarantees in general.

In special cases, however, the outlined connection can hold indeed—even in high dimensions. Recall that the basic requirement for high-dimensional statistics is prior information. In the theories in this section and all of ► Chap. 7, we invoke the most common type of prior information, sparsity, which allows us to sharpen our focus from the entire, typically large, parameter space to a small subspace of it. In fact, we invoke the weaker assumption that the regression vector can be *approximated* by a sparse surrogate: there is an $\boldsymbol{\alpha} \in \mathbb{R}^p$ such that $\boldsymbol{\alpha} \approx \boldsymbol{\beta}$ and $|\text{supp}[\boldsymbol{\alpha}]| \ll n, p$. We call the corresponding linear regression models *approximately sparse*.

approximate sparsity

Approximate sparsity allows us to think in terms of a small set of "relevant" predictors indexed by $\mathcal{S} := \text{supp}[\boldsymbol{\alpha}]$ and a set of "irrelevant" predictors indexed by $\mathcal{S}^{\complement} = \{1, \ldots, p\} \setminus \text{supp}[\boldsymbol{\alpha}]$. If we would know the set $\mathcal{S}$ beforehand, we could replace the original linear regression model by a model of the form

$$\boldsymbol{y} = X_{\mathcal{S}}\boldsymbol{\alpha}_{\mathcal{S}} + \boldsymbol{u}$$

over the much smaller parameter space $\mathbb{R}^{|\mathcal{S}|}$. This implies in particular that approximate sparsity removes any ambiguity from the regression vector as long as the predictors in the *restricted* design matrix $X_{\mathcal{S}} \in \mathbb{R}^{n \times |\mathcal{S}|}$ are linearly independent—compare this to the above example. Moreover, if those predictors are in addition only weakly correlated with all other predictors, we could hope that an estimator can disentangle the relevant predictors (with indexes in $\mathcal{S}$) from the irrelevant predictors (with indexes in $\mathcal{S}^{\complement}$) and, therefore, perform similarly well as if we really knew the true support $\mathcal{S}$ beforehand. Hence, it seems reasonable to expect that accurate prediction implies accurate estimation if the regression model is approximately sparse and the corresponding predictors are only weakly correlated with all other predictors.

The below *compatibility condition* formulates those latter requirements mathematically. Before introducing it, we need to ensure that the prior function is commensurate with the decomposition into relevant and irrelevant predictors.[14]

6

$\mathcal{S}$-decomposability

Definition 6.4.1

$\mathcal{S}$-decomposable Functions Given an index set $\mathcal{S} \subset \{1, \ldots, p\}$ of size $s := |\mathcal{S}|$, a function $\hbar : \mathbb{R}^p \to [0, \infty]$ is called *$\mathcal{S}$-decomposable* if there exist subfunctions[15] $\hbar_{\mathcal{S}} : \mathbb{R}^s \to [0, \infty]$ and $\hbar_{\mathcal{S}^{\complement}} : \mathbb{R}^{p-s} \to [0, \infty]$ such that

$$\hbar[\boldsymbol{a}] = \hbar_{\mathcal{S}}[\boldsymbol{a}_{\mathcal{S}}] + \hbar_{\mathcal{S}^{\complement}}[\boldsymbol{a}_{\mathcal{S}^{\complement}}] \qquad \text{for all } \boldsymbol{a} \in \mathbb{R}^p .$$

Decomposability allows us to separate the prior function into a part that operates on the small number of relevant predictors and a part that operates on all the remaining predictors. A priori, however, it is unknown which predictors are relevant and which ones are irrelevant, so that we typically need to assume $\mathcal{S}$-decomposability for a wide class of index sets $\mathcal{S}$—or even all sets—in practice.

Examples of $\mathcal{S}$-decomposable prior functions include the lasso's ℓ_1-norm (for all $\mathcal{S}$), the group lasso's ℓ_1/ℓ_2-norm (for $\mathcal{S}$ that are compatible with the group structure), and the ridge's squared-ℓ_2-norm (for all $\mathcal{S}$)—see Exercise 6.4.

We can now introduce the compatibility condition.[16]

▪▪ Assumption 6.4.1

compatibility condition

Compatibility Condition Given an index set $\mathcal{S} \subset \{1, \ldots, p\}$, a prior function $\hbar$ that can be decomposed according to Definition 6.4.1, and constants $m \in (0, \infty)$,

$\nu \in (1, \infty)$, we assume that the *compatibility condition* holds:

$$\hbar[\boldsymbol{\delta}] \le \frac{m\|X\boldsymbol{\delta}\|_2}{\sqrt{n}} \qquad \text{for all } \boldsymbol{\delta} \in \mathbb{R}^p : \hbar_{\mathcal{S}^\complement}[\boldsymbol{\delta}_{\mathcal{S}^\complement}] \le \frac{\nu+1}{\nu-1}\hbar_{\mathcal{S}}[\boldsymbol{\delta}_{\mathcal{S}}]\,.$$

We call m the *compatibility constant* for $\mathcal{S}$, $\hbar$.

The requirement on the correlations is captured by the inequality on the left-hand side; the requirement on the sparsity is captured by the inequality in the definition of admissible vectors $\boldsymbol{\delta}$ on the right-hand side. The vectors $\boldsymbol{\delta}$ play the role of $\boldsymbol{\alpha} - \widehat{\boldsymbol{\beta}}$; hence, Assumption 6.4.1 ensures that the correlations in the design are small enough such that the set $\widehat{\mathcal{B}}_m$ of the structural condition contains all vectors $\boldsymbol{\alpha}$ for which $\boldsymbol{\alpha} - \widehat{\boldsymbol{\beta}}$ has limited mass on the set of irrelevant predictors. The following example and Exercise 6.5 illustrate that the compatibility condition indeed relaxes the previous assumption in Example 6.4.1 on the eigenvalues of the Gram matrix in that it allows for arbitrary correlations among irrelevant predictors.

▶ **Example 6.4.2**

Prototypical Cases Where the Compatibility Condition Holds
In this example, we highlight a class of settings where the compatibility condition of Assumption 6.4.1 is met. We consider a set of relevant predictors $\mathcal{S} := \{1, \ldots, s\}$ with $s \in \{1, \ldots, p\}$, a compatibility constant $m \in (0, \infty)$, and a design with scaled Gram matrix of the block-diagonal form

$$\frac{X^\top X}{n} = \begin{pmatrix} A & \\ & B \end{pmatrix},$$

where the smallest eigenvalue of $A \in \mathbb{R}^{s\times s}$ is assumed to be larger or equal to $(2\sqrt{s}\nu/(m(\nu-1)))^2$, and $B \in \mathbb{R}^{(p-s)\times(p-s)}$ is positive semi-definite by construction (see 1. in Exercise 1.2). The lower bound on the eigenvalues of A limits the correlations among the predictors with indexes in $\mathcal{S}$, and the block-diagonal form of the Gram matrix stipulates that those relevant predictors are uncorrelated with all remaining predictors. We then find for all $\boldsymbol{\delta} \in \mathbb{R}^p$

$$\begin{aligned}
\frac{m\|X\boldsymbol{\delta}\|_2}{\sqrt{n}} &= m\sqrt{\frac{\boldsymbol{\delta}^\top X^\top X\boldsymbol{\delta}}{n}} && \text{definition of the } \ell_2\text{-norm}\\
&= m\sqrt{\boldsymbol{\delta}_{\mathcal{S}}{}^\top A\boldsymbol{\delta}_{\mathcal{S}} + \boldsymbol{\delta}_{\mathcal{S}^\complement}{}^\top B\boldsymbol{\delta}_{\mathcal{S}^\complement}} && \text{block-diagonal form of } X^\top X/n\\
&\geq m\sqrt{\left(\frac{2\sqrt{sv}}{m(v-1)}\right)^2 \|\boldsymbol{\delta}_{\mathcal{S}}\|_2^2 + 0} && A\text{'s eigenvalues are equal or larger than } (2\sqrt{sv}/(m(v-1)))^2;\ B \text{ is positive semi-definite}\\
&= \frac{2\sqrt{sv}}{v-1}\|\boldsymbol{\delta}_{\mathcal{S}}\|_2 && \text{consolidating}\\
&\geq \frac{2v}{v-1}\|\boldsymbol{\delta}_{\mathcal{S}}\|_1\,. && \text{Exercise 7.1: first inequality of the first claim with } k=1,\ l=2,\ p=s,\ \boldsymbol{c}=\boldsymbol{\delta}_{\mathcal{S}}
\end{aligned}$$

We now consider as a prior function $\hbar : \boldsymbol{\alpha} \mapsto \|\boldsymbol{\alpha}\|_1$ with decomposition $\hbar_{\mathcal{S}} : \mathbb{R}^s \to \mathbb{R};\ \boldsymbol{\alpha}_{\mathcal{S}} \mapsto \|\boldsymbol{\alpha}_{\mathcal{S}}\|_1$ and $\hbar_{\mathcal{S}^\complement} : \mathbb{R}^{p-s} \to \mathbb{R};\ \boldsymbol{\alpha}_{\mathcal{S}^\complement} \mapsto \|\boldsymbol{\alpha}_{\mathcal{S}^\complement}\|_1$. For every $\boldsymbol{\delta} \in \mathbb{R}^p$ that satisfies $\hbar_{\mathcal{S}^\complement}[\boldsymbol{\delta}_{\mathcal{S}^\complement}] \leq (v+1)\hbar_{\mathcal{S}}[\boldsymbol{\delta}_{\mathcal{S}}]/(v-1)$, that is, $\|\boldsymbol{\delta}_{\mathcal{S}^\complement}\|_1 \leq (v+1)\|\boldsymbol{\delta}_{\mathcal{S}}\|_1/(v-1)$, we then find

$$\begin{aligned}
\hbar[\boldsymbol{\delta}] &= \|\boldsymbol{\delta}\|_1 && \text{choice of } \hbar\\
&= \|\boldsymbol{\delta}_{\mathcal{S}}\|_1 + \|\boldsymbol{\delta}_{\mathcal{S}^\complement}\|_1 && \text{described decomposition of the } \ell_1\text{-norm}\\
&\leq \|\boldsymbol{\delta}_{\mathcal{S}}\|_1 + \frac{v+1}{v-1}\|\boldsymbol{\delta}_{\mathcal{S}}\|_1 && \|\boldsymbol{\delta}_{\mathcal{S}^\complement}\|_1 \leq (v+1)\|\boldsymbol{\delta}_{\mathcal{S}}\|_1/(v-1) \text{ by assumption}\\
&= \frac{2v}{v-1}\|\boldsymbol{\delta}_{\mathcal{S}}\|_1\,. && \text{consolidating}
\end{aligned}$$

Combing the two displays yields

$$\hbar[\boldsymbol{\delta}] \leq \frac{m\|X\boldsymbol{\delta}\|_2}{\sqrt{n}} \qquad \text{for all } \boldsymbol{\delta} \in \mathbb{R}^p : \hbar_{\mathcal{S}^\complement}[\boldsymbol{\delta}_{\mathcal{S}^\complement}] \leq \frac{v+1}{v-1}\hbar_{\mathcal{S}}[\boldsymbol{\delta}_{\mathcal{S}}]\,,$$

as required by Assumption 6.4.1. This means that the compatibility condition is satisfied irrespective of B, that is, irrespective of the correlations among the predictors with indexes in $\mathcal{S}^\complement$. ◀

In the sequel of this section, we show that Assumption 6.4.1 can indeed lead to informative power-two bounds. We first invoke a basic inequality as usual.

Assumption 6.4.2

Generic Basic Inequality Revisited We assume that there is a potentially random quantity $\widehat{w} \in (0, \infty)$ such that the estimator $\widehat{\boldsymbol{\beta}}$ satisfies for all $\boldsymbol{\alpha} \in \mathbb{R}^p$ the basic inequality

$$\|X\boldsymbol{\alpha} - X\widehat{\boldsymbol{\beta}}\|_2^2 \le 2\langle \boldsymbol{y} - X\boldsymbol{\alpha},\, X\widehat{\boldsymbol{\beta}} - X\boldsymbol{\alpha}\rangle + \widehat{w}r\hbar[\boldsymbol{\alpha}] - \widehat{w}r\hbar[\widehat{\boldsymbol{\beta}}]\,.$$

The generic basic inequality here equals the generic basic inequality in Assumption 6.3.1 except that the regression vector $\boldsymbol{\beta}$ is replaced by the general vector $\boldsymbol{\alpha}$ (and accordingly, $\boldsymbol{u} = \boldsymbol{y} - X\boldsymbol{\beta}$ is replaced by $\boldsymbol{y} - X\boldsymbol{\alpha}$). Making these replacements also in ▶ Sect. 6.2 similarly allows one to transfer the sufficient conditions established for the earlier version to the above version. The reason for our switch of focus from $\boldsymbol{\beta}$ to $\boldsymbol{\alpha}$ here is that it will facilitate the inclusion of sparse surrogates of the regression vector in the below treatment of the set $\widehat{\mathcal{B}}_m$.

We finally make assumptions on the prior function.

Assumption 6.4.3

Prior Functions Given an index set $\mathcal{S} \subset \{1, \ldots, p\}$, we impose the following five assumptions on the prior function $\hbar$:

1. $\hbar$ meets the conditions of Theorem 2.4.1 (Hölder inequality).
2. $\hbar$ is $\mathcal{S}$-decomposable according to Definition 6.4.1.
3. $\hbar_{\mathcal{S}}, \hbar_{\mathcal{S}^\complement}$ are positive definite: $\hbar_{\mathcal{S}}, \hbar_{\mathcal{S}^\complement} \ge 0$, $\hbar_{\mathcal{S}}[\boldsymbol{a}] = 0 \Leftrightarrow \boldsymbol{a} = \boldsymbol{0}_s$, and $\hbar_{\mathcal{S}^\complement}[\boldsymbol{a}] = 0 \Leftrightarrow \boldsymbol{a} = \boldsymbol{0}_{p-s}$.
4. $\hbar_{\mathcal{S}}$ satisfies the triangle inequality: $\hbar_{\mathcal{S}}[\boldsymbol{a}+\boldsymbol{b}] \le \hbar_{\mathcal{S}}[\boldsymbol{a}] + \hbar_{\mathcal{S}}[\boldsymbol{b}]$ for all $\boldsymbol{a}, \boldsymbol{b} \in \mathbb{R}^p$.
5. $\hbar_{\mathcal{S}}, \hbar_{\mathcal{S}^\complement}$ are symmetric: $\hbar_{\mathcal{S}}[\boldsymbol{a}] = \hbar_{\mathcal{S}}[-\boldsymbol{a}]$ and $\hbar_{\mathcal{S}^\complement}[\boldsymbol{a}] = \hbar_{\mathcal{S}^\complement}[-\boldsymbol{a}]$ for all $\boldsymbol{a} \in \mathbb{R}^s$, $\boldsymbol{b} \in \mathbb{R}^{p-s}$.

These five properties permit an effective manipulation of the basic inequality, which leads to:

Lemma 6.4.1

Double-Cone Consider an estimator $\widehat{\boldsymbol{\beta}}$ that satisfies the generic basic inequality of Assumption 6.4.2 and whose prior function $\hbar$ satisfies Assumption 6.4.3. Then, it holds for every vector $\boldsymbol{\alpha} \in \mathbb{R}^p$ with $\text{supp}[\boldsymbol{\alpha}] \subset \mathcal{S}$ that

$$\|X\boldsymbol{\alpha} - X\widehat{\boldsymbol{\beta}}\|_2^2 \leq \bigl(2\overline{\hbar}[X^\top(\boldsymbol{y} - X\boldsymbol{\alpha})] + \widehat{wr}\bigr)\hbar_{\mathcal{S}}[\boldsymbol{\alpha}_{\mathcal{S}} - \widehat{\boldsymbol{\beta}}_{\mathcal{S}}] \\ + \bigl(2\overline{\hbar}[X^\top(\boldsymbol{y} - X\boldsymbol{\alpha})] - \widehat{wr}\bigr)\hbar_{\mathcal{S}^\complement}[\boldsymbol{\alpha}_{\mathcal{S}^\complement} - \widehat{\boldsymbol{\beta}}_{\mathcal{S}^\complement}].$$

If additionally $\widehat{wr} \geq 2v\overline{\hbar}[X^\top(\boldsymbol{y} - X\boldsymbol{\alpha})] > 0$ for a constant $v \in (1, \infty)$, we can deduce from the above display that

$$\hbar_{\mathcal{S}^\complement}[\boldsymbol{\alpha}_{\mathcal{S}^\complement} - \widehat{\boldsymbol{\beta}}_{\mathcal{S}^\complement}] \leq \frac{v+1}{v-1}\hbar_{\mathcal{S}}[\boldsymbol{\alpha}_{\mathcal{S}} - \widehat{\boldsymbol{\beta}}_{\mathcal{S}}].$$

An illustration of the second part of the lemma is provided in ◘ Fig. 6.2. The most important consequence of Lemma 6.4.1 is that the error vectors $\boldsymbol{\delta} := \boldsymbol{\alpha} - \widehat{\boldsymbol{\beta}}$ with respect to any sparse surrogate $\boldsymbol{\alpha}$ of the regression vector $\boldsymbol{\beta}$ satisfy the restriction $\hbar_{\mathcal{S}^\complement}[\boldsymbol{\delta}_{\mathcal{S}^\complement}] \leq (v+1)\hbar_{\mathcal{S}}[\boldsymbol{\delta}_{\mathcal{S}}]/(v-1)$ in the compatibility condition of Assumption 6.4.1. In other words, Lemma 6.4.1 and Assumption 6.4.1 taken together guarantee that the set $\widehat{\mathcal{B}}_m$ of the structural condition contains all sparse vectors that describe the data well:

Theorem 6.4.1

$\widehat{\mathcal{B}}_m$ **Under the Compatibility Condition** Under the conditions of Lemma 6.4.1 (double-cone) and Assumption 6.4.1 (compatibility condition), it holds that

$$\widehat{\mathcal{B}}_m \supset \bigl\{\boldsymbol{\alpha} \in \mathbb{R}^p : \text{supp}[\boldsymbol{\alpha}] \subset \mathcal{S},\ \widehat{wr} \geq 2v\overline{\hbar}[X^\top(\boldsymbol{y}-X\boldsymbol{\alpha})] > 0\bigr\}.$$

This theorem summarizes the above result and is the main result of this section. We will exploit it below in deriving effective power-two bounds.

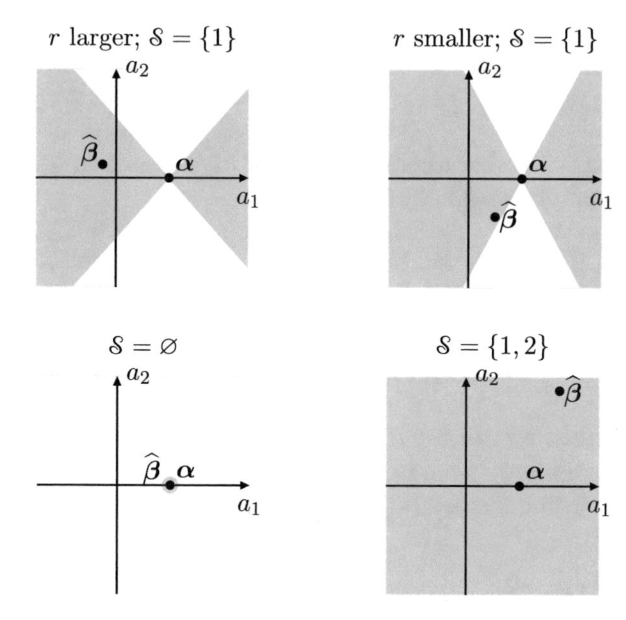

Fig. 6.2 Illustrations of the second part of Lemma 6.4.1 for $p = 2$ and $\hbar$ the ℓ_1-norm from the perspective of the estimator $\widehat{\boldsymbol{\beta}}$. The second part of Lemma 6.4.1 guarantees that the estimator $\widehat{\boldsymbol{\beta}}$ is in an infinite "double-cone" (blue area, *not* white area) with apex $\boldsymbol{\alpha}$:

$$\widehat{\boldsymbol{\beta}} \in \left\{ \boldsymbol{a} \in \mathbb{R}^p \; : \; \|\boldsymbol{\alpha}_{\mathcal{S}^\complement} - \boldsymbol{a}_{\mathcal{S}^\complement}\|_1 \; \le \; \frac{v+1}{v-1}\|\boldsymbol{\alpha}_{\mathcal{S}} - \boldsymbol{a}_{\mathcal{S}}\|_1 \right\}.$$

The smaller this double-cone, the more control we have over the estimator. The size of the cone is determined by the tuning parameter r and the set $\mathcal{S}$: The smaller the tuning parameter r, the smaller values for v need to be chosen, and therefore, the larger the cone (compare the top left panel to the top right panel). The larger $\mathcal{S}$, the more dimensions are covered by $\hbar_{\mathcal{S}}$, and therefore, the larger the cone (compare the bottom left panel to the bottom right panel)

Proof of Lemma 6.4.1 The proof manipulates the basic inequality of Assumption 6.4.2 by exploiting the assumed properties of the prior function.

The inner product term of the basic inequality can be bounded through the Hölder inequality (cf. 1. in Assumption 6.4.3)

$$\begin{aligned} &2\langle \boldsymbol{y} - X\boldsymbol{\alpha},\, X\widehat{\boldsymbol{\beta}} - X\boldsymbol{\alpha}\rangle \\ &= 2\langle X^\top(\boldsymbol{y} - X\boldsymbol{\alpha}),\, \widehat{\boldsymbol{\beta}} - \boldsymbol{\alpha}\rangle \quad \text{property (B.1) of transposition} \\ &\le 2\overline{\hbar}[X^\top(\boldsymbol{y} - X\boldsymbol{\alpha})]\hbar[\widehat{\boldsymbol{\beta}} - \boldsymbol{\alpha}]\,. \qquad \text{Hölder inequality (2.5)} \end{aligned}$$

Plugging this into the basic inequality yields

$$\|X\boldsymbol{\alpha} - X\widehat{\boldsymbol{\beta}}\|_2^2 \leq 2\overline{\hbar}[X^\top(y - X\boldsymbol{\alpha})]\hbar[\widehat{\boldsymbol{\beta}} - \boldsymbol{\alpha}] + \widehat{wr}\hbar[\boldsymbol{\alpha}] - \widehat{wr}\hbar[\widehat{\boldsymbol{\beta}}]\,.$$

Next, with the decomposability of $\hbar$ assumed in 2. of Assumption 6.4.3, we find

$$\begin{aligned}
&\|X\boldsymbol{\alpha} - X\widehat{\boldsymbol{\beta}}\|_2^2 \\
&\leq 2\overline{\hbar}[X^\top(y - X\boldsymbol{\alpha})]\hbar_{\mathcal{S}}[\widehat{\boldsymbol{\beta}}_{\mathcal{S}} - \boldsymbol{\alpha}_{\mathcal{S}}] + 2\overline{\hbar}[X^\top(y - X\boldsymbol{\alpha})]\hbar_{\mathcal{S}^\complement}[\widehat{\boldsymbol{\beta}}_{\mathcal{S}^\complement} - \boldsymbol{\alpha}_{\mathcal{S}^\complement}] \\
&\qquad + \widehat{wr}\hbar_{\mathcal{S}}[\boldsymbol{\alpha}_{\mathcal{S}}] + \widehat{wr}\hbar_{\mathcal{S}^\complement}[\boldsymbol{\alpha}_{\mathcal{S}^\complement}] - \widehat{wr}\hbar_{\mathcal{S}}[\widehat{\boldsymbol{\beta}}_{\mathcal{S}}] - \widehat{wr}\hbar_{\mathcal{S}^\complement}[\widehat{\boldsymbol{\beta}}_{\mathcal{S}^\complement}]\,.
\end{aligned}$$

Further, we can use $\boldsymbol{\alpha}_{\mathcal{S}^\complement} = \mathbf{0}_{|\mathcal{S}^\complement|}$ (since $\operatorname{supp}[\boldsymbol{\alpha}] \subset \mathcal{S}$ by assumption) to modify the last term on the bottom line and to find that $\hbar_{\mathcal{S}^\complement}[\boldsymbol{\alpha}_{\mathcal{S}^\complement}] = 0$ (by 3. of Assumption 6.4.3):

$$\begin{aligned}
&\|X\boldsymbol{\alpha} - X\widehat{\boldsymbol{\beta}}\|_2^2 \\
&\leq 2\overline{\hbar}[X^\top(y - X\boldsymbol{\alpha})]\hbar_{\mathcal{S}}[\widehat{\boldsymbol{\beta}}_{\mathcal{S}} - \boldsymbol{\alpha}_{\mathcal{S}}] + 2\overline{\hbar}[X^\top(y - X\boldsymbol{\alpha})]\hbar_{\mathcal{S}^\complement}[\widehat{\boldsymbol{\beta}}_{\mathcal{S}^\complement} - \boldsymbol{\alpha}_{\mathcal{S}^\complement}] \\
&\qquad + \widehat{wr}\hbar_{\mathcal{S}}[\boldsymbol{\alpha}_{\mathcal{S}}] - \widehat{wr}\hbar_{\mathcal{S}}[\widehat{\boldsymbol{\beta}}_{\mathcal{S}}] - \widehat{wr}\hbar_{\mathcal{S}^\complement}[\widehat{\boldsymbol{\beta}}_{\mathcal{S}^\complement} - \boldsymbol{\alpha}_{\mathcal{S}^\complement}]\,.
\end{aligned}$$

Moreover, we can use the triangle inequality for $\hbar_{\mathcal{S}}$ (see 4. of Assumption 6.4.3) to combine the first and third terms on the bottom line to derive

$$\begin{aligned}
&\|X\boldsymbol{\alpha} - X\widehat{\boldsymbol{\beta}}\|_2^2 \\
&\leq 2\overline{\hbar}[X^\top(y - X\boldsymbol{\alpha})]\hbar_{\mathcal{S}}[\widehat{\boldsymbol{\beta}}_{\mathcal{S}} - \boldsymbol{\alpha}_{\mathcal{S}}] + 2\overline{\hbar}[X^\top(y - X\boldsymbol{\alpha})]\hbar_{\mathcal{S}^\complement}[\widehat{\boldsymbol{\beta}}_{\mathcal{S}^\complement} - \boldsymbol{\alpha}_{\mathcal{S}^\complement}] \\
&\qquad + \widehat{wr}\hbar_{\mathcal{S}}[\boldsymbol{\alpha}_{\mathcal{S}} - \widehat{\boldsymbol{\beta}}_{\mathcal{S}}] - \widehat{wr}\hbar_{\mathcal{S}^\complement}[\widehat{\boldsymbol{\beta}}_{\mathcal{S}^\complement} - \boldsymbol{\alpha}_{\mathcal{S}^\complement}]\,.
\end{aligned}$$

We can finally use the assumed symmetry of $\hbar_{\mathcal{S}}$ and $\hbar_{\mathcal{S}^\complement}$ (see 5. of Assumption 6.4.3) and summarize the terms to

$$\begin{aligned}
\|X\boldsymbol{\alpha} - X\widehat{\boldsymbol{\beta}}\|_2^2 &\leq \big(2\overline{\hbar}[X^\top(y - X\boldsymbol{\alpha})] + \widehat{wr}\big)\hbar_{\mathcal{S}}[\boldsymbol{\alpha}_{\mathcal{S}} - \widehat{\boldsymbol{\beta}}_{\mathcal{S}}] \\
&\quad + \big(2\overline{\hbar}[X^\top(y - X\boldsymbol{\alpha})] - \widehat{wr}\big)\hbar_{\mathcal{S}^\complement}[\boldsymbol{\alpha}_{\mathcal{S}^\complement} - \widehat{\boldsymbol{\beta}}_{\mathcal{S}^\complement}]\,,
\end{aligned}$$

as claimed in the first part of the lemma.

For the second part, we rearrange the above result and use the fact that $\|X\boldsymbol{\alpha} - X\widehat{\boldsymbol{\beta}}\|_2^2 \geq 0$ by the definition of the ℓ_2-norm:

$$\begin{aligned}\big(\widehat{wr} - 2\overline{\hbar}[X^\top(\boldsymbol{y} - X\boldsymbol{\alpha})]\big)\hbar_{\mathcal{S}^\complement}[\boldsymbol{\alpha}_{\mathcal{S}^\complement} - \widehat{\boldsymbol{\beta}}_{\mathcal{S}^\complement}] \\ \leq \big(2\overline{\hbar}[X^\top(\boldsymbol{y} - X\boldsymbol{\alpha})] + \widehat{wr}\big)\hbar_{\mathcal{S}}[\boldsymbol{\alpha}_{\mathcal{S}} - \widehat{\boldsymbol{\beta}}_{\mathcal{S}}]\,.\end{aligned}$$

Now, if $\widehat{wr} \geq 2v\overline{\hbar}[X^\top(\boldsymbol{y} - X\boldsymbol{\alpha})]$, we obtain (recall the non-negativity of $\hbar_{\mathcal{S}}$ and $\hbar_{\mathcal{S}^\complement}$ that follows from 3. of Assumption 6.4.3)

$$\Big(1 - \frac{1}{v}\Big)\widehat{wr}\hbar_{\mathcal{S}^\complement}[\boldsymbol{\alpha}_{\mathcal{S}^\complement} - \widehat{\boldsymbol{\beta}}_{\mathcal{S}^\complement}] \leq \Big(1 + \frac{1}{v}\Big)\widehat{wr}\hbar_{\mathcal{S}}[\boldsymbol{\alpha}_{\mathcal{S}} - \widehat{\boldsymbol{\beta}}_{\mathcal{S}}]\,.$$

Since $1/v < 1$ by assumption on v, we then find

$$\begin{aligned}\widehat{wr}\hbar_{\mathcal{S}^\complement}[\boldsymbol{\alpha}_{\mathcal{S}^\complement} - \widehat{\boldsymbol{\beta}}_{\mathcal{S}^\complement}] &\leq \frac{1 + \frac{1}{v}}{1 - \frac{1}{v}}\widehat{wr}\hbar_{\mathcal{S}}[\boldsymbol{\alpha}_{\mathcal{S}} - \widehat{\boldsymbol{\beta}}_{\mathcal{S}}] \\ &= \frac{v + 1}{v - 1}\widehat{wr}\hbar_{\mathcal{S}}[\boldsymbol{\alpha}_{\mathcal{S}} - \widehat{\boldsymbol{\beta}}_{\mathcal{S}}]\,,\end{aligned}$$

from which the second claim can be derived by dividing through $\widehat{wr} > 0$. □

We now use the compatibility condition together with the double-cone property of high-dimensional estimators to rewrite the power-two bounds of the previous section.

Theorem 6.4.2

Power-Two Bounds Revisited Assume that the estimator $\widehat{\boldsymbol{\beta}}$ of (6.1) satisfies the conditions of Theorem 6.3.2 (power-two bounds) and Lemma 6.4.1 (double-cone). Assume further that the design is weakly correlated in the sense that:

1. The estimator's prior function $\hbar$ satisfies Assumption 6.4.1 (compatibility condition) for an index set $\mathcal{S} \subset \{1, \ldots, p\}$ and constants $m \in (0, \infty)$, $v \in (1, \infty)$.

Assume finally that the model is approximately sparse in the sense that there is a vector $\boldsymbol{\alpha} \in \mathbb{R}^p$ with

2. $\operatorname{supp}[\boldsymbol{\alpha}] \subset \mathcal{S}$ and $\widehat{w}r \geq 2v\overline{\hbar}[X^\top(\boldsymbol{y} - X\boldsymbol{\alpha})] > 0$.
3. $\|X\boldsymbol{\beta} - X\boldsymbol{\alpha}\|_2^2 \leq d\widehat{w}^2 r^2/n$ for a (hopefully small) $d \in [0, \infty]$.

Then,

$$\|X\boldsymbol{\beta} - X\widehat{\boldsymbol{\beta}}\|_2^2 \leq \left(2d + \frac{9m^2(v+1)^2}{2v^2}\right)\frac{\widehat{w}^2 r^2}{n}.$$

This result replaces the minimum over the set $\widehat{\mathcal{B}}_m$ in Theorem 6.3.2 by a more explicit bound. This new bound is essentially a factor times $\widehat{w}^2 r^2/n$, which confirms that the scaled prediction errors $\|X\boldsymbol{\beta} - X\widehat{\boldsymbol{\beta}}\|_2^2/n$ of, say, the lasso/square-root lasso with optimal tuning are at most of order $\sigma \log[p]/n$ (cf. Example 6.3.3) in approximately sparse and weakly correlated regression with Gauss-distributed noise.

Theorem 6.4.2 can be proved in three steps: First, Theorem 6.4.1 implies that $\boldsymbol{\alpha} \in \widehat{\mathcal{B}}_m$. Then, the second part of Theorem 6.3.2 with $b = 2$ and $\boldsymbol{\beta}$ replaced by $\boldsymbol{\alpha}$ (cf. the comments after Assumption 6.4.2) yields a bound for $\|X\boldsymbol{\alpha} - X\widehat{\boldsymbol{\beta}}\|_2^2$. Finally, Lemma B.1.1 ($\|\boldsymbol{a} + \boldsymbol{b}\|_2^2 \leq 2\|\boldsymbol{a}\|_2^2 + 2\|\boldsymbol{b}\|_2^2$) allows one to transfer this bound into a bound for $\|X\boldsymbol{\beta} - X\widehat{\boldsymbol{\beta}}\|_2^2$. We leave the details to the reader.

The major limitation of the above result is the compatibility condition, which stipulates approximate sparsity and weak correlations. Approximate sparsity and weak correlations will also be essential to the development of estimation bounds in the following chapter; in particular, we will show there that the assumptions of Theorem 6.4.2 guarantee estimation accuracy as well. Power-one bounds, in stark contrast, refer to prediction only, which reduce the requirements on sparsity and avoid assumptions on the correlation structure altogether.

6.5 Exercises

6.5.1 Exercises for ▸ Sect. 6.2

Exercise 6.1 ♦ In this exercise, we compare the first-order and second-order basic inequalities in Lemmas 6.2.1

and 6.2.2, respectively. We assume that the conditions of both lemmas are satisfied, that is, the link function is the identity $\mathcal{g} : a \mapsto a$ (cf. Lemma 6.2.1) and the prior function $\mathcal{h}$ is convex (cf. Lemma 6.2.2).

1. Show that the two bounds coincide under the mentioned conditions.
2. Show that Lemma 6.2.1 implies

$$\|X\boldsymbol{\beta} - X\widehat{\boldsymbol{\beta}}\|_2^2 \leq 2\langle \boldsymbol{u},\, X\widehat{\boldsymbol{\beta}} - X\boldsymbol{\beta}\rangle + r\mathcal{h}[\boldsymbol{\beta}] - r\mathcal{h}[\widehat{\boldsymbol{\beta}}]\,,$$

while a slight modification of the proof of Lemma 6.2.2 yields

$$\|X\boldsymbol{\beta} - X\widehat{\boldsymbol{\beta}}\|_2^2 \leq \frac{1}{2}\big(2\langle \boldsymbol{u},\, X\widehat{\boldsymbol{\beta}} - X\boldsymbol{\beta}\rangle + r\mathcal{h}[\boldsymbol{\beta}] - r\mathcal{h}[\widehat{\boldsymbol{\beta}}]\big)\,.$$

This exercise shows that the second-order approach can improve on the first-order approach by a factor 2 if the conditions of both approaches are met and $\boldsymbol{\alpha} = \boldsymbol{\beta}$ (see Claim 2), but the exercise also highlights once more that the two approaches differ mainly in their conditions—identity link function versus convex prior function—rather than in their resulting bounds (see Claim 1).

6.5.2 Exercises for ► Sect. 6.3

Exercise 6.2 ◊◊ In this exercise, we discuss the prior function of the non-negative lasso introduced in Example 6.3.1.

1. Show that the prior function of the non-negative lasso meets 1. and 3. of Assumption 6.3.2.
2. Generalize all bounds of ► Sect. 6.3 such that 2. of Assumption 6.3.2 is not required.
3. Compute the dual function of the non-negative lasso's prior function.
4. Use 3. to specify the bounds derived in 2. for the non-negative lasso.

This exercise highlights the fact that the techniques of ► Sect. 6.3 do not require the prior function to be symmetric or even a norm.

Exercise 6.3 ◊◊ In this exercise, we tailor the probability bounds of ► Sect. 6.3 to the group-lasso estimator (2.3) and the square-root group-lasso estimator. We assume that the groups form a partition of $\{1, \ldots, p\}$, that is, $\cup_{j=1}^k \mathcal{A}_j = \{1, \ldots, p\}$, $\mathcal{A}_j \neq \varnothing$ for all j, and $\mathcal{A}_i \cap \mathcal{A}_j = \varnothing$ for all $i \neq j$.

1. Establish an analog of Example 6.3.2 for the group lasso.
2. Establish an analog of Example 6.3.3 for the group lasso.
3. Compare the group-lasso bounds to the square-root lasso bounds.
4. Repeat 1.–3. for the square-root group-lasso estimator of the form (cf. (2.9))

$$\widehat{\boldsymbol{\beta}}_{\sqrt{\text{group}}} \in \operatorname*{arg\,min}_{\boldsymbol{\alpha} \in \mathbb{R}^p} \left\{ \|\boldsymbol{y} - X\boldsymbol{\alpha}\|_2 + r \sum_{j=1}^{k} \|\boldsymbol{\alpha}_{\mathcal{A}_j}\|_2 \right\}.$$

6.5.3 Exercises for ▶ Sect. 6.4

Exercise 6.4 ♦♦ In this exercise, we study the $\mathcal{S}$-decomposability of Definition 6.4.1 in the context of the group lasso (2.3) (or equivalently the square-root group lasso (2.9)). The corresponding prior function is

$$\hbar : \boldsymbol{a} \mapsto \sum_{j=1}^{k} \|\boldsymbol{a}_{\mathcal{A}_j}\|_2$$

for a fixed integer $k \in \{1, \ldots, p\}$ and a fixed partition $\mathcal{A}_1, \ldots, \mathcal{A}_k$ of $\{1, \ldots, p\}$. As always, $\boldsymbol{a}_{\mathcal{A}_j} \in \mathbb{R}^{|\mathcal{A}_j|}$ summarizes the coordinates of $\boldsymbol{a}$ that have indexes in $\mathcal{A}_j$.

1. Show first that in general, a function is $\mathcal{S}$-decomposable if and only if it is $\mathcal{S}^{\complement}$-decomposable.
2. Show that the prior function $\boldsymbol{a} \mapsto \|\boldsymbol{a}\|_2$ of the edr estimator is a special case of the above prior function.
3. Show that the prior function of the edr estimator is $\mathcal{S}$-decomposable if and only if $\mathcal{S} = \varnothing$ or $\mathcal{S} = \{1, \ldots, p\}$. Show that, in contrast, the prior function $\boldsymbol{a} \mapsto \|\boldsymbol{a}\|_2^2$ of the ridge estimator is decomposable for all $\mathcal{S} \subset \{1, \ldots, p\}$.
4. Show that the prior function $\boldsymbol{a} \mapsto \|\boldsymbol{a}\|_1$ of the lasso estimator is a special case of the above prior function.
5. Show that the prior function of the lasso estimator is $\mathcal{S}$-decomposable for all $\mathcal{S} \subset \{1, \ldots, p\}$.

6. Show that in general, if the above prior function is indeed $\mathcal{S}$-decomposable, the corresponding subfunctions are

$$\hbar_{\mathcal{S}} : \boldsymbol{a}_{\mathcal{S}} \mapsto \sum_{j=1}^{k} \|\boldsymbol{a}_{\mathcal{A}_j \cap \mathcal{S}}\|_2 \quad \text{and} \quad \hbar_{\mathcal{S}^{\complement}} : \boldsymbol{a}_{\mathcal{S}^{\complement}} \mapsto \sum_{j=1}^{k} \|\boldsymbol{a}_{\mathcal{A}_j \cap \mathcal{S}^{\complement}}\|_2 .$$

   Conclude that the above prior function is $\mathcal{S}$-decomposable if and only if for each $j \in \{1, \ldots, k\}$, it holds that either $\mathcal{A}_j \subset \mathcal{S}$ or $\mathcal{A}_j \subset \mathcal{S}^{\complement}$.

We learn in particular that the prior function of the lasso is decomposable for all $\mathcal{S}$, while $\mathcal{S}$ must be commensurate with the group structure in the general case of the group lasso.

Exercise 6.5 ♦♦ In this exercise, we study the compatibility condition of Assumption 6.4.1 in a simple example. We consider the following (scaled) design matrix and the corresponding Gram matrix:

$$\frac{X}{\sqrt{n}} = \begin{pmatrix} 1 & \frac{1}{2} & 0 & 0 \\ 0 & \frac{\sqrt{3}}{2} & 0 & 0 \\ 0 & 0 & 1 & 1 \end{pmatrix} \quad \Rightarrow \quad \frac{X^{\top}X}{n} = \begin{pmatrix} 1 & \frac{1}{2} & 0 & 0 \\ \frac{1}{2} & 1 & 0 & 0 \\ 0 & 0 & 1 & 1 \\ 0 & 0 & 1 & 1 \end{pmatrix} .$$

This means that the first and second predictors are somewhat correlated with each other, the third and fourth predictors are perfectly correlated with each other, and the first and second predictors are uncorrelated with the third and fourth predictors.

We assume that the prior function $\hbar$ is the lasso estimator's ℓ_1-norm. Then, since norms are positive definite, the inequality in Assumption 6.4.1 is clearly satisfied for $\boldsymbol{\delta} = \mathbf{0}_4$, so that we can focus on checking that inequality on the set

$$\mathscr{C} := \left\{ \boldsymbol{\delta} \in \mathbb{R}^4 \ : \ \|\boldsymbol{\delta}_{\mathcal{S}^{\complement}}\|_1 \leq \frac{v+1}{v-1} \|\boldsymbol{\delta}_{\mathcal{S}}\|_1 \right\} \setminus \{\mathbf{0}_4\} .$$

Show the following:

1. Show that for every non-empty set $\mathcal{S} \subset \{1, 2, 3, 4\}$, it holds that

$$\min_{\boldsymbol{\delta} \in \mathscr{C}} \frac{\|X\boldsymbol{\delta}\|_2^2}{n\|\boldsymbol{\delta}\|_1^2} = \min_{\boldsymbol{\delta} \in \mathscr{C}} \frac{\|\boldsymbol{\delta}_{\{1,2\}}\|_1^2}{4\|\boldsymbol{\delta}\|_1^2} .$$

   This identity is the basis for the three following tasks.

2. Conclude from 1. that for $\mathcal{S} = \{1\}$ and $\mathcal{S} = \{2\}$, it holds that

$$\min_{\boldsymbol{\delta} \in \mathcal{C}} \frac{\|X\boldsymbol{\delta}\|_2^2}{n\|\boldsymbol{\delta}\|_1^2} = \frac{(v-1)^2}{16v^2}.$$

This means that the compatibility condition with those sets is satisfied if and only if $m \in [4v/(v-1), \infty)$.

3. Conclude from 1. that for $\mathcal{S} = \{1, 2\}$, it also holds that

$$\min_{\boldsymbol{\delta} \in \mathcal{C}} \frac{\|X\boldsymbol{\delta}\|_2^2}{n\|\boldsymbol{\delta}\|_1^2} = \frac{(v-1)^2}{16v^2}.$$

This means that the compatibility condition with this set is satisfied again if and only if $m \in [4v/(v-1), \infty)$.

4. Conclude from 1. that if $\{3\} \subset \mathcal{S}$ or $\{4\} \subset \mathcal{S}$, it holds that

$$\min_{\boldsymbol{\delta} \in \mathcal{C}} \frac{\|X\boldsymbol{\delta}\|_2^2}{n\|\boldsymbol{\delta}\|_1^2} = 0.$$

This means that the compatibility condition with every such set cannot be satisfied.

The exercise illustrates that the compatibility constant limits correlations (i) among relevant predictors (that is, between any two predictors with indexes in $\mathcal{S}$) and (ii) between relevant and irrelevant predictors (that is, between any predictor with index in $\mathcal{S}$ and any predictor with index in $\mathcal{S}^{\complement}$), but it allows for correlations among irrelevant predictors (that is, between any two predictors with indexes in $\mathcal{S}^{\complement}$).

6.6 Notes and References

1 The term "prediction" is sometimes used differently in the literature: for example, prediction sometimes refers to the data fit $\|\boldsymbol{y} - X\widehat{\boldsymbol{\beta}}\|_2^2$ or to the prediction of an outcome $y_{n+1} \in \mathbb{R}$ for a *new* vector $\boldsymbol{x}_{n+1} \in \mathbb{R}^p$.

2 The terms "power-one/power-two" relate to the tuning parameters. Lederer et al. (2019), in contrast, speak of *sparsity bounds* and *penalty bounds*, respectively, since the constant m is connected to sparsity (see our ▶ Sect. 6.4) and $\|\boldsymbol{\alpha}\|_1$ to the prior term—which is also called penalty.

3 Since the effective noise $2\|X^\top \boldsymbol{u}\|_\infty$ is unobserved and usually even has an unknown distribution, this is not a practical proposal. For tuning-parameter calibration in practice, refer to ► Chap. 4.
4 This is true under minimal assumptions: see Lederer et al. (2019), especially their Lemma A.3 on p. 1238.
5 The square-root lasso has been introduced in Belloni et al. (2011, Definition (8) on p. 792); the closely related *scaled lasso* has been introduced in Sun and Zhang (2012, (3), (4), and (5) on p. 881) based on work by Antoniadis (2010), Städler et al. (2010), Sun and Zhang (2010). Further theoretical guarantees and algorithms, as well as the version (2.9) with grouped variables, have been established in Bunea et al. (2014).
6 The proof of the second-order basic inequality is along the lines of Lederer et al. (2019, Proof of Theorem 2.1 on pp. 1249ff). That paper also discusses the factor two (see 2.in Exercise 6.1) that can be different between the two approaches, and it discusses different proof techniques more generally.
7 Finite sample guarantees in high-dimensional statistics are often called *oracle inequalities* because they involve quantities (such as $\boldsymbol{\beta}$ or aspects of it) that in practice would be known only by an *oracle*, that is, “a person (such as a priestess of ancient Greece) through whom a deity is believed to speak” (Merriam-Webster.com, 2019).
8 Our proofs in this section, as well as in the following sections, do not require that the estimators be of the form (6.1): in principle, one can take any estimator that satisfies Assumption 6.3.1 for a function $\hbar$ that satisfies (a subset of) the conditions in Assumption 6.3.2. However, it is easier to follow the derivations when one has the specific type of estimators (6.1) in mind.
9 This is the Lagrange version of Efron et al. (2004, Program (3.18) on p. 421). While Efron et al. (2004) call the estimator *positive lasso*, we use the name non-negative lasso to clarify that the prior function is infinite only if a parameter value is *strictly* smaller than zero. Refer to Meinshausen (2013) and references therein for more information about regression with non-negative parameters.
10 One can also generalize the second-order basic inequality in Lemma 6.2.2 such that it applies to the non-negative lasso by generalizing the notion of convexity in Definition 2.5.1 from the real line to the extended real line. We omit the details and refer to Hiriart-Urruty and Lemaréchal (2004) for background information on convexity.
11 The existence of such a tuning parameter is proved in Lederer et al. (2019, Lemma 2.1 on p. 1230).
12 In fact, the tuning is the only difference between the lasso and the square-root lasso: one can show that any lasso estimator for a given tuning parameter equals a square-root lasso estimator for some (usually different) tuning parameter and vice versa—we omit the details. A heuristic concept for the square-root lasso’s differences to the lasso is established in Lederer and Müller (2015, p. 2730). That concept is also developed further into the *trex estimator*, which attempts ℓ_1-regularized regression without any tuning parameters. Further details on that estimator can be found in Bien et al. (2018a,b).

13 This is why power-one bounds are often called *slow-rate bounds* and power-two bounds *fast-rate bounds*. However, this naming is misleading: for example, Dalalyan et al. (2017, Chapter 5 on pp. 562ff) develop refined power-one prediction bounds for the lasso that have an $1/n$-rate under certain conditions. Since the square-root lasso and the lasso differ only in the tuning, these bounds also apply to the square-root lasso. In general, the issue of how prediction performances depend on the design of the regression model is intricate: this was pointed out by Hebiri and Lederer (2013) and van de Geer and Lederer (2013) and studied in depth in that mentioned paper by Dalalyan et al. (2017).

14 Decomposability has been discussed in Negahban et al. (2012, Section 2.2) and Wainwright (2014, Section 3.2). Our corresponding Definition 6.4.1 is a special case of Negahban et al. (2012, Definition 1 on p. 4) for $\mathcal{M} := \overline{\mathcal{M}} := \{\boldsymbol{\alpha} \in \mathbb{R}^p : \operatorname{supp}[\boldsymbol{\alpha}] \subset \mathcal{S}\}$ and of Wainwright (2014, Equation (22) on p. 244) for $\mathcal{M} := \{\boldsymbol{\alpha} \in \mathbb{R}^p : \operatorname{supp}[\boldsymbol{\alpha}] \subset \mathcal{S}\}$.

15 If $\mathcal{S} = \varnothing$, we set $\hbar_{\mathcal{S}} \equiv 0$ and $\hbar_{\mathcal{S}^\complement} \equiv \hbar$; the set of admissible $\boldsymbol{\delta}$ in the display of Assumption 6.4.1 is then $\{\boldsymbol{\delta} : \hbar[\boldsymbol{\delta}] \leq 0\}$. Similarly, if $\mathcal{S} = \{1, \ldots, p\}$, we set $\hbar_{\mathcal{S}} \equiv \hbar$ and $\hbar_{\mathcal{S}^\complement} \equiv 0$; the set of admissible $\boldsymbol{\delta}$ in the display of Assumption 6.4.1 is then $\{\boldsymbol{\delta} : \hbar[\boldsymbol{\delta}] \geq 0\}$.

16 Our compatibility condition is a modified and extended version of the one introduced in van de Geer (2007, Section 2.1). The closely related *restricted eigenvalue condition* was introduced in Bickel et al. (2009, p. 1710). Comparisons among different conditions for the lasso can be found in van de Geer and Bühlmann (2009). A geometric interpretation of compatibility constants and relationships to entropy can be found in van de Geer and Lederer (2013). A generalization of the restricted eigenvalue beyond regression-type data is *restricted strong convexity*, introduced and discussed in Negahban et al. (2012, Section 2.4) and Wainwright (2014, Section 3.1). A refined version of compatibility constants and ideas for how to obtain bounds for them in practice are discussed in Dalalyan et al. (2017, Equation (10) on p. 557 and Appendix on pp. 578ff).

Theory II: Estimation and Support Recovery

Contents

J. Lederer, *Fundamentals of High-Dimensional Statistics*, Springer Texts in Statistics,
https://doi.org/10.1007/978-3-030-73792-4_7

The regression model (1.1) in ▶ Sect. 1.1 relates blood levels of a biomarker with characteristics of the subjects' genomes. Corresponding data allow us to analyze this relationship from a variety of different perspectives: For example, we can study how the biomarker levels depend on the *ensemble of genes*, we can study the role of each *individual gene*, or we can study *which genes* influence the biomarker levels in the first place. Summarizing the data in the vector-valued Eq. (1.2), the three different perspectives concern the three different quantities $X\boldsymbol{\beta}$; $\boldsymbol{\beta}$; and $\text{supp}[\boldsymbol{\beta}]$, respectively, which motivate the prediction error $\|X\boldsymbol{\beta} - X\widehat{\boldsymbol{\beta}}\|_2^2$, estimation errors such as $\|\boldsymbol{\beta} - \widehat{\boldsymbol{\beta}}\|_2$, and support recovery errors such as false negatives $|\{j \in \{1, \ldots, p\} : \beta_j \neq 0, \widehat{\beta}_j = 0\}|$, respectively. The prediction error is the focus of the previous chapter; in this chapter, we develop theory in terms of estimation and support recovery errors. The statistical framework remains the same: We consider the linear regression model (2.1) and the regularized least-squares estimators (6.1).

7.1 Overview

The power-one bounds in ▶ Sect. 6.3 illustrate the fact that prediction is almost always possible. The reason is that prediction views the regression vector through the lens of the design matrix, which essentially reduces the complexity of the problem. Estimation and support recovery, in contrast, concern the regression vector directly. All theories in this chapter, therefore, hinge on strict conditions, namely sparsity and weak correlations.

For an illustration, consider again the genome application from ▶ Sect. 1.1. The predictors $\boldsymbol{x}_4, \boldsymbol{x}_6, \boldsymbol{x}_8 \in \{0, 1, \ldots\}^{\times 7}$ that contain the copy numbers of the fourth, sixth, and eighth gene in the seven subjects are linearly dependent: $\boldsymbol{x}_4 = \boldsymbol{x}_6 + \boldsymbol{x}_8$. Therefore, the "true" regression vector $\boldsymbol{\beta}$ and every alternate $\widetilde{\boldsymbol{\beta}}$ with $\widetilde{\beta}_4 + \widetilde{\beta}_6 = \beta_4 + \beta_6$, $\widetilde{\beta}_4 + \widetilde{\beta}_8 = \beta_4 + \beta_8$, and $\widetilde{\beta}_j = \beta_j$ for $j \notin \{4, 6, 8\}$ form the same data-generating process: $\boldsymbol{y} = X\boldsymbol{\beta} + \boldsymbol{u} = X\widetilde{\boldsymbol{\beta}} + \boldsymbol{u}$. Simply put, the correlations among the predictors make the regression vector ill-defined. Since $X\boldsymbol{\beta} = X\widetilde{\boldsymbol{\beta}}$ still holds, this fuzziness in the modeling is irrelevant for prediction, but it precludes estimation and support recovery. To make estimation and support recovery possible, we need to impose additional assumptions such as sparsity: Assume that $|\text{supp}[\boldsymbol{\beta}]| \leq 1$;

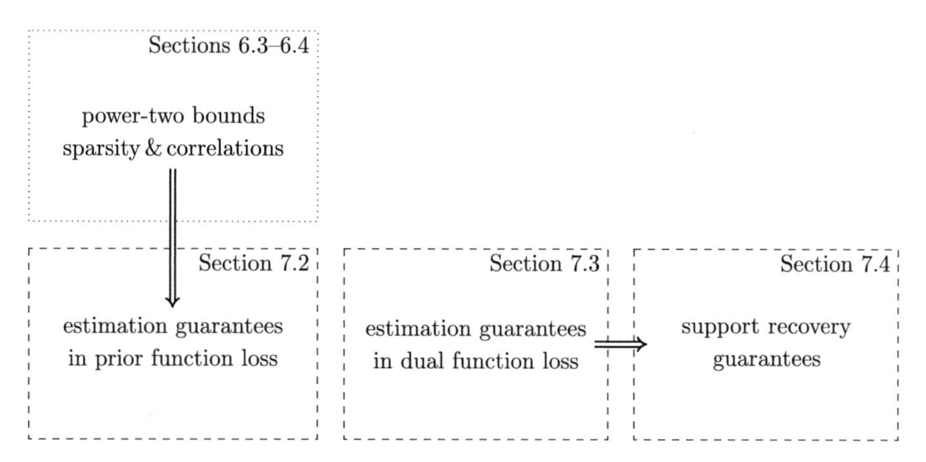

Fig. 7.1 Overview of this chapter. In ▶ Sect. 7.2, we transform the prediction guarantees of ▶ Sects. 6.3 and 6.4 into estimation guarantees in $\hbar$-loss. In ▶ Sect. 7.3, we introduce the primal-dual witness technique, which allows us to derive estimation guarantees in $\overline{\hbar}$-loss. In ▶ Sect. 7.4, we turn specific dual function bounds into support recovery guarantees

then, $\widetilde{\boldsymbol{\beta}} = \boldsymbol{\beta}$ is the only vector that satisfies the above equations and $|\text{supp}[\widetilde{\boldsymbol{\beta}}]| \leq 1$. This means that the sparsity counterbalances the correlations such that the target for estimation $\boldsymbol{\beta}$ and the target for support recovery $\text{supp}[\boldsymbol{\beta}]$ become well-defined.

In this chapter, we formalize such interplay between sparsity and correlations to establish guarantees for estimation and support recovery. The outline is depicted in ◘ Fig. 7.1: In ▶ Sect. 7.2, we use the power-two bounds and the compatibility condition introduced in ▶ Sections 6.3 and 6.4, respectively, to derive estimation bounds in the error induced by the prior function. In ▶ Sect. 7.3, we define the irrepresentability condition to derive estimation bounds in the error induced by the prior function's dual. In ▶ Sect. 7.3, we finally exploit specific examples of these bounds to derive bounds in terms of support recovery.

7.2 Estimation Guarantees in $\hbar$-loss

In this section, we transform power-two prediction bounds into estimation bounds. The facilitator in this transformation is the compatibility condition, because it connects prediction terms $\|X\boldsymbol{\delta}\|_2^2$ with estimation terms $\hbar[\boldsymbol{\delta}]$.

This involvement of the compatibility condition stipulates again—cf. ► Sect. 6.4—sparsity and weak correlations.

Our estimation bounds are as follows:

Theorem 7.2.1

Prior Function Bounds Assume that the estimator $\widehat{\boldsymbol{\beta}}$ of (6.1) satisfies the conditions of Theorem 6.3.2 (power-two bounds) and Lemma 6.4.1 (double-cone). Assume further that the design is weakly correlated in the sense that

1. The estimator's prior function $\hbar$ satisfies Assumption 6.4.1 (compatibility condition) for an index set $\mathcal{S} \subset \{1, \ldots, p\}$ and constants $m \in (0, \infty)$, $v \in (1, \infty)$.

Assume finally that the model is approximately sparse in the sense that there is a vector $\boldsymbol{\alpha} \in \mathbb{R}^p$ with

2. $\operatorname{supp}[\boldsymbol{\alpha}] \subset \mathcal{S}$ and $\widehat{w}r \geq 2v\overline{\hbar}[X^\top(\boldsymbol{y} - X\boldsymbol{\alpha})] > 0$;
3. $\hbar[\boldsymbol{\beta} - \boldsymbol{\alpha}] \leq d\widehat{w}r/n$ for a (hopefully small) $d \in [0, \infty]$.

Then,

$$\hbar[\boldsymbol{\beta} - \widehat{\boldsymbol{\beta}}] \leq \left(d + \frac{\sqrt{2}m^2(v+1)}{v}\right)\frac{\widehat{w}r}{n}.$$

This bound guarantees accuracy in terms of the estimation error $\hbar[\boldsymbol{\beta} - \widehat{\boldsymbol{\beta}}]$, which is induced by the prior function $\hbar$; similar bounds can also be established for other estimation errors (see Exercise 7.1). The assumptions parallel those in Theorem 6.4.2 for the power-two prediction bounds. This analogy is no coincidence, as our proof relates estimation and prediction through the compatibility condition, and it highlights that power-two prediction bounds essentially entail estimation bounds.

► Example 7.2.1

ℓ_1-Estimation Bound for the Lasso In this example, we derive explicit estimation bounds for the standard lasso (2.2). Assume that $r = 4\|X^\top \boldsymbol{u}\|_\infty$ and that the requirements of Theorem 7.2.1 above are met for $\widehat{w} = 1$ (cf. ► Sect. 6.2) and $\boldsymbol{\alpha} = \boldsymbol{\beta}$ (which allows us to set $v = 2$ and $d = 0$). The estimation bound in the theorem is then

$$\|\boldsymbol{\beta} - \widehat{\boldsymbol{\beta}}_{\text{lasso}}\|_1 \leq \frac{\sqrt{72}m^2}{n}\|X^\top \boldsymbol{u}\|_\infty.$$

To exemplify this bound, we consider Gauss-distributed noise and normalized design: $\boldsymbol{u} \sim \mathcal{N}_n[\mathbf{0}_n, \sigma^2 \mathrm{I}_{n\times n}]$ for some standard deviation $\sigma \in (0,\infty)$, and $(X^\top X)_{jj} = n$ for all $j \in \{1,\ldots,p\}$. We can then derive similarly as in the overview section of ► Chap. 6 that for every $t \in (0,1]$

$$\begin{aligned}
&\mathbb{P}\left\{\|\boldsymbol{\beta} - \widehat{\boldsymbol{\beta}}_{\text{lasso}}\|_1 \le 12m^2\sigma\sqrt{\frac{\log[p/t]}{n}}\right\}\\
&\ge \mathbb{P}\left\{\frac{\sqrt{72}m^2}{n}\|X^\top \boldsymbol{u}\|_\infty \le 12m^2\sigma\sqrt{\frac{\log[p/t]}{n}}\right\} && \text{above bound}\\
&\ge \mathbb{P}\left\{2\|X^\top \boldsymbol{u}\|_\infty \le \sigma\sqrt{8mn\log[p/t]}\right\}\\
&\qquad \text{consolidating; } m = \max_{j\in\{1,\ldots,p\}}(X^\top X)_{jj}/n = 1 \text{ by assumption}\\
&\ge 1-t\,. && \text{Lemma 4.2.1 (Gauss-distributed noise)}
\end{aligned}$$

In the completely uncorrelated case, where $X^\top X/n = \mathrm{I}_{p\times p}$, this bound can be processed further. The scaled Gram matrix's smallest eigenvalue in this case is 1, so that according to Example 6.4.2 (shuffle the predictors if necessary and set $A = X_{\mathcal{S}}^\top X_{\mathcal{S}}/n = \mathrm{I}_{|\mathcal{S}|\times|\mathcal{S}|}$ and $B = X_{\mathcal{S}^\complement}^\top X_{\mathcal{S}^\complement}/n = \mathrm{I}_{|\mathcal{S}^\complement|\times|\mathcal{S}^\complement|}$), the compatibility condition holds for all $m \in (0,\infty)$ such that $(2\sqrt{s}v/(m(v-1)))^2 \le 1$, where $s := |\mathcal{S}|$. Here $v = 2$, so that $m = 4\sqrt{s}$ works, and the above bound becomes

$$\mathbb{P}\left\{\|\boldsymbol{\beta} - \widehat{\boldsymbol{\beta}}_{\text{lasso}}\|_1 \ge 192\sigma s\sqrt{\frac{\log[p/t]}{n}}\right\} \le t\,.$$

Similar bounds can be derived for designs that have some small correlations—we omit the details.

Hence, in the case of Gaussian linear regression models with weakly correlated predictors, we can expect the ℓ_1-estimation error of a lasso with properly calibrated tuning parameter to be bounded by a universal constant times $\sigma s\sqrt{\log[p]/n}$. The latter factor is linear in the number of relevant model parameters s but only logarithmic in the total number of model parameters p, which illustrates once more the lasso's potential for sparse, high-dimensional regression.

◄

Proof of Theorem 7.2.1 We first show that the vectors in question are feasible in terms of the compatibility condition. We then use the compatibility condition to transform the estimation problem into a prediction problem. We finally treat this prediction problem via a power-two bound from the previous chapter.

Step 1 Lemma 6.4.1 (double-cone) implies directly that for the $\boldsymbol{\alpha}$ described in the theorem (see especially the 2. assumption)

$$\hbar_{\mathcal{S}^{\mathsf{C}}}[\boldsymbol{\alpha}_{\mathcal{S}^{\mathsf{C}}} - \widehat{\boldsymbol{\beta}}_{\mathcal{S}^{\mathsf{C}}}] \leq \frac{v+1}{v-1}\hbar_{\mathcal{S}}[\boldsymbol{\alpha}_{\mathcal{S}} - \widehat{\boldsymbol{\beta}}_{\mathcal{S}}].$$

This means that $\boldsymbol{\delta} := \boldsymbol{\alpha} - \widehat{\boldsymbol{\beta}}$ is part of the set in question for the compatibility condition in Assumption 6.4.1.

Step 2 We now use Step 1 and the compatibility condition to derive the inequality

$$\hbar[\boldsymbol{\beta} - \widehat{\boldsymbol{\beta}}] \leq \frac{d\widehat{w}r}{n} + \frac{m\|X\boldsymbol{\alpha} - X\widehat{\boldsymbol{\beta}}\|_2}{\sqrt{n}}.$$

This inequality relates the estimator's estimation accuracy to its prediction accuracy.

We find for $\boldsymbol{\alpha}$ as described in the theorem that

$$\begin{aligned}
&\hbar[\boldsymbol{\beta} - \widehat{\boldsymbol{\beta}}] \\
&= \hbar[\boldsymbol{\beta} - \boldsymbol{\alpha} + \boldsymbol{\alpha} - \widehat{\boldsymbol{\beta}}] && \text{adding a zero-valued term} \\
&\leq \hbar[\boldsymbol{\beta} - \boldsymbol{\alpha}] + \hbar[\boldsymbol{\alpha} - \widehat{\boldsymbol{\beta}}] && \text{triangle inequality for } \hbar \text{ (3. of Assumption 6.3.2, which is stipulated in Theorem 6.3.2)} \\
&\leq d\widehat{w}r/n + \hbar[\boldsymbol{\alpha} - \widehat{\boldsymbol{\beta}}]. && \text{3. assumption in the theorem}
\end{aligned}$$

Hence, it remains to bound $\hbar[\boldsymbol{\alpha} - \widehat{\boldsymbol{\beta}}]$. According to Step 1, the vector $\boldsymbol{\delta} = \boldsymbol{\alpha} - \widehat{\boldsymbol{\beta}}$ is a candidate for the compatibility condition in Assumption 6.4.1, so that we can use the inequality in that condition to derive

$$\hbar[\boldsymbol{\alpha} - \widehat{\boldsymbol{\beta}}] \leq \frac{m\|X\boldsymbol{\alpha} - X\widehat{\boldsymbol{\beta}}\|_2}{\sqrt{n}}.$$

Plugging this into the foregoing inequality yields

$$\hbar[\boldsymbol{\beta} - \widehat{\boldsymbol{\beta}}] \leq \frac{d\widehat{w}r}{n} + \frac{m\|X\boldsymbol{\alpha} - X\widehat{\boldsymbol{\beta}}\|_2}{\sqrt{n}},$$

as desired.

Step 3 We now combine Step 2 with a slightly modified version of Theorem 6.3.2 (power-two bounds) to show that

$$\hbar[\boldsymbol{\beta} - \widehat{\boldsymbol{\beta}}] \leq \left(d + \frac{\sqrt{2}m^2(v+1)}{v}\right)\frac{\widehat{w}r}{n}.$$

This is the bound stated in the theorem.

Theorem 6.3.2 bounds the prediction error with respect to the regression vector: $\|X\boldsymbol{\beta} - X\widehat{\boldsymbol{\beta}}\|_2^2$. However, replacing the assumption $\widehat{w}r \geq 2v\overline{\hbar}[X^\top \boldsymbol{u}]$ by $\widehat{w}r \geq 2v\overline{\hbar}[X^\top(\boldsymbol{y} - X\boldsymbol{\alpha})]$, we can take the exact same steps as in the proof of that theorem to bound the prediction error with respect to $\boldsymbol{\alpha}$:

$$\|X\boldsymbol{\alpha} - X\widehat{\boldsymbol{\beta}}\|_2^2 \leq \frac{(b+1)^2 m^2 (v+1)^2 \widehat{w}^2 r^2}{4(b-1)v^2 n}.$$

Details

1. In a sense, this corresponds to writing the linear regression model (2.1) in the form $\boldsymbol{y} = X\boldsymbol{\alpha} + \widetilde{\boldsymbol{u}}$ with $\widetilde{\boldsymbol{u}} := \boldsymbol{u} + X\boldsymbol{\beta} - X\boldsymbol{\alpha}$; in particular, this reformulation of the model implies $2v\overline{\hbar}[X^\top(\boldsymbol{y} - X\boldsymbol{\alpha})] = 2v\overline{\hbar}[X^\top \widetilde{\boldsymbol{u}}]$.
2. The prefactor in the above bound can be reduced by modifying the proof of Theorem 6.3.2 slightly—we leave this to the reader.

Since b is arbitrary in $(1, \infty]$, we can set $b = 3$ (which minimizes $(b+1)^2/(b-1)$ over $(1, \infty]$) to find

$$\|X\boldsymbol{\alpha} - X\widehat{\boldsymbol{\beta}}\|_2^2 \leq \frac{2m^2(v+1)^2\widehat{w}^2 r^2}{v^2 n}.$$

Plugging this inequality into the one derived in Step 2 and consolidating yields

$$\begin{aligned}\hbar[\boldsymbol{\beta} - \widehat{\boldsymbol{\beta}}] &\leq \frac{d\widehat{w}r}{n} + \frac{m\frac{\sqrt{2}m(v+1)\widehat{w}r}{v\sqrt{n}}}{\sqrt{n}} \\ &= \left(d + \frac{\sqrt{2}m^2(v+1)}{v}\right)\frac{\widehat{w}r}{n},\end{aligned}$$

as desired. □

7.3 Estimation Guarantees in $\overline{\mathscr{h}}$-loss

In this section, we derive bounds for $\overline{\mathscr{h}}[\boldsymbol{\beta} - \widehat{\boldsymbol{\beta}}]$ by using the *primal-dual witness technique*.[1] This technique establishes conditions for a solution of an optimization problem that is restricted to a subset of the model's parameter space to be a solution also of the original, full optimization problem. Since it is computationally infeasible to verify these conditions for each potential subset, the primal-dual technique is not a viable algorithm for solving optimization problems. Instead, the primal-dual technique provides "theoretical witnesses" for the existence of sparse solutions.

We consider estimators of the form (6.1) with, for simplicity, the link function equal to the identity: $\mathscr{g}[a] = a$ for all $a \in [0, \infty)$. We assume that the prior function $\mathscr{h} : \mathbb{R}^p \to [0, \infty]$ is convex and $\mathcal{S}$-decomposable according to Definition 6.4.1 for a given index set $\mathcal{S} \subset \{1, \ldots, p\}$. The convexity of the prior function enables us to apply the KKT conditions—see ▶ Sect. 2.5. The decomposability enables us to study the subspaces corresponding to $\mathcal{S}$ and $\mathcal{S}^{\complement}$ essentially separately. If an $\mathcal{S}$-decomposable prior function $\mathscr{h}$ is convex, also its subfunctions $\mathscr{h}_{\mathcal{S}}, \mathscr{h}_{\mathcal{S}^{\complement}}$ are convex—see Exercise 7.2.

We now proceed in three steps: We first construct primal-dual pairs to restricted problems. We then establish conditions under which these pairs are solutions of the full problems as well. We then use this connection between the restricted and full problems as a basis for deriving a dual analog of Theorem 7.2.1.

7.3.1 Step 1: Construction of Primal-Dual Pairs

Our first step is to construct a primal-dual pair for a version of the optimization problem (6.1) that is restricted to model parameters with zero-valued coordinates outside a given index set $\mathcal{S} \subset \{1, \ldots, p\}$. The primal vector is the solution of the restricted problem; the dual vector is its counterpart in terms of the KKT conditions.

primal-dual witness construction

Definition 7.3.1

Primal-Dual Witness Construction Given an index set $\mathcal{S} \subset \{1,\ldots,p\}$ of size $s := |\mathcal{S}|$ and a prior function $\hbar$ that is convex (see Definition 2.5.1) and $\mathcal{S}$-decomposable (see Definition 6.4.1), construct a pair of vectors $\widehat{\boldsymbol{\gamma}} = (\widehat{\boldsymbol{\gamma}}_{\mathcal{S}}^\top, \widehat{\boldsymbol{\gamma}}_{\mathcal{S}^\complement}^\top)^\top, \widehat{\boldsymbol{v}} = (\widehat{\boldsymbol{v}}_{\mathcal{S}}^\top, \widehat{\boldsymbol{v}}_{\mathcal{S}^\complement}^\top)^\top \in \mathbb{R}^p$ as follows:
(Primal 1) Define $\widehat{\boldsymbol{\gamma}}_{\mathcal{S}} \in \mathbb{R}^s$ such that

$$\widehat{\boldsymbol{\gamma}}_{\mathcal{S}} \in \underset{\boldsymbol{\theta}\in\mathbb{R}^s}{\arg\min}\left\{ \|\boldsymbol{y} - X_{\mathcal{S}}\boldsymbol{\theta}\|_2^2 + r\hbar_{\mathcal{S}}[\boldsymbol{\theta}]\right\};$$

(Primal 2) Define $\widehat{\boldsymbol{\gamma}}_{\mathcal{S}^\complement} := \boldsymbol{0}_{p-s}$;
(Dual 1) Define $\widehat{\boldsymbol{v}}_{\mathcal{S}} \in \mathbb{R}^s$ such that

$$-2X_{\mathcal{S}}^\top(\boldsymbol{y} - X_{\mathcal{S}}\widehat{\boldsymbol{\gamma}}_{\mathcal{S}}) + r\widehat{\boldsymbol{v}}_{\mathcal{S}} = \boldsymbol{0}_s;$$

(Dual 2) Define $\widehat{\boldsymbol{v}}_{\mathcal{S}^\complement} \in \mathbb{R}^{p-s}$ such that

$$-2X_{\mathcal{S}^\complement}^\top(\boldsymbol{y} - X_{\mathcal{S}}\widehat{\boldsymbol{\gamma}}_{\mathcal{S}}) + r\widehat{\boldsymbol{v}}_{\mathcal{S}^\complement} = \boldsymbol{0}_{p-s}.$$

We call $\widehat{\boldsymbol{\gamma}}$ the *primal vector* and $\widehat{\boldsymbol{v}}$ the *Lagrange dual vector* or simply the *dual vector*.

Recall that $X_{\mathcal{S}}$ (and similarly $X_{\mathcal{S}^\complement}$) consists of the columns of X that have indexes in $\mathcal{S}$ (in $\mathcal{S}^\complement$) and that $X_{\mathcal{S}}^\top := (X_{\mathcal{S}})^\top$ (and $X_{\mathcal{S}^\complement}{}^\top := (X_{\mathcal{S}^\complement})^\top$). The convexity of the prior function allows us to think in terms of KKT conditions; the $\mathcal{S}$-decomposability of the prior function allows us to separate the restricted problem from the full problem.

The vector $\widehat{\boldsymbol{\gamma}}_{\mathcal{S}}$ is not necessarily unique, but given $\widehat{\boldsymbol{\gamma}}_{\mathcal{S}}$ and $r > 0$, all other vectors are uniquely defined.

The dual vector's coordinates are usually all different from zero, while by construction, the primal vector is sparse if $s = |\mathcal{S}|$ is small. The hope is that Definition 7.3.1 returns a $\widehat{\boldsymbol{\gamma}}$ that is sparse and yet a solution of the full problem (6.1), which would allow us to remove a large part of the model's parameter space from the theoretical analyses. We will show that this is indeed the case if the design is only weakly correlated, the tuning parameters are large enough, and there is a sparse surrogate vector for the regression vector by showing that $\widehat{\boldsymbol{v}}$ is a subgradient[2] of $\hbar$ at $\widehat{\boldsymbol{\gamma}}$, that is, $\widehat{\boldsymbol{v}} \in \partial\hbar[\widehat{\boldsymbol{\gamma}}]$.

Just as we use the shorthand *dual functions* for *Hölder dual* functions, we use the shorthand *dual vectors* for

Lagrange dual vectors. But the full names should remind us that the two concepts are very different: dual vectors are related to Lagrange dual functions; dual functions are related to the Hölder inequality (see ▶ Sect. 2.4).[3]

7.3.2 Step 2: Establishing Conditions for a Successful Construction

Having introduced the primal vector through a solution of a restricted optimization problem in the first step, we show in this second step that this vector is also a solution of the full problem (6.1) (recall that in this section, $\mathscr{g}$ is the identity function and $\mathscr{h}$ convex and decomposable) under two conditions: 1. The "relevant" predictors indexed by $\mathcal{S}$ and the "irrelevant" predictors indexed by $\mathcal{S}^{\complement}$ are not too much correlated, so that these two groups can be distinguished based on data; 2. the tuning parameters are large enough to overrule the effective noise.

irrepresentability condition

We formulate 1. in terms of the *irrepresentability condition*.

▪▪ Assumption 7.3.1

Irrepresentability Condition Given an index set $\mathcal{S} \subset \{1, \ldots, p\}$, a prior function $\mathscr{h}$ that is convex and can be decomposed according to Definition 6.4.1, a corresponding primal-dual pair $(\widehat{\boldsymbol{\gamma}}, \widehat{\boldsymbol{\nu}})$, and a constant $c \in (0, \infty)$, we assume that the *irrepresentability condition* holds: $X_{\mathcal{S}}^\top X_{\mathcal{S}}$ is invertible and

$$\sup_{\boldsymbol{a}\in\partial\mathscr{h}_{\mathcal{S}}[\widehat{\boldsymbol{\gamma}}_{\mathcal{S}}]} \overline{\mathscr{h}}_{\mathcal{S}^{\complement}}\big[X_{\mathcal{S}^{\complement}}^\top X_{\mathcal{S}}(X_{\mathcal{S}}^\top X_{\mathcal{S}})^{-1}\boldsymbol{a}\big] \le 1 - c\,,$$

where $\overline{\mathscr{h}}_{\mathcal{S}^{\complement}} := \overline{\mathscr{h}_{\mathcal{S}^{\complement}}}$ is the dual function of $\mathscr{h}_{\mathcal{S}^{\complement}}$ (see Definition 2.4.1). We call c the *irrepresentability constant* for $\mathcal{S}$, $\mathscr{h}$.

The irrepresentability condition limits the correlations between relevant predictors (the columns of $X_{\mathcal{S}}$) and irrelevant predictors (the columns of $X_{\mathcal{S}^{\complement}}$). Essentially, it ensures that the columns of $X_{\mathcal{S}}$ cannot be expressed through the columns of $X_{\mathcal{S}^{\complement}}$: Exercise 7.3, for example, shows that for $\mathscr{h}$ equal to the lasso's ℓ_1-norm, the assumption is satisfied if $X_{\mathcal{S}}^\top X_{\mathcal{S}}$ is invertible and $\max_{j\in\mathcal{S}^{\complement}} \|\widehat{\boldsymbol{\beta}}_{\mathrm{ls}}^j\|_1 \le 1-c$, where $\widehat{\boldsymbol{\beta}}_{\mathrm{ls}}^j \equiv \widehat{\boldsymbol{\beta}}_{\mathrm{ls}}^j[X_j, X_{\mathcal{S}}]$ is the least-squares estimator that regresses the jth predictor onto the predictors with indexes in $\mathcal{S}$.

In ▶ Sect. 6.4, we have introduced another measure for the correlations in the design: the compatibility condition in Assumption 6.4.1.[4] Both the compatibility condition and the irrepresentability condition are tailored for mathematical convenience rather than for plausibility in applications; therefore, results based on these assumptions should be taken with a grain of salt.

The following theorem is now the main result of Step 2.

Theorem 7.3.1

Successful Primal-Dual Construction Assume that the design is weakly correlated in the sense that

1. The estimator's prior function $\hbar$ satisfies Assumption 7.3.1 (irrepresentability condition) for an index set $\mathcal{S} \subset \{1, \ldots, p\}$ and a constant $c \in (0, \infty)$.

Assume that the tuning parameter is large enough in the sense that

2. $r > 2\overline{\hbar}_{\mathcal{S}^\complement}\big[X_{\mathcal{S}^\complement}^\top\big(\mathrm{I}_{n\times n} - X_{\mathcal{S}}(X_{\mathcal{S}}^\top X_{\mathcal{S}})^{-1}X_{\mathcal{S}}^\top\big)y\big]/c$.

Assume also that $\hbar_{\mathcal{S}^\complement}$ is a norm (cf. Exercise 2.3, Claim 6) and that $(\widehat{\gamma}, \widehat{v})$ is a primal-dual pair constructed according to Definition 7.3.1. Then, $\widehat{\gamma}$ is also a solution of the full problem (6.1), that is,

$$\widehat{\gamma} \in \underset{\alpha\in\mathbb{R}^p}{\arg\min}\left\{\|y - X\alpha\|_2^2 + r\hbar[\alpha]\right\}.$$

We then say that the primal-dual construction was successful.

Assuming that the predictors are not too much correlated and the tuning parameter not too small, the theorem ensures a successful primal-dual construction, which means that the primal vector is also a solution of the original problem (6.1). Since the primal vector is supported on the set $\mathcal{S}$ (see *(Primal 2)* in Definition 7.3.1), the theorem guarantees that under the mentioned assumptions, there exists an $\mathcal{S}$-sparse solution of (6.1). This solution is unique under additional conditions—see Exercise 7.4.

In order to establish a proof of Theorem 7.3.1, we first introduce an auxiliary lemma.

Lemma 7.3.1

Sufficient Condition on the Dual Vector Let $(\widehat{\gamma}, \widehat{v})$ be a primal-dual pair constructed according to Definition 7.3.1. If $\hbar_{\mathcal{S}^\complement}$ satisfies the conditions of the Hölder inequality in Theorem 2.4.1 and $r > 0$, then $\overline{\hbar}_{\mathcal{S}^\complement}[\widehat{v}_{\mathcal{S}^\complement}] \leq 1$ implies $\widehat{v} \in \partial\hbar[\widehat{\gamma}]$.

Proof of Lemma 7.3.1 The functions $\hbar_{\mathcal{S}}$ and $\hbar_{\mathcal{S}^\complement}$ are convex according to Exercise 7.2. Hence, in view of Exercise 2.8, a sufficient condition for $\widehat{v} \in \partial\hbar[\widehat{\gamma}]$ is that both (i) $\widehat{v}_{\mathcal{S}} \in \partial\hbar_{\mathcal{S}}[\widehat{\gamma}_{\mathcal{S}}]$ and (ii) $\widehat{v}_{\mathcal{S}^\complement} \in \partial\hbar_{\mathcal{S}^\complement}[\widehat{\gamma}_{\mathcal{S}^\complement}]$. We show Parts (i) and (ii) in order.

To prove Part (i), we apply the KKT conditions to the restricted problem: since $\widehat{\gamma}_{\mathcal{S}}$ is a solution of the optimization problem *(Primal 1)* in Definition 7.3.1, the KKT conditions (see Example 2.5.3) say that there is a $\widehat{\kappa} \in \partial\hbar_{\mathcal{S}}[\widehat{\gamma}_{\mathcal{S}}]$ such that

$$-2X_{\mathcal{S}}^\top \left(y - X_{\mathcal{S}}\widehat{\gamma}_{\mathcal{S}}\right) + r\widehat{\kappa} \;=\; \mathbf{0}_s\,.$$

Comparing to *(Dual 1)* and noting that $r \in (0, \infty)$ by assumption, we find that $\widehat{\kappa} = \widehat{v}_{\mathcal{S}}$, as desired.

Part (ii) is more involved, because *(Dual 2)* does not relate to a minimization problem directly. However, assuming $\overline{\hbar}_{\mathcal{S}^\complement}[\widehat{v}_{\mathcal{S}^\complement}] \leq 1$, we find for every $c \in \mathbb{R}^{p-s}$

$$\begin{aligned}
&\langle \widehat{v}_{\mathcal{S}^\complement},\, c - \widehat{\gamma}_{\mathcal{S}^\complement}\rangle \\
&= \langle \widehat{v}_{\mathcal{S}^\complement},\, c\rangle && \widehat{\gamma}_{\mathcal{S}^\complement} = \mathbf{0}_{p-s} \text{ by (Primal 2)} \\
&\leq \overline{\hbar}_{\mathcal{S}^\complement}[\widehat{v}_{\mathcal{S}^\complement}]\hbar_{\mathcal{S}^\complement}[c] && \text{Hölder inequality (2.5)} \\
&\leq \hbar_{\mathcal{S}^\complement}[c] && \hbar \text{ non-negative by the assumptions of Theorem 2.4.1;} \\
& && \overline{\hbar}_{\mathcal{S}^\complement}[\widehat{v}_{\mathcal{S}^\complement}] \leq 1 \text{ by the above assumption} \\
&= \hbar_{\mathcal{S}^\complement}[c] - \hbar_{\mathcal{S}^\complement}[\widehat{\gamma}_{\mathcal{S}^\complement}]\,. && \hbar_{\mathcal{S}^\complement}[\widehat{\gamma}_{\mathcal{S}^\complement}] = \hbar_{\mathcal{S}^\complement}[\mathbf{0}_{p-s}] = 0 \text{ by} \\
& && \text{the assumptions of Theorem 2.4.1}
\end{aligned}$$

Rearranging this display yields

$$\hbar_{\mathcal{S}^\complement}[c] \;\geq\; \hbar_{\mathcal{S}^\complement}[\widehat{\gamma}_{\mathcal{S}^\complement}] + \langle \widehat{v}_{\mathcal{S}^\complement},\, c - \widehat{\gamma}_{\mathcal{S}^\complement}\rangle$$

for all $c \in \mathbb{R}^{p-s}$, which means by the definition of subdifferentials in ► Sect. 2.5 that $\widehat{v}_{\mathcal{S}^\complement} \in \partial\hbar_{\mathcal{S}^\complement}[\widehat{\gamma}_{\mathcal{S}^\complement}]$, as desired.

□

We can now conclude with the proof of Theorem 7.3.1.

Proof of Theorem 7.3.1 *(Primal 2)*, *(Dual 1)*, and *(Dual 2)* taken together yield

$$-2X^\top(\boldsymbol{y} - X\widehat{\boldsymbol{\gamma}}) + r\widehat{\boldsymbol{v}} \;=\; \mathbf{0}_p\,.$$

Hence, Example 2.5.3 ensures that $\widehat{\boldsymbol{\gamma}}$ is a solution of the full problem if $\widehat{\boldsymbol{v}} \in \partial\hbar[\widehat{\boldsymbol{\gamma}}]$. Since $\overline{\hbar}_{\mathcal{S}^\complement}$ is a norm, it meets the assumptions for the Hölder inequality, and since c and $\overline{\hbar}_{\mathcal{S}^\complement}$ are non-negative (see 4. or 6. in Exercise 2.3), it holds that $r > 0$, so that in view of Lemma 7.3.1, it remains to show that $\overline{\hbar}_{\mathcal{S}^\complement}[\widehat{\boldsymbol{v}}_{\mathcal{S}^\complement}] \leq 1$.

Now, *(Dual 1)* is

$$-2X_{\mathcal{S}}^\top(\boldsymbol{y} - X_{\mathcal{S}}\widehat{\boldsymbol{\gamma}}_{\mathcal{S}}) + r\widehat{\boldsymbol{v}}_{\mathcal{S}} \;=\; \mathbf{0}_s\,.$$

Rearranging this gives

$$2X_{\mathcal{S}}^\top X_{\mathcal{S}}\widehat{\boldsymbol{\gamma}}_{\mathcal{S}} \;=\; 2X_{\mathcal{S}}^\top\boldsymbol{y} - r\widehat{\boldsymbol{v}}_{\mathcal{S}}\,,$$

which, since the matrix $X_{\mathcal{S}}^\top X_{\mathcal{S}}$ is invertible by the irrepresentability condition 7.3.1, can be solved for $\widehat{\boldsymbol{\gamma}}_{\mathcal{S}}$:

$$\widehat{\boldsymbol{\gamma}}_{\mathcal{S}} \;=\; (X_{\mathcal{S}}^\top X_{\mathcal{S}})^{-1}X_{\mathcal{S}}^\top\boldsymbol{y} - r(X_{\mathcal{S}}^\top X_{\mathcal{S}})^{-1}\widehat{\boldsymbol{v}}_{\mathcal{S}}/2\,.$$

Next, *(Dual 2)* is

$$-2X_{\mathcal{S}^\complement}^\top(\boldsymbol{y} - X_{\mathcal{S}}\widehat{\boldsymbol{\gamma}}_{\mathcal{S}}) + r\widehat{\boldsymbol{v}}_{\mathcal{S}^\complement} \;=\; \mathbf{0}_{p-s}\,.$$

Plugging in the above expression for $\widehat{\boldsymbol{\gamma}}_{\mathcal{S}}$ gives

$$-2X_{\mathcal{S}^\complement}^\top\big(\boldsymbol{y} - X_{\mathcal{S}}\big((X_{\mathcal{S}}^\top X_{\mathcal{S}})^{-1}X_{\mathcal{S}}^\top\boldsymbol{y} - r(X_{\mathcal{S}}^\top X_{\mathcal{S}})^{-1}\widehat{\boldsymbol{v}}_{\mathcal{S}}/2\big)\big) + r\widehat{\boldsymbol{v}}_{\mathcal{S}^\complement} \;=\; \mathbf{0}_{p-s}\,,$$

which can be rearranged to

$$r\widehat{\boldsymbol{v}}_{\mathcal{S}^\complement} \;=\; 2X_{\mathcal{S}^\complement}^\top\big(\mathrm{I}_{n\times n} - X_{\mathcal{S}}(X_{\mathcal{S}}^\top X_{\mathcal{S}})^{-1}X_{\mathcal{S}}^\top\big)\boldsymbol{y} + rX_{\mathcal{S}^\complement}^\top X_{\mathcal{S}}(X_{\mathcal{S}}^\top X_{\mathcal{S}})^{-1}\widehat{\boldsymbol{v}}_{\mathcal{S}}\,.$$

We can now apply the function $\overline{\hbar}_{\mathcal{S}^\complement}$ on both sides and invoke the triangle inequality and the absolute homogeneity of norms (see 6. in Exercise 2.3)

$$r\overline{\hbar}_{\mathcal{S}^{\complement}}[\widehat{\boldsymbol{\nu}}_{\mathcal{S}^{\complement}}] \leq 2\overline{\hbar}_{\mathcal{S}^{\complement}}\big[X_{\mathcal{S}^{\complement}}^{\top}\big(\mathrm{I}_{n\times n} - X_{\mathcal{S}}(X_{\mathcal{S}}^{\top}X_{\mathcal{S}})^{-1}X_{\mathcal{S}}^{\top}\big)\boldsymbol{y}\big] \\ + r\overline{\hbar}_{\mathcal{S}^{\complement}}\big[X_{\mathcal{S}^{\complement}}^{\top}X_{\mathcal{S}}(X_{\mathcal{S}}^{\top}X_{\mathcal{S}})^{-1}\widehat{\boldsymbol{\nu}}_{\mathcal{S}}\big].$$

By assumption on r, the first term on the right-hand side is bounded by

$$2\overline{\hbar}_{\mathcal{S}^{\complement}}\big[X_{\mathcal{S}^{\complement}}^{\top}(\mathrm{I}_{n\times n} - X_{\mathcal{S}}(X_{\mathcal{S}}^{\top}X_{\mathcal{S}})^{-1}X_{\mathcal{S}}^{\top})\boldsymbol{y}\big] < rc\,.$$

By the assumed irrepresentability condition, and since $\widehat{\boldsymbol{\nu}}_{\mathcal{S}} \in \partial\hbar_{\mathcal{S}}[\widehat{\boldsymbol{\gamma}}]$ (see (i) in the above proof of Lemma 7.3.1), the second term on the right-hand side is bounded by

$$r\overline{\hbar}_{\mathcal{S}^{\complement}}\big[X_{\mathcal{S}^{\complement}}^{\top}X_{\mathcal{S}}(X_{\mathcal{S}}^{\top}X_{\mathcal{S}})^{-1}\widehat{\boldsymbol{\nu}}_{\mathcal{S}}\big] \leq r(1-c)\,.$$

Collecting terms gives

$$r\overline{\hbar}_{\mathcal{S}^{\complement}}[\widehat{\boldsymbol{\nu}}_{\mathcal{S}^{\complement}}] \leq rc + r(1-c) \;=\; r\,,$$

which implies in view of $r \in (0,\infty)$ ($r > 0$ according to an earlier part of the proof; $r < \infty$ by assumption) that

$$\overline{\hbar}_{\mathcal{S}^{\complement}}[\widehat{\boldsymbol{\nu}}_{\mathcal{S}^{\complement}}] \leq 1\,,$$

as desired. □

7.3.3 Step 3: Deriving Dual Bounds

We finally show that successful primal-dual constructions can lead to guarantees in $\overline{\hbar}$-loss, which is induced by the dual of the prior function.

Theorem 7.3.2

Dual Function Bounds Assume that the primal-dual witness construction (see Step 1) was successful (see Step 2). Assume also that $\hbar_{\mathcal{S}}$ and $\hbar_{\mathcal{S}^{\complement}}$ are norms and that $X_{\mathcal{S}}^{\top}X_{\mathcal{S}}/n$ is invertible. Assume finally that the model is approximately sparse in the sense that there is a vector $\boldsymbol{\alpha} \in \mathbb{R}^p$ with

1. $\operatorname{supp}[\boldsymbol{\alpha}] \subset \mathcal{S}$ and $\overline{\hbar}_{\mathcal{S}}[(X_{\mathcal{S}}^{\top}X_{\mathcal{S}}/n)^{-1}\widehat{\boldsymbol{\nu}}_{\mathcal{S}}]r \geq 2v\overline{\hbar}_{\mathcal{S}}[(X_{\mathcal{S}}^{\top}X_{\mathcal{S}}/n)^{-1}X_{\mathcal{S}}^{\top}(\boldsymbol{y} - X\boldsymbol{\alpha})]$ for a $v \in (0,\infty)$;
2. $\overline{\hbar}[\boldsymbol{\beta} - \boldsymbol{\alpha}] \leq dr/n$ for a (hopefully small) $d \in [0,\infty]$.

Then, (6.1) has a solution $\widehat{\boldsymbol{\beta}}$ that satisfies $\text{supp}[\widehat{\boldsymbol{\beta}}] \subset \mathcal{S}$ and

$$\overline{\hbar}[\boldsymbol{\beta} - \widehat{\boldsymbol{\beta}}] \leq \left(d + \frac{\overline{\hbar}_{\mathcal{S}}[(X_{\mathcal{S}}^\top X_{\mathcal{S}}/n)^{-1}\widehat{\boldsymbol{v}}_{\mathcal{S}}](v+1)}{2v}\right)\frac{r}{n}.$$

These bounds resemble the ones of Theorem 7.2.1, especially since both m and $\overline{\hbar}_{\mathcal{S}}[(X_{\mathcal{S}}^\top X_{\mathcal{S}}/n)^{-1}\widehat{\boldsymbol{v}}_{\mathcal{S}}]$ can be viewed as measures for the design correlations. Nevertheless, the bounds here differ from those earlier ones in three main aspects: they limit the correlations among the predictors through the irrepresentability condition (via Step 2) rather than through the restricted eigenvalue condition; they concern the dual of the prior function rather than the original prior function; they also guarantee that the estimated support is included in the true support. The latter two features make Theorem 7.2.1 particularly interesting for support recovery—see the following section.

▶ Example 7.3.1

ℓ_∞-Estimation Bound for the Lasso In this example, we show that Theorems 7.3.1 and 7.3.2 generalize the ℓ_∞-bound for the lasso estimator (2.2) that follows from the lasso's explicit expression for orthogonal design. For orthogonal design, that is, $X^\top X = n\mathrm{I}_{p\times p}$, the least-squares estimator (1.3) satisfies the explicit expression (1.4) (since $X^\top X = n\mathrm{I}_{n\times n}$ implies that $X^\top X$ is invertible) and, therefore,

$$\begin{aligned}
&\|\boldsymbol{\beta} - \widehat{\boldsymbol{\beta}}_{\mathrm{ls}}\|_\infty \\
&= \|\boldsymbol{\beta} - (X^\top X)^{-1}X^\top \boldsymbol{y}\|_\infty && \text{Eq. (1.4)} \\
&= \|\boldsymbol{\beta} - (X^\top X)^{-1}X^\top(X\boldsymbol{\beta} + \boldsymbol{u})\|_\infty && \text{linear model (2.1)} \\
&= \|-(X^\top X)^{-1}X^\top \boldsymbol{u}\|_\infty && (X^\top X)^{-1}X^\top X\boldsymbol{\beta} = \boldsymbol{\beta} \\
&= \|(X^\top X/n)^{-1}X^\top \boldsymbol{u}\|_\infty/n && \text{absolute homogeneity of norms} \\
&= \|X^\top \boldsymbol{u}\|_\infty/n\,, && X^\top X/n = \mathrm{I}_{n\times n} \text{ by assumption}
\end{aligned}$$

and more generally, the lasso satisfies the explicit expression (2.8) and, therefore, (we leave the details to the reader)

$$\|\boldsymbol{\beta} - \widehat{\boldsymbol{\beta}}_{\mathrm{lasso}}\|_\infty \leq \|X^\top \boldsymbol{u}\|_\infty/n + r/(2n)\,.$$

For our usual tuning parameter $r = 4\|X^\top \boldsymbol{u}\|_\infty$, the latter inequality becomes

$$\|\boldsymbol{\beta} - \widehat{\boldsymbol{\beta}}_{\text{lasso}}\|_\infty \leq \frac{3}{n}\|X^\top \boldsymbol{u}\|_\infty .$$

We now show that the same bound follows from Theorems 7.3.1 and 7.3.2. Recall that the lasso's prior function $\hbar$ and its subfunctions $\hbar_{\mathcal{S}}$ and $\hbar_{\mathcal{S}^\complement}$ in Definition 6.4.1 are the ℓ_1-norms on $\mathbb{R}^p$, $\mathbb{R}^s$, and $\mathbb{R}^{p-s}$, respectively (cf. Example 6.4.2) and that the corresponding dual functions $\overline{\hbar}$, $\overline{\hbar}_{\mathcal{S}}$, and $\overline{\hbar}_{\mathcal{S}^\complement}$ are the ℓ_∞-norms on $\mathbb{R}^p$, $\mathbb{R}^s$, and $\mathbb{R}^{p-s}$, respectively (see 3. in Exercise 2.2). For orthogonal design, the irrepresentability constant in Assumption 7.3.1 can be set to $c = 1$ according to

$$\sup_{a\in\partial\hbar_{\mathcal{S}}[\widehat{\boldsymbol{\gamma}}_{\mathcal{S}}]} \overline{\hbar}_{\mathcal{S}^\complement}\bigl[X_{\mathcal{S}^\complement}^\top X_{\mathcal{S}}(X_{\mathcal{S}}^\top X_{\mathcal{S}})^{-1}\mathbf{a}\bigr]$$

$$= \sup_{a\in\partial\hbar_{\mathcal{S}}[\widehat{\boldsymbol{\gamma}}_{\mathcal{S}}]} \overline{\hbar}_{\mathcal{S}^\complement}\bigl[\mathbf{0}_{(p-s)\times s}(X_{\mathcal{S}}^\top X_{\mathcal{S}})^{-1}\mathbf{a}\bigr]$$

$X^\top X = n\mathrm{I}_{p\times p}$ entails $X_{\mathcal{S}^\complement}{}^\top X_{\mathcal{S}} = \mathbf{0}_{(p-s)\times s}$

$$= \sup_{a\in\partial\hbar_{\mathcal{S}}[\widehat{\boldsymbol{\gamma}}_{\mathcal{S}}]} \overline{\hbar}_{\mathcal{S}^\complement}\bigl[\mathbf{0}_{p-s}\bigr]$$

linearity of matrix–vector multiplications

$$= \sup_{a\in\partial\|\widehat{\boldsymbol{\gamma}}_{\mathcal{S}}\|_1} \|\mathbf{0}_{p-s}\|_\infty$$

$\hbar$ is the ℓ_1-norm

$$= \sup_{a\in\partial\|\widehat{\boldsymbol{\gamma}}_{\mathcal{S}}\|_1} 0$$

norms are positive definite

$$= 0 = 1 - 1 ,$$

subdifferentials of convex functions are not empty (cf. Page 57)

and the correlation measure $\overline{\hbar}_{\mathcal{S}}[(X_{\mathcal{S}}^\top X_{\mathcal{S}}/n)^{-1}\widehat{\boldsymbol{\nu}}_{\mathcal{S}}]$ in Theorem 7.3.2 is equal to one according to

$$\overline{\hbar}_{\mathcal{S}}\bigl[(X_{\mathcal{S}}^\top X_{\mathcal{S}}/n)^{-1}\widehat{\boldsymbol{\nu}}_{\mathcal{S}}\bigr]$$

$$= \|\widehat{\boldsymbol{\nu}}_{\mathcal{S}}\|_\infty$$

$X^\top X = n\mathrm{I}_{p\times p}$ entails $X_{\mathcal{S}}^\top X_{\mathcal{S}}/n = \mathrm{I}_{s\times s}$; $\hbar$ is the ℓ_1-norm

$$= 1 ,$$

$\widehat{\boldsymbol{\nu}}_{\mathcal{S}} \in \partial\|\widehat{\boldsymbol{\gamma}}_{\mathcal{S}}\|_1$ (see Lemma 7.3.1 and its proof); $|(\widehat{\nu}_{\mathcal{S}})_j| \leq 1$ and $|(\widehat{\nu}_{\mathcal{S}})_j| = |\mathrm{sign}[(\widehat{\gamma}_{\mathcal{S}})_j]| = 1$ if $(\widehat{\gamma}_{\mathcal{S}})_j \neq 0$ (see Example 2.5.3) where we have assumed $\widehat{\gamma} \neq \mathbf{0}_p$ in the last step to avoid mathematical subtleties, and $\mathcal{S}$ was arbitrary throughout.

Now, take $\mathcal{S} := \operatorname{supp}[\boldsymbol{\beta}]$. Then, the tuning parameter $r = 4\|X^\top \boldsymbol{u}\|_\infty$ satisfies the assumptions of Theorems 7.3.1 and 7.3.2:

$$
\begin{aligned}
&2\overline{\hbar}_{\mathcal{S}^{\complement}}\big[{X_{\mathcal{S}^{\complement}}}^\top\big(\mathrm{I}_{n\times n} - X_{\mathcal{S}}(X_{\mathcal{S}}^\top X_{\mathcal{S}})^{-1}X_{\mathcal{S}}^\top\big)\boldsymbol{y}\big]/c \\
&= 2\overline{\hbar}_{\mathcal{S}^{\complement}}\big[{X_{\mathcal{S}^{\complement}}}^\top \boldsymbol{y}\big]/c \quad && X^\top X = n\mathrm{I}_{p\times p} \text{ entails } {X_{\mathcal{S}^{\complement}}}^\top X_{\mathcal{S}} = \mathbf{0}_{(p-s)\times s} \\
&= 2\overline{\hbar}_{\mathcal{S}^{\complement}}\big[{X_{\mathcal{S}^{\complement}}}^\top (X\boldsymbol{\beta} + \boldsymbol{u})\big]/c && \text{linear model (2.1)} \\
&= 2\overline{\hbar}_{\mathcal{S}^{\complement}}\big[{X_{\mathcal{S}^{\complement}}}^\top (X_{\mathcal{S}}\boldsymbol{\beta}_{\mathcal{S}} + \boldsymbol{u})\big]/c && \mathcal{S} = \operatorname{supp}[\boldsymbol{\beta}] \text{ by definition} \\
&= 2\overline{\hbar}_{\mathcal{S}^{\complement}}\big[{X_{\mathcal{S}^{\complement}}}^\top \boldsymbol{u}\big]/c && X^\top X = n\mathrm{I}_{p\times p} \text{ entails } {X_{\mathcal{S}^{\complement}}}^\top X_{\mathcal{S}} = \mathbf{0}_{(p-s)\times s} \\
&= 2\|{X_{\mathcal{S}^{\complement}}}^\top \boldsymbol{u}\|_\infty && \hbar \text{ is the } \ell_1\text{-norm; } c = 1 \text{ by above} \\
&\le 2\|X^\top \boldsymbol{u}\|_\infty && \text{definition of the } \ell_\infty\text{-norm} \\
&< 4\|X^\top \boldsymbol{u}\|_\infty \;=\; r\,, && \text{choice of } r
\end{aligned}
$$

where we have assumed $\|X^\top \boldsymbol{u}\|_\infty \neq 0$ in the last step to avoid mathematical subtleties again, and, for $\boldsymbol{\alpha} = \boldsymbol{\beta}$ (which allows us to set $d = 0$) and $v = 2$,

$$
\begin{aligned}
&2v\overline{\hbar}_{\mathcal{S}}\big[(X_{\mathcal{S}}^\top X_{\mathcal{S}}/n)^{-1}X_{\mathcal{S}}^\top(\boldsymbol{y} - X\boldsymbol{\alpha})\big] \\
&= 2v\overline{\hbar}_{\mathcal{S}}\big[X_{\mathcal{S}}^\top(\boldsymbol{y} - X\boldsymbol{\alpha})\big] \quad && X^\top X = n\mathrm{I}_{p\times p} \text{ entails } X_{\mathcal{S}}^\top X_{\mathcal{S}}/n = \mathrm{I}_{s\times s} \\
&= 4\overline{\hbar}_{\mathcal{S}}\big[X_{\mathcal{S}}^\top \boldsymbol{u}\big] && v = 2;\ \boldsymbol{\alpha} = \boldsymbol{\beta};\ \text{linear model (2.1)} \\
&= 4\|{X_{\mathcal{S}^{\complement}}}^\top \boldsymbol{u}\|_\infty && \hbar \text{ is the } \ell_1\text{-norm} \\
&\le 4\|X^\top \boldsymbol{u}\|_\infty && \max_{j\in\mathcal{S}^{\complement}}|a_j| \le \max_{j\in\{1,\dots,p\}}|a_j| \\
&= \overline{\hbar}_{\mathcal{S}}\big[(X_{\mathcal{S}}^\top X_{\mathcal{S}}/n)^{-1}\widehat{\boldsymbol{v}}_{\mathcal{S}}\big]r\,. \\
& && \overline{\hbar}_{\mathcal{S}}[(X_{\mathcal{S}}^\top X_{\mathcal{S}}/n)^{-1}\widehat{\boldsymbol{v}}_{\mathcal{S}}] = 1 \text{ according to above; choice of r}
\end{aligned}
$$

Hence, the assumptions of Theorems 7.3.1 and 7.3.2 are met. The bound in Theorem 7.3.2 then ensures that the lasso solution $\widehat{\boldsymbol{\beta}}_{\text{lasso}}$ (which is unique in view of the explicit expression mentioned above) satisfies

$$
\|\boldsymbol{\beta} - \widehat{\boldsymbol{\beta}}_{\text{lasso}}\|_\infty \le \frac{3}{n}\|X^\top \boldsymbol{u}\|_\infty\,,
$$

which equals the bound derived above. However, while the derivation based on the explicit expression of the lasso requires exact orthogonality, the derivation based on Theorems 7.3.1 and 7.3.2 can be relaxed readily to approximate orthogonality.

For Gauss-distributed noise $\boldsymbol{u} \sim \mathcal{N}_n[\mathbf{0}_n, \sigma^2 \mathrm{I}_{n\times n}]$, the bound can be combined with Lemma 4.2.1 as usual to obtain

$$\mathbb{P}\left\{ \|\boldsymbol{\beta} - \widehat{\boldsymbol{\beta}}_{\text{lasso}}\|_\infty \le \sigma\sqrt{\frac{18\log[p/t]}{n}} \right\} \ \ge\ 1 - t\,.$$

We can thus expect that in a sparse,[5] weakly correlated regression with Gauss-distributed noise, the sup-norm error of the lasso estimator is bounded by $\sigma\sqrt{\log[p]/n}$ with high probability. ◀

We conclude this section with the proof of Theorem 7.3.2.

Proof of Theorem 7.3.2 Since the primal-dual construction is assumed successful, the primal vector $\widehat{\boldsymbol{\beta}} := \widehat{\boldsymbol{\gamma}}$ constructed in Definition 6.4.1 is a solution of the full problem (6.1). In view of *(Primal 2)* in Definition 6.4.1, it thus holds that $\text{supp}[\widehat{\boldsymbol{\beta}}] \subset \mathcal{S}$. We establish the remaining bound in three parts: first, we show that dual function $\overline{\hbar}$ can be decomposed into a function on $\mathcal{S}$ and a function on $\mathcal{S}^{\complement}$; then, we derive a bound on the set $\mathcal{S}$; finally, we combine Parts 1 and 2 and the assumptions of the theorem to deduce the bound in the theorem.

Part 1 We first show that under the conditions stated in the theorem, the function $\overline{\hbar}$ is $\mathcal{S}$-"sub-"decomposable:

$$\overline{\hbar}[\boldsymbol{a}] \le \overline{\hbar}_{\mathcal{S}}[\boldsymbol{a}_{\mathcal{S}}] + \overline{\hbar}_{\mathcal{S}^{\complement}}[\boldsymbol{a}_{\mathcal{S}^{\complement}}] \qquad \text{for all } \boldsymbol{a} \in \mathbb{R}^p\,.$$

The decomposability of the prior function $\hbar$ is a main restriction in this section. The subdecomposability of the dual $\overline{\hbar}$, on the other hand, then follows "automatically" from the definition of dual functions and the Hölder inequality: we find for every $\boldsymbol{a} \in \mathbb{R}^p$

$$\overline{\hbar}[\boldsymbol{a}] = \sup\left\{ \langle \boldsymbol{a},\, \boldsymbol{c}\rangle \ :\ \boldsymbol{c} \in \mathbb{R}^p,\ \hbar[\boldsymbol{c}] \le 1 \right\}$$

Definition 2.4.1 (dual functions)

$$= \sup\left\{ \langle \boldsymbol{a},\, \boldsymbol{c}\rangle \ :\ \boldsymbol{c}_{\mathcal{S}} \in \mathbb{R}^s,\ \boldsymbol{c}_{\mathcal{S}^{\complement}} \in \mathbb{R}^{p-s},\right.$$

$$\hbar_{\mathcal{S}}[\boldsymbol{c}_{\mathcal{S}}] + \hbar_{\mathcal{S}^{\complement}}[\boldsymbol{c}_{\mathcal{S}^{\complement}}] \leq 1\Big\}$$

$\hbar$ is $\mathcal{S}$-decomposable by assumption (cf. Definition 6.4.1)

$$= \sup\Big\{\langle \boldsymbol{a}_{\mathcal{S}}, \boldsymbol{c}_{\mathcal{S}}\rangle + \langle \boldsymbol{a}_{\mathcal{S}^{\complement}}, \boldsymbol{c}_{\mathcal{S}^{\complement}}\rangle :$$

$$\boldsymbol{c}_{\mathcal{S}} \in \mathbb{R}^{s},\ \boldsymbol{c}_{\mathcal{S}^{\complement}} \in \mathbb{R}^{p-s},\ \hbar_{\mathcal{S}}[\boldsymbol{c}_{\mathcal{S}}] + \hbar_{\mathcal{S}^{\complement}}[\boldsymbol{c}_{\mathcal{S}^{\complement}}] \leq 1\Big\}$$

linearity of the standard inner product

$$\leq \sup\Big\{\overline{\hbar}_{\mathcal{S}}[\boldsymbol{a}_{\mathcal{S}}]\hbar_{\mathcal{S}}[\boldsymbol{c}_{\mathcal{S}}] + \overline{\hbar}_{\mathcal{S}^{\complement}}[\boldsymbol{a}_{\mathcal{S}^{\complement}}]\hbar_{\mathcal{S}}[\boldsymbol{c}_{\mathcal{S}^{\complement}}] :$$

$$\boldsymbol{c}_{\mathcal{S}} \in \mathbb{R}^{s},\ \boldsymbol{c}_{\mathcal{S}^{\complement}} \in \mathbb{R}^{p-s},\ \hbar_{\mathcal{S}}[\boldsymbol{c}_{\mathcal{S}}] + \hbar_{\mathcal{S}^{\complement}}[\boldsymbol{c}_{\mathcal{S}^{\complement}}] \leq 1\Big\}$$

Hölder inequality (2.5) ($\hbar_{\mathcal{S}}$ and $\hbar_{\mathcal{S}^{\complement}}$ are norms)

$$\leq \sup\Big\{\overline{\hbar}_{\mathcal{S}}[\boldsymbol{a}_{\mathcal{S}}] + \overline{\hbar}_{\mathcal{S}^{\complement}}[\boldsymbol{a}_{\mathcal{S}^{\complement}}] :$$

$$\boldsymbol{c}_{\mathcal{S}} \in \mathbb{R}^{s}, \boldsymbol{c}_{\mathcal{S}^{\complement}} \in \mathbb{R}^{p-s},\ \hbar_{\mathcal{S}}[\boldsymbol{c}_{\mathcal{S}}] + \hbar_{\mathcal{S}^{\complement}}[\boldsymbol{c}_{\mathcal{S}^{\complement}}] \leq 1\Big\}$$

$\hbar_{\mathcal{S}}, \hbar_{\mathcal{S}^{\complement}}$ are non-negative since they are norms,
and therefore, $\hbar_{\mathcal{S}}[\boldsymbol{c}_{\mathcal{S}}], \hbar_{\mathcal{S}^{\complement}}[\boldsymbol{c}_{\mathcal{S}^{\complement}}] \leq 1$;
$\overline{\hbar}_{\mathcal{S}}, \overline{\hbar}_{\mathcal{S}^{\complement}} \geq 0$ by 4. or 6. in Exercise 2.3

$$= \overline{\hbar}_{\mathcal{S}}[\boldsymbol{a}_{\mathcal{S}}] + \overline{\hbar}_{\mathcal{S}^{\complement}}[\boldsymbol{a}_{\mathcal{S}^{\complement}}],$$

argument of the supremum does not depend on $\boldsymbol{c}_{\mathcal{S}}, \boldsymbol{c}_{\mathcal{S}^{\complement}}$

where we have used for the last equality again the fact that $\hbar_{\mathcal{S}}$ and $\hbar_{\mathcal{S}^{\complement}}$ are norms, which ensures that $\hbar_{\mathcal{S}}[\mathbf{0}_s] = \hbar_{\mathcal{S}^{\complement}}[\mathbf{0}_{p-s}] = 0$, and thus, that the supremum is over a non-empty set. This concludes the proof of Part 1.

Part 2 We now establish a bound for $\widehat{\boldsymbol{\beta}}_{\mathcal{S}} = \widehat{\boldsymbol{\gamma}}_{\mathcal{S}}$ in $\overline{\hbar}_{\mathcal{S}}$:

$$\overline{\hbar}_{\mathcal{S}}\big[\boldsymbol{\alpha}_{\mathcal{S}} - \widehat{\boldsymbol{\beta}}_{\mathcal{S}}\big] \leq \overline{\hbar}_{\mathcal{S}}\big[(X_{\mathcal{S}}^{\top}X_{\mathcal{S}}/n)^{-1}\widehat{\boldsymbol{v}}_{\mathcal{S}}\big]r/(2n) + \overline{\hbar}_{\mathcal{S}}\big[(X_{\mathcal{S}}^{\top}X_{\mathcal{S}}/n)^{-1}X_{\mathcal{S}}^{\top}(\boldsymbol{y} - X_{\mathcal{S}}\boldsymbol{\alpha}_{\mathcal{S}})\big]/n\,.$$

We base our derivation on the primal-dual construction in Definition 7.3.1. *(Dual 1)* ensures that

$$-2X_{\mathcal{S}}^{\top}(\boldsymbol{y} - X_{\mathcal{S}}\widehat{\boldsymbol{\beta}}_{\mathcal{S}}) + r\widehat{\boldsymbol{v}}_{\mathcal{S}} = \mathbf{0}_s\,.$$

Adding a zero-valued term on the left-hand side gives

$$-2X_{\mathcal{S}}^{\top}(\boldsymbol{y} - X_{\mathcal{S}}\boldsymbol{\alpha}_{\mathcal{S}} + X_{\mathcal{S}}\boldsymbol{\alpha}_{\mathcal{S}} - X_{\mathcal{S}}\widehat{\boldsymbol{\beta}}_{\mathcal{S}}) + r\widehat{\boldsymbol{v}}_{\mathcal{S}} = \mathbf{0}_s\,,$$

and rearranging then gives

$$-2X_{\mathcal{S}}^{\top}X_{\mathcal{S}}(\boldsymbol{\alpha}_{\mathcal{S}} - \widehat{\boldsymbol{\beta}}_{\mathcal{S}}) = -r\widehat{\boldsymbol{v}}_{\mathcal{S}} + 2X_{\mathcal{S}}^{\top}(\boldsymbol{y} - X_{\mathcal{S}}\boldsymbol{\alpha}_{\mathcal{S}})\,.$$

Since the restricted Gram matrix $X_{\mathcal{S}}^\top X_{\mathcal{S}}$ is invertible by assumption, we find

$$\boldsymbol{\alpha}_{\mathcal{S}} - \widehat{\boldsymbol{\beta}}_{\mathcal{S}} = r(X_{\mathcal{S}}^\top X_{\mathcal{S}})^{-1}\widehat{\boldsymbol{v}}_{\mathcal{S}}/2 + (X_{\mathcal{S}}^\top X_{\mathcal{S}})^{-1} X_{\mathcal{S}}^\top (X_{\mathcal{S}}\boldsymbol{\alpha}_{\mathcal{S}} - \boldsymbol{y}).$$

We apply the function $\overline{\hbar}_{\mathcal{S}}$ on both sides and invoke the triangle inequality (1. in Exercise 2.3) and the absolute homogeneity (3. or 6. in Exercise 2.3) on the right-hand side to derive

$$\begin{aligned}\overline{\hbar}_{\mathcal{S}}[\boldsymbol{\alpha}_{\mathcal{S}} - \widehat{\boldsymbol{\beta}}_{\mathcal{S}}] \le\ & \overline{\hbar}_{\mathcal{S}}\big[(X_{\mathcal{S}}^\top X_{\mathcal{S}}/n)^{-1}\widehat{\boldsymbol{v}}_{\mathcal{S}}\big] r/(2n) \\ & + \overline{\hbar}_{\mathcal{S}}\big[(X_{\mathcal{S}}^\top X_{\mathcal{S}}/n)^{-1} X_{\mathcal{S}}^\top (\boldsymbol{y} - X_{\mathcal{S}}\boldsymbol{\alpha}_{\mathcal{S}})\big]/n,\end{aligned}$$

as desired.

Part 3 We finally derive the desired bound for $\widehat{\boldsymbol{\beta}} = \widehat{\boldsymbol{\gamma}}$ in $\overline{\hbar}$:

$$\overline{\hbar}[\boldsymbol{\beta} - \widehat{\boldsymbol{\beta}}] \le \left(d + \frac{\overline{\hbar}_{\mathcal{S}}\big[(X_{\mathcal{S}}^\top X_{\mathcal{S}}/n)^{-1}\widehat{\boldsymbol{v}}_{\mathcal{S}}\big](v+1)}{2v}\right)\frac{r}{n}.$$

We use the subdecomposability of $\overline{\hbar}$ established in Part 1 and the bound in $\overline{\hbar}_{\mathcal{S}}$ established in Part 2 to find

$$\begin{aligned}
&\overline{\hbar}[\boldsymbol{\beta} - \widehat{\boldsymbol{\beta}}] \\
&= \overline{\hbar}[\boldsymbol{\beta} - \boldsymbol{\alpha} + \boldsymbol{\alpha} - \widehat{\boldsymbol{\beta}}] && \text{adding a zero-valued term} \\
&\le \overline{\hbar}[\boldsymbol{\beta} - \boldsymbol{\alpha}] + \overline{\hbar}[\boldsymbol{\alpha} - \widehat{\boldsymbol{\beta}}] && \text{triangle inequality (1. in Exercise 2.3)} \\
&\le \overline{\hbar}[\boldsymbol{\beta} - \boldsymbol{\alpha}] + \overline{\hbar}_{\mathcal{S}}[\boldsymbol{\alpha}_{\mathcal{S}} - \widehat{\boldsymbol{\beta}}_{\mathcal{S}}] + \overline{\hbar}_{\mathcal{S}^{\complement}}[\boldsymbol{\alpha}_{\mathcal{S}^{\complement}} - \widehat{\boldsymbol{\beta}}_{\mathcal{S}^{\complement}}] && \text{Part 1 applied to the second term} \\
&\le \overline{\hbar}[\boldsymbol{\beta} - \boldsymbol{\alpha}] + \overline{\hbar}_{\mathcal{S}}\big[(X_{\mathcal{S}}^\top X_{\mathcal{S}}/n)^{-1}\widehat{\boldsymbol{v}}_{\mathcal{S}}\big] r/(2n) \\
&\quad + \overline{\hbar}_{\mathcal{S}}\big[(X_{\mathcal{S}}^\top X_{\mathcal{S}}/n)^{-1} X_{\mathcal{S}}^\top (\boldsymbol{y} - X_{\mathcal{S}}\boldsymbol{\alpha}_{\mathcal{S}})\big]/n \\
&\quad + \overline{\hbar}_{\mathcal{S}^{\complement}}[\boldsymbol{\alpha}_{\mathcal{S}^{\complement}} - \widehat{\boldsymbol{\beta}}_{\mathcal{S}^{\complement}}] && \text{Part 2 applied to the second term} \\
&= \overline{\hbar}[\boldsymbol{\beta} - \boldsymbol{\alpha}] + \overline{\hbar}_{\mathcal{S}}\big[(X_{\mathcal{S}}^\top X_{\mathcal{S}}/n)^{-1}\widehat{\boldsymbol{v}}_{\mathcal{S}}\big] r/(2n) \\
&\quad + \overline{\hbar}_{\mathcal{S}}\big[(X_{\mathcal{S}}^\top X_{\mathcal{S}}/n)^{-1} X_{\mathcal{S}}^\top (\boldsymbol{y} - X\boldsymbol{\alpha})\big]/n \\
&\quad + \overline{\hbar}_{\mathcal{S}^{\complement}}[\mathbf{0}_{p-s}] && \boldsymbol{\alpha}_{\mathcal{S}^{\complement}} = \widehat{\boldsymbol{\beta}}_{\mathcal{S}^{\complement}} = \mathbf{0}_{p-s} \text{ by the 2. assumption} \\
& && \text{in the theorem and (Primal 2), respectively}
\end{aligned}$$

$$= \overline{\hbar}[\boldsymbol{\beta} - \boldsymbol{\alpha}] + \overline{\hbar}_{\mathcal{S}}\big[(X_{\mathcal{S}}^\top X_{\mathcal{S}}/n)^{-1}\widehat{\boldsymbol{v}}_{\mathcal{S}}\big]r/(2n)$$
$$+ \overline{\hbar}_{\mathcal{S}}\big[(X_{\mathcal{S}}^\top X_{\mathcal{S}}/n)^{-1}X_{\mathcal{S}}^\top(\boldsymbol{y} - X\boldsymbol{\alpha})\big]/n$$

$\overline{\hbar}_{\mathcal{S}^\complement}[\boldsymbol{0}_{p-s}] = 0$ by 6. in Exercise 2.3

$$= dr/n + \overline{\hbar}_{\mathcal{S}}\big[(X_{\mathcal{S}}^\top X_{\mathcal{S}}/n)^{-1}\widehat{\boldsymbol{v}}_{\mathcal{S}}\big]r/(2n)$$
$$+ \overline{\hbar}_{\mathcal{S}}\big[(X_{\mathcal{S}}^\top X_{\mathcal{S}}/n)^{-1}\widehat{\boldsymbol{v}}_{\mathcal{S}}\big]r/(2vn)$$

1. and 2. assumptions of the theorem

$$= \left(d + \frac{\overline{\hbar}_{\mathcal{S}}\big[(X_{\mathcal{S}}^\top X_{\mathcal{S}}/n)^{-1}\widehat{\boldsymbol{v}}_{\mathcal{S}}\big](v+1)}{2v}\right)\frac{r}{n}, \qquad \text{consolidating}$$

as desired. □

7.4 Support Recovery Guarantees

We have discussed in ▶ Sect. 6.4 the fact that for approximately sparse models, it makes sense to speak of relevant predictors (predictors that correspond to non-zero-valued variables in the sparse vector) and irrelevant predictors (predictors that correspond to zero-valued variables in the sparse vector). In this section, we aim to differentiate these two groups of predictors based on data. This task is called *support recovery*, *variable selection*, or *feature selection*.

How well an estimator $\widehat{\boldsymbol{\beta}} \in \mathbb{R}^p$ performs this task is typically measured in terms of *false negatives* and *false positives*. False negatives are falsely omitted predictors, and false positives are falsely selected predictors; accordingly, given a sparse surrogate vector $\boldsymbol{\alpha} \in \mathbb{R}^p$, the number of false negatives is $\text{fn} := |\{j \in \{1, \dots, p\} : \widehat{\beta}_j = 0 \text{ and } \alpha_j \neq 0\}|$, and the number of false positives is $\text{fp} := |\{j \in \{1, \dots, p\} : \widehat{\beta}_j \neq 0 \text{ and } \alpha_j = 0\}|$. The smaller these two numbers, the better the estimator's performance at support recovery.

false negatives

false positives

The following approach to support recovery is based on an accurate estimation of each of the surrogate vector's coordinate values. We thus assume the following:

▪▪ Assumption 7.4.1

Generic Sup-Norm Bound We assume that for a sparse surrogate vector $\boldsymbol{\alpha}$ of the regression vector $\boldsymbol{\beta}$ and for a (potentially random) value $b \in [0, \infty)$, the estimator $\widehat{\boldsymbol{\beta}}$ satisfies the bound

$$\|\boldsymbol{\alpha} - \widehat{\boldsymbol{\beta}}\|_\infty \leq b\,.$$

For orthogonal design, Example 7.3.1 provides such a bound with $\boldsymbol{\alpha} = \boldsymbol{\beta}$ and $b = 3\|X^\top \boldsymbol{u}\|_\infty/n$ for a lasso with optimal tuning parameter, and Example 4.4.1 provides such a bound with $\boldsymbol{\alpha} = \boldsymbol{\beta}$ and $b = 9\|X^\top \boldsymbol{u}\|_\infty/n$ for a lasso with a data-driven tuning parameter. In general, such bounds can be expected only if the correlations among the predictors are weak.

The generic ℓ_∞-bound in Assumption 7.4.1 ensures that $\widehat{\boldsymbol{\beta}}$ captures all "reasonably" large predictors: it holds for all $j \in \{1, \dots, p\}$ with $|\alpha_j| > b$ that

$$
\begin{aligned}
|\widehat{\beta}_j| &= |\alpha_j - \alpha_j + \widehat{\beta}_j| + |\alpha_j - \widehat{\beta}_j| - |\alpha_j - \widehat{\beta}_j| && \text{adding zero-valued terms}\\
&\geq |\alpha_j| - |\alpha_j - \widehat{\beta}_j| && \text{triangle inequality applied to the first two terms}\\
&\geq |\alpha_j| - \|\boldsymbol{\alpha} - \widehat{\boldsymbol{\beta}}\|_\infty && \|\boldsymbol{a}\|_\infty = \max_{i\in\{1,\dots,p\}}|a_i| \geq |a_j| \text{ by definition of the } \ell_\infty\text{-norm}\\
&> b - b = 0\,. && |\alpha_j| > b \text{ by assumption; } \|\boldsymbol{\alpha} - \widehat{\boldsymbol{\beta}}\|_\infty \leq b \text{ by Assumption 7.4.1}
\end{aligned}
$$

This means that if most coordinate values of the sparse surrogate vector are either exactly zero or sufficiently large in absolute value, Assumption 7.4.1 guarantees that the estimator $\widehat{\boldsymbol{\beta}}$ performs well at support recovery in that it has a small number of false negatives.

On the other hand, Assumption 7.4.1 does not directly guarantee that $\widehat{\boldsymbol{\beta}}$ has a small number of false positives.[6] However, such a guarantee follows when $\widehat{\boldsymbol{\beta}}$ is complemented with a thresholding step (2.4). A sufficiently large cutoff c together with Assumption 7.4.1 ensures that all irrelevant predictors are discarded: If $c \geq b$, it holds for all $j \in \{1, \dots, p\}$ with $\alpha_j = 0$ that

$$
\begin{aligned}
|\widehat{\beta}_j| &= |\alpha_j - \widehat{\beta}_j| && \alpha_j = 0 \text{ by assumption}\\
&\leq \|\boldsymbol{\alpha} - \widehat{\boldsymbol{\beta}}\|_\infty && \|\boldsymbol{a}\|_\infty = \max_{i\in\{1,\dots,p\}}|a_i| \geq |a_j| \text{ by definition of the } \ell_\infty\text{-norm}\\
&\leq b && \|\boldsymbol{\alpha} - \widehat{\boldsymbol{\beta}}\|_\infty \leq b \text{ by Assumption 7.4.1}\\
&\leq c\,, && c \geq b \text{ by assumption}
\end{aligned}
$$

which implies in view of the definition of thresholding that $(\widehat{\beta}^c)_j = 0$. This means that if the cutoff is large enough, Assumption 7.4.1 guarantees that the thresholded estimator $\widehat{\boldsymbol{\beta}}^c$ performs well at support recovery in that it has a small number of false positives.

The following theorem refines these insights:

Theorem 7.4.1

Sign Consistent Support Recovery Consider a thresholded estimator $\widehat{\boldsymbol{\beta}}^c$ as defined in (2.4) based on an initial estimator $\widehat{\boldsymbol{\beta}}$ that satisfies Assumption 7.4.1 (generic sup-norm bound). It then holds:

1. For every cutoff $c \in [0, \infty]$, the thresholded estimator correctly identifies the signs of all sufficiently large variables of the sparse surrogate vector:

$$\text{sign}\left[(\widehat{\beta}^c)_j\right] = \text{sign}[\alpha_j]$$

for all $j \in \{1, \ldots, p\}$ with $|\alpha_j| > b + c$.

2. For every cutoff $c \in [b, \infty]$, the thresholded estimator also finds all zero-valued variables of the sparse surrogate vector:

$$\text{sign}\left[(\widehat{\beta}^c)_j\right] = \text{sign}[\alpha_j] = 0$$

for all $j \in \{1, \ldots, p\}$ with $\alpha_j = 0$.

The first part of the theorem limits false negatives; the second part limits false positives. If the cutoff is selected appropriately and there is no "ambiguous signal," that is, if $c \geq b$ and $\alpha_1, \ldots, \alpha_p \notin [-b - c, b + c]$, the two parts together guarantee perfect support recovery: $\text{fn} = \text{fp} = 0$. The thresholded estimator is then even sign consistent, which means that it identifies also the correct signs of all of the surrogate vector's coordinates values. But again, such perfect support recovery requires 1. the non-zero parameters to be sufficiently large, 2. a well-chosen cutoff, and 3. a suitable bound to start with; therefore, it is often unrealistic in practice.

The condition $|\alpha_j| > b + c$ for ruling out false negatives suggests small cutoffs or no thresholding altogether, while the condition $c \geq b$ for ruling out false positives suggests large cutoffs. Hence in practice, the size of the cutoff c needs to reflect the analyst's objective: A small cutoff is in order for *variable screening*, that is, the detection of all signals (for example, if one just wants to decrease the dimensionality of the problem for a subsequent treatment). For sparse estimators such as the lasso, $c = 0$ may work. A large cutoff is in order when predictors should be selected conservatively (for example, if it is expensive to study predictors further). A possible compromise between these two aspects is provided by adaptive validation as discussed in ► Sect. 4.4:

► Example 7.4.1

Thresholding the Lasso via Adaptive Validation In this example, we apply thresholding for support recovery with the lasso estimator (2.2). This requires the calibration of two tuning parameters: the lasso's original tuning parameter r and the cutoff c. Because both parameters affect support recovery, they need to be in sync.

Adaptive validation provides such a synchronized calibration. First, adaptive validation suggests $\widehat{r}_{\text{av}}$ in (4.4) for the lasso's original tuning parameter. This choice ensures

$$\|\boldsymbol{\beta} - \widehat{\boldsymbol{\beta}}_{\text{lasso}}[\widehat{r}_{\text{av}}]\|_\infty \leq \frac{9}{n}\|X^\top \boldsymbol{u}\|_\infty$$

for orthogonal designs (and similar guarantees for weakly correlated designs)—see Example 4.4.1. Hence, Assumption 7.4.1 is satisfied with $\boldsymbol{\alpha} = \boldsymbol{\beta}$ and $b = 9\|X^\top \boldsymbol{u}\|_\infty/n$.

Then, adaptive validation prompts the cutoff $c := 9\widehat{r}_{\text{av}}/(4n)$. This choice ensures that $(\widehat{\beta^c})_j \neq 0$ for all $\beta_j > 18\|X^\top \boldsymbol{u}\|_\infty/n$—see 1. in Theorem 7.4.1 and note that $b + c = 9\|X^\top \boldsymbol{u}\|_\infty/n + 9\widehat{r}_{\text{av}}/(4n) \geq 18\|X^\top \boldsymbol{u}\|_\infty/n$ in view of the bound $\widehat{r}_{\text{av}} \leq 4\|X^\top \boldsymbol{u}\|_\infty$ in Example 4.4.1—which means that all sufficiently large predictors are selected. For Gauss-distributed noise $\boldsymbol{u} \sim \mathcal{N}_n[\mathbf{0}_n, \sigma^2 \mathrm{I}_{n\times n}]$, for example, this essentially includes all predictors that are larger than $\sigma\sqrt{\log[p]/n}$—see again Example 4.4.1. In this sense, adaptive validation allows us to threshold "safely."◄

Finally, bear in mind that thresholding typically benefits only support recovery (and not prediction and estimation).

Proof of Theorem 7.4.1 The proof of 1. is a refinement of the above derivations: If $\alpha_j \geq b + c$,

$$\begin{aligned} \widehat{\beta}_j &= \alpha_j - \alpha_j + \widehat{\beta}_j && \text{adding a zero-valued term} \\ &\geq \alpha_j - |\alpha_j - \widehat{\beta}_j| && -|a| \leq a \end{aligned}$$

$$\geq \alpha_j - \|\boldsymbol{\alpha} - \widehat{\boldsymbol{\beta}}\|_\infty \qquad \|\boldsymbol{a}\|_\infty = \max_{i\in\{1,\dots,p\}}|a_i| \geq |a_j| \text{ by definition of the } \ell_\infty\text{-norm}$$

$$> b + c - b = c, \qquad \alpha_j > b + c \text{ by assumption; } \|\boldsymbol{\alpha} - \widehat{\boldsymbol{\beta}}\|_\infty \leq b \text{ by Assumption 7.4.1}$$

which means in view of the definition of the thresholded estimator in (2.4) that $(\widehat{\beta}^c)_j = \widehat{\beta}_j > 0$, as desired. The case $\alpha_j \leq -b - c$ follows along the same lines.

The proof of 2. has already been stated above the theorem in its entirety. □

7.5 Exercises

7.5.1 Exercises for ► Sect. 7.2

Exercise 7.1 ♦♦ In this exercise, we show that the lasso's ℓ_1-estimation bounds in Example 7.2.1 also entail estimation bounds with respect to other norms. We proceed in two steps.

1. Use the classical Hölder inequality (2.6) to show that for all $\boldsymbol{c} \in \mathbb{R}^p$ and $k, l \in [1, \infty]$ with $k < l$, it holds that

   $$\|\boldsymbol{c}\|_k \leq p^{1/k-1/l}\|\boldsymbol{c}\|_l ,$$

   and to show that for all $\boldsymbol{c} \in \mathbb{R}^p$ and $k, l \in [1, \infty]$ with $k \geq l$, it holds that

   $$\|\boldsymbol{c}\|_k \leq \|\boldsymbol{c}\|_l .$$

2. Conclude from Claim 1 and Example 7.2.1 that for every $q \in [1, \infty]$, it holds that

   $$\mathbb{P}\left\{ \|\boldsymbol{\beta} - \widehat{\boldsymbol{\beta}}_{\text{lasso}}\|_q \geq 192\sigma s\sqrt{\frac{\log[p/t]}{n}} \right\} \leq t$$

   under the conditions of the example.

The compatibility condition in Assumption 6.4.1 is tailored, in a sense, to estimation in $\hbar$-loss function, that is, ℓ_1-loss in the lasso case. Replacing that condition with (slightly more restrictive) versions that better capture the specifics of other ℓ_q-loss functions can reduce the dependence on the sparsity level from s to $s^{1/q}$. We omit the details.

7.5.2 Exercises for ▶ Sect. 7.3

Exercise 7.2 ◇◇ In this exercise, we study the convexity of subfunctions of convex prior functions. Consider a finite, $\mathcal{S}$-decomposable prior function $\hbar$ with subfunctions $\hbar_{\mathcal{S}}$ and $\hbar_{\mathcal{S}^\complement}$ (cf. Definition 6.4.1). Show that $\hbar$ is convex if and only if both $\hbar_{\mathcal{S}}$ and $\hbar_{\mathcal{S}^\complement}$ are convex (cf. Definition 2.5.1).

Exercise 7.3 ◆◆ In this exercise, we study the irrepresentability condition of Assumption 7.3.1 for the lasso's ℓ_1-prior function. Show that

$$\sup_{\boldsymbol{a}\in\partial\hbar_{\mathcal{S}}[\widehat{\boldsymbol{\gamma}}_{\mathcal{S}}]} \overline{\hbar}_{\mathcal{S}^\complement}\big[{X_{\mathcal{S}^\complement}}^\top X_{\mathcal{S}}(X_{\mathcal{S}}^\top X_{\mathcal{S}})^{-1}\boldsymbol{a}\big] \le \max_{j\in\mathcal{S}^\complement} \|(X_{\mathcal{S}}^\top X_{\mathcal{S}})^{-1}X_{\mathcal{S}}^\top \boldsymbol{x}_j\|_1\,,$$

where $\hbar$ is the ℓ_1-norm and $\boldsymbol{x}_1,\ldots,\boldsymbol{x}_p\in\mathbb{R}^n$ the columns of the design matrix: $X=(\boldsymbol{x}_1,\ldots,\boldsymbol{x}_p)$.

The vector $(X_{\mathcal{S}}^\top X_{\mathcal{S}})^{-1}X_{\mathcal{S}}^\top \boldsymbol{x}_j$ is the least-squares estimator for regressing the irrelevant predictor $\boldsymbol{x}_j$ on the matrix of relevant predictors $X_{\mathcal{S}}$ (cf. Eq. (1.4)); hence, the right-hand side of the above inequality is yet another measure for how much the relevant predictors are correlated with the irrelevant ones.

Exercise 7.4 ◆◆◆ In this exercise, we study the uniqueness of the lasso estimator (2.2). Given a corresponding primal-dual pair $(\widehat{\boldsymbol{\gamma}},\widehat{\boldsymbol{v}})$ constructed according to Definition 7.3.1, show the following three claims:

1. The restricted primal vector $\widehat{\boldsymbol{\gamma}}_{\mathcal{S}}$ is the unique solution of the restricted lasso problem in *(Primal 1)* if the restricted Gram matrix $X_{\mathcal{S}}^\top X_{\mathcal{S}}$ is invertible.
2. The primal vector $\widehat{\boldsymbol{\gamma}}$ is not necessarily the unique solution of the full lasso problem (2.2) even if $X_{\mathcal{S}}^\top X_{\mathcal{S}}$ is invertible and the primal-dual witness construction was successful. (In contrast, the primal-dual pairs in Definition 7.3.1 are then uniquely defined.)
3. The primal vector $\widehat{\boldsymbol{\gamma}}$ is the unique solution of the full lasso problem if $X_{\mathcal{S}}^\top X_{\mathcal{S}}$ is invertible, $\|\widehat{\boldsymbol{v}}_{\mathcal{S}^\complement}\|_\infty<1$, and

$r \in (0, \infty)$. Conclude that this implies in particular that the lasso solution is supported on $\mathcal{S}$, which relates to the discussion of false positives in ▶ Sect. 7.4.

This exercise shows that uniqueness of the lasso estimator requires the *strict* dual feasibility condition $\|\widehat{\boldsymbol{v}}_{\mathcal{S}^\complement}\|_\infty < 1$ rather than the dual feasibility condition $\|\widehat{\boldsymbol{v}}_{\mathcal{S}^\complement}\|_\infty \leq 1$ that is used in the main text (cf. Lemma 7.3.1, for example).[7]

7.6 Notes and References

1 The primal-dual witness technique was introduced in Wainwright (2009). Our treatment generalizes the discussion in Hastie et al. (2015, Chapter 11.4 on pp. 301ff) beyond the lasso.

2 We could, therefore, call the approach *primal-subgradient witness technique* instead. In any case, we use the terms *subgradient* and *dual* interchangeably, because subgradients and solutions of the "dual problem" are intimately related—see books on optimization, such as Boyd and Vandenberghe (2004), for details.

3 A definition of Lagrange dual functions can be found in Hiriart-Urruty and Lemaréchal (2004, Display (5.2.5) on p. 197). Our definition of Hölder dual functions generalizes the concept of *dual norms*; a definition of those can be found in Hiriart-Urruty and Lemaréchal (2004, Section C.3.2 on p. 146).

4 See van de Geer and Bühlmann (2009) for a comparison among such conditions.

5 When the orthogonality is exact, sparsity is not needed: The derivation via the explicit expression of the lasso does not involve $\mathcal{S}$, and the derivation via the theorems also works with $\mathcal{S} := \{1, \ldots, p\}$. In general, however, it is important to keep track of $\mathcal{S}$: For designs that are only approximately orthogonal (for example, if $p > n$), the set $\mathcal{S}$ must be small to meet the irrespresentability condition and, more generally, to avoid that the quantities that involve correlations, such as $(X_{\mathcal{S}}^\top X_{\mathcal{S}}/n)^{-1}$, render the bounds ineffective. The rate $\sigma\sqrt{\log[p]/n}$, on the other hand, remains the same across different sparsity levels $s = |\mathcal{S}|$ (in contrast to the rate $\sigma s\sqrt{\log[p]/n}$ in Example 7.2.1).

6 Assumption 7.4.1 can be complemented with further assumptions to guarantee small fp or even fp $=$ 0 without any thresholding—see, for example, 3. in Exercise 7.4 or Zhao and Yu (2006). However, as always, the more assumptions, the less plausible the theoretical framework.

7 The uniqueness of the lasso estimator is discussed from a different standpoint in Tibshirani (2013); Schneider and Ewald (2017).

Supplementary Information

J. Lederer, *Fundamentals of High-Dimensional Statistics*, Springer Texts in Statistics, https://doi.org/10.1007/978-3-030-73792-4

A Solutions

A.1 Solutions for ▶ Chap. 1

Solutions for ▶ Sect. 1.1

Solution 1.1 See the R file on the book homepage.

Solutions for ▶ Sect. 1.2

Solution 1.2 We prove the claims in order.

1. The proof of the first claim follows from basic linear algebra:

$$\begin{aligned} &\boldsymbol{\alpha}^\top X^\top X\boldsymbol{\alpha} \\ &= \|X\boldsymbol{\alpha}\|_2^2 && \text{definition of the } \ell_2\text{-norm on Page IX} \\ &\geq 0\,, && \text{norms are non-negative according to Page IX} \end{aligned}$$

   as desired.

2. The proof of the second claim follows again from basic linear algebra.

   Write $X = (\boldsymbol{x}_1, \ldots, \boldsymbol{x}_p)$ with columns $\boldsymbol{x}_1, \ldots, \boldsymbol{x}_p \in \mathbb{R}^n$. If $p > n$, we know by linear algebra that the columns must be linearly dependent. For example, there are $a_1, \ldots, a_{p-1} \in \mathbb{R}$ such that $\boldsymbol{x}_p = \sum_{j=1}^{p-1} a_j\boldsymbol{x}_j$. Then, for $\boldsymbol{w} := (a_1, \ldots, a_{p-1}, -1)^\top \in \mathbb{R}^p$, it holds that $\boldsymbol{w} \neq \boldsymbol{0}_n$ and

$$X\boldsymbol{w} = \sum_{j=1}^{p} w_j\boldsymbol{x}_j = \sum_{j=1}^{p-1} w_j\boldsymbol{x}_j + w_p\boldsymbol{x}_p = \sum_{j=1}^{p-1} a_j\boldsymbol{x}_j - \boldsymbol{x}_p = \boldsymbol{0}_n\,.$$

Hence,

$$\begin{aligned} \boldsymbol{w}^\top X^\top X\boldsymbol{w} &= (X\boldsymbol{w})^\top X\boldsymbol{w} && (AB)^\top = B^\top A^\top \\ &= \|X\boldsymbol{w}\|_2^2 && \text{definition of the } \ell_2\text{-norm} \\ &= \|\mathbf{0}_n\|_2^2 && \text{above display} \\ &= 0 && \text{positive definiteness of norms} \end{aligned}$$

for $\boldsymbol{w} \neq \mathbf{0}_n$, which means that $X^\top X$ is not invertible.

3. We again resort to linear algebra.

   $\Rightarrow$: Assume that $X\boldsymbol{\gamma} = \mathbf{0}_n$ for a $\boldsymbol{\gamma} \neq \mathbf{0}_p$. Then, for every $\widehat{\boldsymbol{\beta}}_{\text{ls}} \in \arg\min_{\boldsymbol{\alpha}\in\mathbb{R}^p} \|\boldsymbol{y} - X\boldsymbol{\alpha}\|_2^2$, also $\widehat{\boldsymbol{\beta}}_{\text{ls}} + \boldsymbol{\gamma} \in \arg\min_{\boldsymbol{\alpha}\in\mathbb{R}^p} \|\boldsymbol{y} - X\boldsymbol{\alpha}\|_2^2$. Hence, $\widehat{\boldsymbol{\beta}}_{\text{ls}}$ is not unique.

   $\Leftarrow$: Assume that $\arg\min_{\boldsymbol{\alpha}\in\mathbb{R}^p} \|\boldsymbol{y} - X\boldsymbol{\alpha}\|_2^2$ is not unique. Then, there are least-squares estimators $\widehat{\boldsymbol{\gamma}}_{\text{ls}}, \widehat{\boldsymbol{\beta}}_{\text{ls}}$ such that $\widehat{\boldsymbol{\gamma}}_{\text{ls}} \neq \widehat{\boldsymbol{\beta}}_{\text{ls}}$ but

$$\|\boldsymbol{y} - X\widehat{\boldsymbol{\gamma}}_{\text{ls}}\|_2^2 = \|\boldsymbol{y} - X\widehat{\boldsymbol{\beta}}_{\text{ls}}\|_2^2 .$$

   However, since $\boldsymbol{a} \mapsto \|\boldsymbol{y} - \boldsymbol{a}\|_2^2$ is *strictly* convex, this means that $X\widehat{\boldsymbol{\gamma}}_{\text{ls}} = X\widehat{\boldsymbol{\beta}}_{\text{ls}}$, which in turn means that $X\boldsymbol{\gamma} = \mathbf{0}_n$ for $\boldsymbol{\gamma} := \widehat{\boldsymbol{\gamma}}_{\text{ls}} - \widehat{\boldsymbol{\beta}}_{\text{ls}} \neq \mathbf{0}_p$.
   The stated conclusion now follows from the fact that $X\boldsymbol{\gamma} \neq \mathbf{0}_n$ for all $\boldsymbol{\gamma} \in \mathbb{R}^p \setminus \{\mathbf{0}_p\}$ if and only if $X^\top X$ is invertible.

4. We use again that the function $\boldsymbol{a} \mapsto \|\boldsymbol{y} - \boldsymbol{a}\|_2^2$ is *strictly* convex.

   Assume that $X\widehat{\boldsymbol{\gamma}}_{\text{ls}} \neq X\widehat{\boldsymbol{\beta}}_{\text{ls}}$. Then, for every $a \in (0, 1)$,

$$\begin{aligned} &\|\boldsymbol{y} - X\big(a\widehat{\boldsymbol{\gamma}}_{\text{ls}} + (1-a)\widehat{\boldsymbol{\beta}}_{\text{ls}}\big)\|_2^2 \\ &= \|\boldsymbol{y} - aX\widehat{\boldsymbol{\gamma}}_{\text{ls}} + (1-a)X\widehat{\boldsymbol{\beta}}_{\text{ls}}\|_2^2 \\ &\qquad \text{multiplying out the design-related part} \\ &< a\|\boldsymbol{y} - X\widehat{\boldsymbol{\gamma}}_{\text{ls}}\|_2^2 + (1-a)\|\boldsymbol{y} - X\widehat{\boldsymbol{\beta}}_{\text{ls}}\|_2^2 \\ &\qquad \text{strict convexity of the mentioned function;} \\ &\qquad \text{use the function values} \\ &\qquad \boldsymbol{a} = aX\widehat{\boldsymbol{\gamma}}_{\text{ls}} \text{ and } \boldsymbol{a} = (1-a)X\widehat{\boldsymbol{\beta}}_{\text{ls}}\text{, respectively} \\ &= a\|\boldsymbol{y} - X\widehat{\boldsymbol{\beta}}_{\text{ls}}\|_2^2 + (1-a)\|\boldsymbol{y} - X\widehat{\boldsymbol{\beta}}_{\text{ls}}\|_2^2 \\ &\qquad \text{both } \widehat{\boldsymbol{\gamma}}_{\text{ls}} \text{ and } \widehat{\boldsymbol{\beta}}_{\text{ls}} \text{ are least-squares solutions} \\ &= \|\boldsymbol{y} - X\widehat{\boldsymbol{\beta}}_{\text{ls}}\|_2^2 , \qquad \text{consolidating terms} \end{aligned}$$

which means that $a\widehat{\boldsymbol{\gamma}}_{\mathrm{ls}} + (1 - a)\widehat{\boldsymbol{\beta}}_{\mathrm{ls}}$ yields a strictly smaller value in the objective function than $\widehat{\boldsymbol{\beta}}_{\mathrm{ls}}$. This contradicts that $\widehat{\boldsymbol{\beta}}_{\mathrm{ls}}$ is a least-squares solution.

5. The proof is short: we just need to use the properties of the Moore–Penrose inverse.

According to ▶ Sect. 1.2, we have to show that $X^\top X(X^+\boldsymbol{y}) = X^\top \boldsymbol{y}$. For this, we compute

$$\begin{aligned} X^\top X(X^+\boldsymbol{y}) &= X^\top (XX^+)^\top \boldsymbol{y} && \text{Part 3 in the definition of Moore–Penrose inverses} \\ &= (XX^+X)^\top \boldsymbol{y} && \text{3. in Lemma B.2.1 (reversion of transposition)} \\ &= X^\top \boldsymbol{y}\,, && \text{Part 1 in the definition of Moore–Penrose inverses} \end{aligned}$$

as desired.

Alternatively, we could show that for all $\boldsymbol{\alpha} \in \mathbb{R}^p$,

$$\|\boldsymbol{y} - X\boldsymbol{\alpha}\|_2^2 \ \geq\ \|\boldsymbol{y} - X\widehat{\boldsymbol{\beta}}_{\mathrm{ls}}\|_2^2\,.$$

For this, we first observe that

$$\begin{aligned} &2\langle(\mathrm{I}_{n\times n} - XX^+)\boldsymbol{y},\ X(X^+\boldsymbol{y} - \boldsymbol{\alpha})\rangle \\ &= 2\langle\boldsymbol{y},\ (\mathrm{I}_{n\times n} - XX^+)^\top X(X^+\boldsymbol{y} - \boldsymbol{\alpha})\rangle && \text{property (B.1 of transposition)} \\ &= 2\langle\boldsymbol{y},\ (\mathrm{I}_{n\times n} - XX^+)X(X^+\boldsymbol{y} - \boldsymbol{\alpha})\rangle && \text{3. in the definition of Moore–Penrose inverses} \\ &= 2\langle\boldsymbol{y},\ (X - XX^+X)(X^+\boldsymbol{y} - \boldsymbol{\alpha})\rangle && \text{reorganizing} \\ &= 0\,. && \text{1. in the definition of Moore–Penrose inverses} \end{aligned}$$

Using this, we find for every $\boldsymbol{\alpha} \in \mathbb{R}^p$

$$\begin{aligned} &\|\boldsymbol{y} - X\boldsymbol{\alpha}\|_2^2 \\ &= \|(\mathrm{I}_{n\times n} - XX^+)\boldsymbol{y} + XX^+\boldsymbol{y} - X\boldsymbol{\alpha}\|_2^2 && \text{adding a zero-valued term} \\ &= \|(\mathrm{I}_{n\times n} - XX^+)\boldsymbol{y} + X(X^+\boldsymbol{y} - \boldsymbol{\alpha})\|_2^2 && \text{factorizing X} \\ &= \|(\mathrm{I}_{n\times n} - XX^+)\boldsymbol{y}\|_2^2 + \|X(X^+\boldsymbol{y} - \boldsymbol{\alpha})\|_2^2 \\ &\quad + 2\langle(\mathrm{I}_{n\times n} - XX^+)\boldsymbol{y},\ X(X^+\boldsymbol{y} - \boldsymbol{\alpha})\rangle && \text{expanding the square} \\ &= \|(\mathrm{I}_{n\times n} - XX^+)\boldsymbol{y}\|_2^2 + \|X(X^+\boldsymbol{y} - \boldsymbol{\alpha})\|_2^2 && \text{previous display} \\ &= \|\boldsymbol{y} - XX^+\boldsymbol{y}\|_2^2 + \|XX^+\boldsymbol{y} - X\boldsymbol{\alpha}\|_2^2 && \text{expanding the bracket in the second term} \\ &= \|\boldsymbol{y} - X\widehat{\boldsymbol{\beta}}_{\mathrm{ls}}\|_2^2 + \|X\widehat{\boldsymbol{\beta}}_{\mathrm{ls}} - X\boldsymbol{\alpha}\|_2^2 && \text{definition of } \widehat{\boldsymbol{\beta}}_{\mathrm{ls}} \end{aligned}$$

$$\geq \|y - X\widehat{\beta}_{ls}\|_2^2 , \qquad \text{positive definiteness of norms}$$

as desired.

6. Each of the three claims is a brief exercise in linear algebra.
   (i) One needs to verify that X^+ satisfies the four properties of the definition of Moore–Penrose inverses on Page 19. The first property can be derived as follows:

$$(DD^+D)_{ij}$$

$$= \sum_{k=1}^{p} D_{ik} \sum_{l=1}^{n} D^+_{kl} D_{lj} \qquad \text{explicit form of matrix–matrix multiplications}$$

$$= D_{ii} D^+_{ij} D_{jj} \qquad D \text{ diagonal by assumption}$$

$$= \begin{cases} D_{ii} D^+_{ii} D_{ii} = D_{ii} & \text{for } i = j \\ 0 & \text{for } i \neq j \end{cases} \qquad \text{definition of } D^+ \text{ in the exercise text}$$

$$= D_{ij} . \qquad D \text{ diagonal by assumption}$$

   The remaining three properties are proved similarly.

   (ii) Observe first that

$$(DD^+)_{ij}$$

$$= \sum_{k=1}^{p} D_{ik} D^+_{kj} \qquad \text{explicit form of matrix–matrix multiplication}$$

$$= D_{ii} D^+_{ij} \qquad D \text{ diagonal}$$

$$= \begin{cases} D_{ii} D^+_{ii} = 1 & \text{for } i = j,\ D_{ii} \neq 0 ; \\ D_{ii} D^+_{ii} = 0 & \text{for } i = j,\ D_{ii} = 0 ; \\ 0 & \text{for } i \neq j . \end{cases} \qquad \text{definition of } D^+$$

   Therefore, DD^+ is diagonal with zeros and ones as entries, and the number of ones is $|\{i \in \{1, \ldots, \min\{n, p\}\} : D_{ii} \neq 0\}| = \text{rank}[D]$. Since U, V are orthogonal (see Definition B.2.8), $\text{rank}[D] = \text{rank}[X]$, from which we can conclude the claim.

(iii) We need to verify that X^+ satisfies the four properties of the definition of Moore–Penrose inverses on Page 19. The first property can be derived as follows:

$$
\begin{aligned}
& XX^+X \\
&= UDV^\top(VD^+U^\top)UDV^\top && \text{SVD and definition of } X^+ \\
&= UDD^+DV^\top && U, V \text{ orthogonal by assumption} \\
&= UDV^\top && D^+ \text{ is a Moore–Penrose inverse of } D \text{ by assumption} \\
&= X\,. && \text{SVD}
\end{aligned}
$$

The other three properties can be verified similarly.

7. The short proof is based on the previous findings.

   We first note that, in view of Claim 3, it is sufficient to show the equality for *one* least-squares solution. We opt for $\widehat{\boldsymbol{\beta}}_{\text{ls}} = X^+\boldsymbol{y}$ motivated by Claim 4. We then find

$$
\begin{aligned}
& \|X\boldsymbol{\beta} - X\widehat{\boldsymbol{\beta}}_{\text{ls}}\|_2^2 \\
&= \|X\boldsymbol{\beta} - XX^+\boldsymbol{y}\|_2^2 && \text{our choice of } \widehat{\boldsymbol{\beta}}_{\text{ls}} \\
&= \|X\boldsymbol{\beta} - XX^+(X\boldsymbol{\beta} + \boldsymbol{u})\|_2^2 && \text{model assumptions: } \boldsymbol{y} = X\boldsymbol{\alpha} + \boldsymbol{u} \\
&= \|XX^+\boldsymbol{u}\|_2^2 && \text{1. in the definition of Moore–Penrose inverses and consolidating} \\
&= \|UDV^\top VD^+U^\top\boldsymbol{u}\|_2^2 && \text{SVD and 5.(iii) above} \\
&= \|UDD^+U^\top\boldsymbol{u}\|_2^2\,, && V \text{ orthogonal (Definition B.2.8)}
\end{aligned}
$$

   as desired.

8. After some simple calculations, the claim follows from the above results and the properties of Chi-squared distributions.

   We first rewrite the right-hand side of the display in 6. as

$$
\begin{aligned}
& \|UDD^+U^\top\boldsymbol{u}\|_2^2 \\
&= (UDD^+U^\top\boldsymbol{u})^\top UDD^+U^\top\boldsymbol{u} && \text{definition of the } \ell_2\text{-norm}
\end{aligned}
$$

$$= (U^\top \boldsymbol{u})^\top (DD^+)^\top U^\top U DD^+ U^\top \boldsymbol{u}$$

Lemma B.2.1 (reversion of transposition)

$$= (U^\top \boldsymbol{u})^\top (DD^+)^\top DD^+ U^\top \boldsymbol{u}$$

U orthogonal (Definition B.2.8)

$$= (U^\top \boldsymbol{u})^\top DD^+ DD^+ U^\top \boldsymbol{u}$$

5.(i) and 3. in the definition of Moore–Penrose inverses

$$= (U^\top \boldsymbol{u})^\top DD^+ U^\top \boldsymbol{u}\,.$$

4.(i) and 1. or 2. in the definition of Moore–Penrose inverses

Setting $\boldsymbol{\gamma} := U^\top \boldsymbol{u}/\sigma$ and combining with 6. yield

$$\|X\boldsymbol{\beta} - X\widehat{\boldsymbol{\beta}}_{\mathrm{ls}}\|_2^2 \sim \sigma^2 \boldsymbol{\gamma}^\top DD^+ \boldsymbol{\gamma}\,,$$

and thus, dividing both sides by n,

$$\frac{\|X\boldsymbol{\beta} - X\widehat{\boldsymbol{\beta}}_{\mathrm{ls}}\|_2^2}{n} \sim \frac{\sigma^2 \boldsymbol{\gamma}^\top DD^+ \boldsymbol{\gamma}}{n}\,.$$

Since U is orthogonal, $\boldsymbol{\gamma} \sim \mathcal{N}_n[\mathbf{0}_n, \mathrm{I}_{n\times n}]$. Moreover, according to 4.(ii), DD^+ has rank$[X]$ ones on its diagonal and zeros everywhere else. These two observations imply that $\boldsymbol{\gamma}^\top DD^+ \boldsymbol{\gamma} \sim \chi^2_{\mathrm{rank}[X]}$. The claim now follows from the fact that the mean of a Chi-squared random distribution equals its degrees of freedom—see 1. in Exercise 5.4.

9. We confirm the properties of Moore–Penrose matrices.

All four properties in the definition of Moore–Penrose inverses on Page 19 can be approached similarly, so that we focus only on 1.:

$$X(X^\top X)^+ X^\top X = X\,.$$

For this, we consider first general $A \in \mathbb{R}^{p\times p}$, $B \in \mathbb{R}^{n\times p}$ that satisfy $B^\top BA = \mathbf{0}_{p\times p}$. Then,

$$B^\top BA = \mathbf{0}_{p\times p}$$

$$\Rightarrow \quad A^\top B^\top BA = \mathbf{0}_{p\times p}$$

multiplying both sides of the assumed equality by $A^\top$ from the left

$$\Rightarrow \quad (BA)^\top (BA) = \mathbf{0}_{p\times p}$$

3. in Lemma B.2.1 (reversion of transposition)

$$\Rightarrow \quad \left((BA)^\top (BA)\right)_{jj} = 0 \quad \text{for all } j \in \{1, \ldots, p\}$$

definition of matrix–matrix multiplication

$$\Rightarrow \quad \sum_{i=1}^{n} ((BA)^\top)_{ji} (BA)_{ij} = 0 \quad \text{for all } j \in \{1, \ldots, p\}$$

definition of matrix–matrix multiplication

$$\Rightarrow \quad \sum_{i=1}^{n} ((BA)_{ij})^2 = 0 \quad \text{for all } j \in \{1, \ldots, p\}$$

Definition B.2.1 of transposition

$$\Rightarrow \quad (BA)_{ij} = 0 \quad \text{for all } i \in \{1, \ldots, n\},\ j \in \{1, \ldots, p\}$$

squared terms are non-negative

$$\Rightarrow \quad BA = \mathbf{0}_{n\times p}\,. \qquad \text{definition of matrices}$$

Now, we use the definition of Moore–Penrose inverses for $(X^\top X)^+$ and the above display with $A = (XX^\top)^+ X^\top - \mathrm{I}_{p\times p}$ and $B = X^\top$ to find

$$X^\top X (X^\top X)^+ X^\top X = X^\top X$$

1. in the definition of Moore–Penrose inverses applied to $(X^\top X)^+$

$$\Rightarrow \quad X^\top X\left((X^\top X)^+ X^\top X - \mathrm{I}_{p\times p}\right) = \mathbf{0}_{n\times n}$$

factorizing $X^\top X$

$$\Rightarrow \quad X\left((X^\top X)^+ X^\top X - \mathrm{I}_{p\times p}\right) = \mathbf{0}_{n\times p}$$

previous display

$$\Rightarrow \quad X(X^\top X)^+ X^\top X = X\,,$$

multiplying the bracket out and rearranging terms

as desired.

Solutions for ▶ Sect. 1.3

Solution 1.3 The proofs are straightforward calculations.

1. By assumption, $f_{\boldsymbol{\alpha}}$ is the density of $\mathcal{N}_n[X\boldsymbol{\alpha}, \sigma^2 \mathrm{I}_{n\times n}]$, and g the density of $\mathcal{N}_p[\mathbf{0}_p, \tau^2 \mathrm{I}_{p\times p}]$, that is,

$$f_{\boldsymbol{\alpha}}[\boldsymbol{y}] = \frac{1}{(2\pi\sigma^2)^{n/2}} e^{-\|\boldsymbol{y}-X\boldsymbol{\alpha}\|_2^2/(2\sigma^2)}$$

and

$$g[\boldsymbol{\alpha}] = \frac{1}{(2\pi\tau^2)^{p/2}} e^{-\|\boldsymbol{\alpha}\|_2^2/(2\tau^2)} .$$

Using these formulae and the properties of the logarithm yields

$$\begin{aligned}
&\log\left[f_{\boldsymbol{\alpha}}[\boldsymbol{y}]g[\boldsymbol{\alpha}]\right] \\
&= \log\left[\frac{1}{(2\pi\sigma^2)^{n/2}} e^{-\|\boldsymbol{y}-X\boldsymbol{\alpha}\|_2^2/(2\sigma^2)} \frac{1}{(2\pi\tau^2)^{p/2}} e^{-\|\boldsymbol{\alpha}\|_2^2/(2\tau^2)}\right] \\
&= -\frac{n}{2}\log[2\pi\sigma^2] - \frac{1}{2\sigma^2}\|\boldsymbol{y} - X\boldsymbol{\alpha}\|_2^2 - \frac{p}{2}\log[2\pi\tau^2] - \frac{1}{2\tau^2}\|\boldsymbol{\alpha}\|_2^2 .
\end{aligned}$$

Then,

$$\begin{aligned}
&\underset{\boldsymbol{\alpha}\in\mathbb{R}^p}{\arg\max}\, \ell[\boldsymbol{\alpha} \mid \boldsymbol{y}] \\
&= \underset{\boldsymbol{\alpha}\in\mathbb{R}^p}{\arg\min}\left\{\frac{n}{2}\log[2\pi\sigma^2] + \frac{1}{2\sigma^2}\|\boldsymbol{y} - X\boldsymbol{\alpha}\|_2^2 \right. \\
&\qquad\qquad \left. + \frac{p}{2}\log[2\pi\tau^2] + \frac{1}{2\tau^2}\|\boldsymbol{\alpha}\|_2^2\right\} \\
&\qquad\qquad\qquad \text{hint and above display} \\
&= \underset{\boldsymbol{\alpha}\in\mathbb{R}^p}{\arg\min}\left\{\frac{1}{2\sigma^2}\|\boldsymbol{y} - X\boldsymbol{\alpha}\|_2^2 + \frac{1}{2\tau^2}\|\boldsymbol{\alpha}\|_2^2\right\} \\
&\qquad\qquad\qquad \text{omitting terms that do not depend on } \boldsymbol{\alpha} \\
&= \underset{\boldsymbol{\alpha}\in\mathbb{R}^p}{\arg\min}\left\{\|\boldsymbol{y} - X\boldsymbol{\alpha}\|_2^2 + \frac{\sigma^2}{\tau^2}\|\boldsymbol{\alpha}\|_2^2\right\} . \\
&\qquad\qquad\qquad \text{multiplying through by } 2\sigma^2 \text{ and noting} \\
&\qquad\qquad\qquad \text{that this does not affect any minimizer}
\end{aligned}$$

Hence, $\widehat{\boldsymbol{\beta}}_{\text{map}} = \widehat{\boldsymbol{\beta}}_{\text{ridge}}$ for $r = \sigma^2/\tau^2$, as desired.

2. Now,

$$\mathscr{g}[\boldsymbol{\alpha}] = \frac{1}{(2\tau)^p} e^{-\|\boldsymbol{\alpha}\|_1/\tau},$$

but we can proceed as above otherwise. In particular, we find

$$\begin{aligned}
&\log\left[\mathscr{f}_{\boldsymbol{\alpha}}[\boldsymbol{y}]\mathscr{g}[\boldsymbol{\alpha}]\right] \\
&= \log\left[\frac{1}{(2\pi\sigma^2)^{n/2}} e^{-\|\boldsymbol{y}-X\boldsymbol{\alpha}\|_2^2/(2\sigma^2)} \frac{1}{(2\tau)^p} e^{-\|\boldsymbol{\alpha}\|_1/\tau}\right] \\
&= -\frac{n}{2}\log[2\pi\sigma^2] - \frac{1}{2\sigma^2}\|\boldsymbol{y} - X\boldsymbol{\alpha}\|_2^2 - p\log[2\tau] - \frac{1}{\tau}\|\boldsymbol{\alpha}\|_1
\end{aligned}$$

and

$$\begin{aligned}
&\underset{\boldsymbol{\alpha}\in\mathbb{R}^p}{\arg\max}\, \mathscr{f}[\boldsymbol{\alpha} \mid \boldsymbol{y}] \\
&= \underset{\boldsymbol{\alpha}\in\mathbb{R}^p}{\arg\min}\left\{\frac{n}{2}\log[2\pi\sigma^2] + \frac{1}{2\sigma^2}\|\boldsymbol{y} - X\boldsymbol{\alpha}\|_2^2 + p\log[2\tau] + \frac{1}{\tau}\|\boldsymbol{\alpha}\|_1\right\} \\
&= \underset{\boldsymbol{\alpha}\in\mathbb{R}^p}{\arg\min}\left\{\frac{1}{2\sigma^2}\|\boldsymbol{y} - X\boldsymbol{\alpha}\|_2^2 + \frac{1}{\tau}\|\boldsymbol{\alpha}\|_1\right\} \\
&= \underset{\boldsymbol{\alpha}\in\mathbb{R}^p}{\arg\min}\left\{\|\boldsymbol{y} - X\boldsymbol{\alpha}\|_2^2 + \frac{2\sigma^2}{\tau}\|\boldsymbol{\alpha}\|_1\right\}
\end{aligned}$$

by following the same lines as above. Hence, $\widehat{\boldsymbol{\beta}}_{\text{map}} = \widehat{\boldsymbol{\beta}}_{\text{lasso}}$ for $r = 2\sigma^2/\tau$, as desired.
3. The proof follows the exact same scheme as above.

Solutions for ▶ Sect. 1.4

Solution 1.4 The solutions are simple applications of the definitions of convexity and strict convexity.
1. There is a number of ways to prove this claim: we choose a route that requires minimal knowledge about calculus.

   With $\mathscr{f} : \boldsymbol{a} \mapsto \|\boldsymbol{y} - X\boldsymbol{a}\|_2^2$, we find

$$\begin{aligned}
&\mathscr{f}[w\boldsymbol{a} + (1-w)\boldsymbol{b}] - w\mathscr{f}[\boldsymbol{a}] - (1-w)\mathscr{f}[\boldsymbol{b}] \\
&= \|\boldsymbol{y} - X(w\boldsymbol{a} + (1-w)\boldsymbol{b})\|_2^2 \\
&\quad - w\|\boldsymbol{y} - X\boldsymbol{a}\|_2^2 - (1-w)\|\boldsymbol{y} - X\boldsymbol{b}\|_2^2 \qquad \text{choice of } \mathscr{f} \\
&= \|w(\boldsymbol{y} - X\boldsymbol{a}) + (1-w)(\boldsymbol{y} - X\boldsymbol{b})\|_2^2
\end{aligned}$$

$$
\begin{aligned}
&-w\|\boldsymbol{y}-X\boldsymbol{a}\|_2^2-(1-w)\|\boldsymbol{y}-X\boldsymbol{b}\|_2^2 \\
&\qquad\qquad\qquad\text{linearity of matrix–vector multiplications} \\
&=\|w(\boldsymbol{y}-X\boldsymbol{a})\|_2^2+\|(1-w)(\boldsymbol{y}-X\boldsymbol{b})\|_2^2 \\
&\quad+2\langle w(\boldsymbol{y}-X\boldsymbol{a}),\,(1-w)(\boldsymbol{y}-X\boldsymbol{b})\rangle \\
&\quad-w\|\boldsymbol{y}-X\boldsymbol{a}\|_2^2-(1-w)\|\boldsymbol{y}-X\boldsymbol{b}\|_2^2 \\
&\qquad\qquad\qquad\|\boldsymbol{a}+\boldsymbol{b}\|_2^2=\|\boldsymbol{a}\|_2^2+\|\boldsymbol{b}\|_2^2+2\langle\boldsymbol{a},\,\boldsymbol{b}\rangle \\
&=w^2\|\boldsymbol{y}-X\boldsymbol{a}\|_2^2+(1-w)^2\|\boldsymbol{y}-X\boldsymbol{b}\|_2^2 \\
&\quad+2w(1-w)\langle\boldsymbol{y}-X\boldsymbol{a},\,\boldsymbol{y}-X\boldsymbol{b}\rangle \\
&\quad-w\|\boldsymbol{y}-X\boldsymbol{a}\|_2^2-(1-w)\|\boldsymbol{y}-X\boldsymbol{b}\|_2^2 \\
&\qquad\qquad\qquad\text{absolute homogeneity of norms and } w,\,1-w\in[0,1]; \\
&\qquad\qquad\qquad\text{linearity of inner products} \\
&=w^2\big(\|\boldsymbol{y}-X\boldsymbol{a}\|_2^2+\|\boldsymbol{y}-X\boldsymbol{b}\|_2^2-2\langle\boldsymbol{y}-X\boldsymbol{a},\,\boldsymbol{y}-X\boldsymbol{b}\rangle\big) \\
&\quad-w\big(\|\boldsymbol{y}-X\boldsymbol{a}\|_2^2+\|\boldsymbol{y}-X\boldsymbol{b}\|_2^2-2\langle\boldsymbol{y}-X\boldsymbol{a},\,\boldsymbol{y}-X\boldsymbol{b}\rangle\big) \\
&\qquad\qquad\qquad\text{sorting with respect to } w \\
&=w^2\|\boldsymbol{y}-X\boldsymbol{a}-(\boldsymbol{y}-X\boldsymbol{b})\|_2^2-w\|\boldsymbol{y}-X\boldsymbol{a}-(\boldsymbol{y}-X\boldsymbol{b})\|_2^2 \\
&\qquad\qquad\qquad\|\boldsymbol{a}+\boldsymbol{b}\|_2^2=\|\boldsymbol{a}\|_2^2+\|\boldsymbol{b}\|_2^2+2\langle\boldsymbol{a},\,\boldsymbol{b}\rangle \\
&=(w^2-w)\|X\boldsymbol{b}-X\boldsymbol{a}\|_2^2 \qquad\qquad\text{consolidating} \\
&\le 0\,, \qquad\qquad w^2\le w \text{ for } w\in[0,1];\text{ norms are non-negative}
\end{aligned}
$$

as desired.

2. This claim can be proved along the same lines as 1., but for the sake of illustration, we present a different route.

   A smooth function $\mathbb{R}^p \to \mathbb{R}$ is strictly convex if and only if its *Hesse matrix*, which is the matrix of second-order derivatives, is positive definite everywhere. In our case, $\boldsymbol{a} \mapsto \|\boldsymbol{y}-X\boldsymbol{a}\|_2^2$ is indeed smooth, and its Hesse matrix is

   $$\nabla^2\|\boldsymbol{y}-X\boldsymbol{a}\|_2^2 = 2X^\top X\,.$$

   Hence, the function in question is strictly convex if and only if $X^\top X$ is positive definite. Since $X^\top X$ is symmetric, and positive definiteness and invertibility are equivalent for symmetric matrices, this yields the desired claim.

3. There is a plethora of such functions; we just look at two simple examples.

   Considering functions $\mathbb{R}^p \to \mathbb{R}$, a simple example for the first case is the constant function $\boldsymbol{a} \mapsto 0$, for which every point is a minimum; a simple example for the second case is $\boldsymbol{a} \mapsto \|\boldsymbol{a}\|_1$, for which $\mathbf{0}_p$ is the only minimum.

   For the bonus question, the answer is no. Indeed, naming the function in question f and $\boldsymbol{a} := (1,0)^\top$, $\boldsymbol{b} := (0,1)^\top$ and assuming that f is convex, we find

$$\begin{aligned}
1 &= f\big[(1,1)^\top\big] && \text{definition of } f\\
&= f\big[(2,0)^\top/2 + (0,2)^\top/2\big] && \text{basic vector algebra}\\
&\le f\big[(2,0)^\top\big]/2 + f\big[(0,2)^\top\big]/2 && \text{assumed convexity}\\
&= 0/2 + 0/2 && \text{definition of } f\\
&= 0\,, && \text{consolidating}
\end{aligned}$$

   which is a contradiction.

4. We prove this by a simple contradiction.

   Assume that $\boldsymbol{a}$ and $\boldsymbol{b}$ are two distinct minima of f. The presumed strict convexity implies for every intermediate point $w\boldsymbol{a} + (1-w)\boldsymbol{b}$, $w \in (0,1)$, that

$$f\big[w\boldsymbol{a} + (1-w)\boldsymbol{b}\big] \;<\; wf[\boldsymbol{a}] + (1-w)f[\boldsymbol{b}]\,.$$

   Since both $\boldsymbol{a}$ and $\boldsymbol{b}$ are minima of f, it holds that $f[\boldsymbol{a}] = f[\boldsymbol{b}]$. Plugging this into the display and collecting terms yield

$$f\big[w\boldsymbol{a} + (1-w)\boldsymbol{b}\big] \;<\; wf[\boldsymbol{a}] + (1-w)f[\boldsymbol{a}] \;=\; f[\boldsymbol{a}]\,,$$

   which means that $\boldsymbol{a}$ is not a minimum of f as assumed initially. This is the desired contradiction.

Solution 1.6 The proof follows readily from the explicit form of the ridge estimator.

► Sect. 1.4 provides us with

$$\widehat{\boldsymbol{\beta}}_{\text{ridge}}[r] \;=\; \frac{1}{4 - 8d + 4d^2 + (9 + d^2)r + r^2}\begin{pmatrix} 4 - 8d + 4d^2 + 5r \\ (4+d)r \end{pmatrix}$$

for all $r \in (0, \infty)$ and $d \in \mathbb{R}$, and therefore, for $d = 1$,

$$\widehat{\boldsymbol{\beta}}_{\text{ridge}}[r] = \frac{1}{10r + r^2}\begin{pmatrix}5r\\5r\end{pmatrix} = \frac{1}{1 + r/10}\begin{pmatrix}1/2\\1/2\end{pmatrix}.$$

From here, a straightforward calculation gives

$$\begin{aligned}
&\|\widehat{\boldsymbol{\beta}}_{\text{ridge}}[r] - (1/2, 1/2)^\top\|_2\\
&= \sqrt{\Bigl(\frac{1/2}{1 + r/10} - \frac{1}{2}\Bigr)^2 + \Bigl(\frac{1/2}{1 + r/10} - \frac{1}{2}\Bigr)^2}\\
&= \sqrt{\frac{1}{2}\Bigl(\frac{1}{1 + r/10} - 1\Bigr)^2}\\
&= \sqrt{\frac{1}{2}\Bigl(\frac{r/10}{1 + r/10}\Bigr)^2}\\
&= \sqrt{\frac{1}{2}\Bigl(\frac{r}{10 + r}\Bigr)^2}\\
&= \frac{r}{\sqrt{2}(10 + r)},
\end{aligned}$$

as desired.

This result and the fact that $r/(\sqrt{2}(10 + r))$ continuously approaches 0 as $r \to 0$ ensure that the ridge estimator continuously approaches the least-squares solution $(1 - a, a)^\top$ with $a = 1/2$ as $r \to 0$.

Solution 1.7 We prove the eleven claims in order.

1. The proof of the first claim simply consists of plugging in the values for $\boldsymbol{y}$ and X and some reformulations.

   We first derive

$$\begin{aligned}
&\boldsymbol{y} - X\boldsymbol{\alpha}\\
&= \begin{pmatrix}1\\2\end{pmatrix} - \begin{pmatrix}1 & d\\2 & 2\end{pmatrix}\begin{pmatrix}\alpha_1\\\alpha_2\end{pmatrix} && \text{definitions of } \boldsymbol{y} \text{ and } X \text{ in Table 1.3}\\
&= \begin{pmatrix}1\\2\end{pmatrix} - \begin{pmatrix}\alpha_1 + d\alpha_2\\2\alpha_1 + 2\alpha_2\end{pmatrix} && \text{matrix–vector multiplication}\\
&= \begin{pmatrix}1 - \alpha_1 - d\alpha_2\\2 - 2\alpha_1 - 2\alpha_2\end{pmatrix} && \text{vector–vector addition}
\end{aligned}$$

$$= -\begin{pmatrix} \alpha_1 - 1 + d\alpha_2 \\ 2(\alpha_1 - 1) + 2\alpha_2 \end{pmatrix}. \qquad \text{rearranging the quantities}$$

Hence,

$$\begin{aligned} &\|\boldsymbol{y} - X\boldsymbol{\alpha}\|_2^2 \\ &= \big(\alpha_1 - 1 + d\alpha_2\big)^2 + \big(2(\alpha_1 - 1) + 2\alpha_2\big)^2 \\ &\qquad \text{invoking the above display and the definition of the } \ell_2\text{-norm} \\ &= 5(\alpha_1 - 1)^2 + (4 + d^2)\alpha_2^2 + 2(4 + d)(\alpha_1 - 1)\alpha_2\,, \\ &\qquad \text{expanding and summarizing terms} \end{aligned}$$

as desired.

2. This proof follows from 1. by plugging in d.
   Indeed, we find

$$\begin{aligned} &\|\boldsymbol{y} - X\boldsymbol{\alpha}\|_2^2 \\ &= 5(\alpha_1 - 1)^2 + (4 + d^2)\alpha_2^2 + 2(4 + d)(\alpha_1 - 1)\alpha_2 \\ &\qquad \text{1. just above} \\ &= 5\big((\alpha_1 - 1)^2 + \alpha_2^2 + 2(\alpha_1 - 1)\alpha_2\big) \\ &\qquad \text{using that } d = 1 \text{ and summarizing terms} \\ &= 5(\alpha_1 - 1 + \alpha_2)^2\,, \qquad \text{binomial theorem} \end{aligned}$$

as desired.

3. The proof follows from rewriting the terms in 2.
   We find

$$\begin{aligned} \|\boldsymbol{y} - X\boldsymbol{\alpha}\|_2^2 &= c \\ \Leftrightarrow \quad 5(\alpha_1 - 1 + \alpha_2)^2 &= c \qquad \text{2. just above} \\ \Leftrightarrow \quad \alpha_1 - 1 + \alpha_2 &= \pm\sqrt{\frac{c}{5}} \\ &\qquad \text{dividing both sides by 5 and taking square-roots} \\ \Leftrightarrow \quad \alpha_2 &= 1 - \alpha_1 \pm \sqrt{\frac{c}{5}}\,, \\ &\qquad \text{rearranging terms} \end{aligned}$$

as desired.

4. The proof consists of plugging in the values and taking limits.

   We find

$$\frac{\big((\cos\omega)(\alpha_1-1)+(\sin\omega)\alpha_2\big)^2}{a^2} + \frac{\big(-(\sin\omega)(\alpha_1-1)+(\cos\omega)\alpha_2\big)^2}{b^2}$$

$$\to 10\big((\cos 45^\circ)(\alpha_1-1)+(\sin 45^\circ)\alpha_2\big)^2 + \frac{\big(-(\sin 45^\circ)(\alpha_1-1)+(\cos 45^\circ)\alpha_2\big)^2}{b^2}$$

plugging in the values for ω and a

$$= \frac{10(\alpha_1-1+\alpha_2)^2}{2} + \frac{(\alpha_1-1+\alpha_2)^2}{2b^2}$$

$\sin 45^\circ = \cos 45^\circ = 1/\sqrt{2}$

$$\to 5(\alpha_1-1+\alpha_2)^2 .$$

consolidating and taking the limit $b\to\infty$

   In view of the comment in the exercise, this means that the level sets converge to the specified limit. We conclude with 2. that the straight lines that form the level sets of the least-squares can be interpreted as degenerate ellipses.

5. Just expand the squared terms and summarize the factors.
6. This is a simple algebra exercise.

   We find

$$\frac{(\cos\omega)^2}{a^2} + \frac{(\sin\omega)^2}{b^2} = 5$$

comparing the (α_1-1)-terms

$$\Rightarrow \quad \frac{(\cos\omega)^2}{a^2} + \frac{1-(\cos\omega)^2}{b^2} = 5$$

$(\sin\omega)^2 + (\cos\omega)^2 = 1$

$$\Rightarrow \quad (\cos\omega)^2\Big(\frac{1}{a^2} - \frac{1}{b^2}\Big) = 5 - \frac{1}{b^2}$$

factorizing and rearranging terms

$$\Rightarrow \quad (\cos\omega)^2 = \frac{5 - \frac{1}{b^2}}{\frac{1}{a^2} - \frac{1}{b^2}},$$

dividing both sides by $1/a^2 - 1/b^2$ under the assumption $a \neq b$

as desired.

7. This works as above.

   We find

$$\frac{(\sin\omega)^2}{a^2} + \frac{(\cos\omega)^2}{b^2} = 4 + d^2$$

comparing the α_2-terms

$$\Rightarrow \quad \frac{1 - (\cos\omega)^2}{a^2} + \frac{(\cos\omega)^2}{b^2} = 4 + d^2$$

$(\sin\omega)^2 + (\cos\omega)^2 = 1$

$$\Rightarrow \quad (\cos\omega)^2\left(\frac{1}{b^2} - \frac{1}{a^2}\right) + \frac{1}{a^2} = 4 + d^2$$

factorizing terms

$$\Rightarrow \quad \frac{5 - \frac{1}{b^2}}{\frac{1}{a^2} - \frac{1}{b^2}}\left(\frac{1}{b^2} - \frac{1}{a^2}\right) + \frac{1}{a^2} = 4 + d^2 \qquad \text{Claim 6}$$

$$\Rightarrow \quad \frac{1}{b^2} - 5 + \frac{1}{a^2} = 4 + d^2$$

simplifying the left-hand side

$$\Rightarrow \quad \frac{1}{a^2} + \frac{1}{b^2} = 9 + d^2,$$

consolidating

as desired.

8. The proof combines the results from the two previous proof steps.

   We first observe that

$$(\cos\omega)^2 = \frac{5 - \frac{1}{b^2}}{\frac{1}{a^2} - \frac{1}{b^2}} \qquad \text{Claim 6}$$

$$= \frac{5 - \frac{1}{b^2}}{\frac{1}{a^2} + \frac{1}{b^2} - \frac{2}{b^2}} \qquad \text{adding a zero-valued term}$$

$$= \frac{5 - \frac{1}{b^2}}{9 + d^2 - \frac{2}{b^2}} \qquad \text{Claim 7}$$

$$= \frac{5b^2 - 1}{(9 + d^2)b^2 - 2}, \qquad \text{multiplying through by } b^2$$

and similarly,

$$1 - (\cos\omega)^2 = 1 - \frac{5b^2 - 1}{(9 + d^2)b^2 - 2} \qquad \text{previous display}$$

$$= \frac{(9 + d^2)b^2 - 2 - 5b^2 + 1}{(9 + d^2)b^2 - 2}$$

putting the two terms on a common denominator

$$= \frac{(4 + d^2)b^2 - 1}{(9 + d^2)b^2 - 2}. \qquad \text{consolidating}$$

Using that $(\sin\omega)^2 + (\cos\omega)^2$ and combining the two displays yield

$$\begin{aligned}(\cos\omega)^2(\sin\omega)^2 &= (\cos\omega)^2(1 - (\cos\omega)^2)\\ &= \frac{(5b^2 - 1)\big((4 + d^2)b^2 - 1\big)}{\big((9 + d^2)b^2 - 2\big)^2}\\ &= \frac{5(4 + d^2)b^4 - (9 + d^2)b^2 + 1}{(9 + d^2)^2b^4 - 4(9 + d^2)b^2 + 4},\end{aligned}$$

as desired.

9. We do a proof by contradiction.
   Assume that $a = b$. Similarly as in 6., we then find

$$\frac{(\cos\omega)^2}{a^2} + \frac{(\sin\omega)^2}{b^2} = 5$$

comparing the $(\alpha_1 - 1)$-terms as in 6.

$$\Rightarrow \quad \frac{1}{a^2} = 5 \qquad a = b;\ (\sin\omega)^2 + (\cos\omega)^2 = 1$$

$$\Rightarrow \quad a = b = \frac{1}{\sqrt{5}}.$$

solving for a; using again that $a = b$

Then, similarly as in 7.,

$$\frac{(\sin\omega)^2}{a^2}+\frac{(\cos\omega)^2}{b^2} = 4+d^2$$

comparing the α_2-terms as in 7.

$$\Rightarrow \quad 5 = 4+d^2$$

$a = 1/\sqrt{5}$ according to the previous display; $(\sin\omega)^2+(\cos\omega)^2=1$

$$\Rightarrow \quad d = \pm 1\,.$$

consolidating

The case $d = 1$ is excluded by assumption. For $d = -1$, we find

$$2\left(\frac{1}{a^2}-\frac{1}{b^2}\right)(\cos\omega)(\sin\omega) = 2(4+d)$$

comparing the $(1-\alpha_1)\alpha_2$-terms

$$\Rightarrow \quad 0 = 6\,,$$

$a = b$ by assumption; $d = -1$

which means that $a = b$ cannot be true if $d = -1$ either. Thus, we have contradicted $a = b$, as desired.

10. We proceed similarly as before.

    Observe that

$$2\left(\frac{1}{a^2}-\frac{1}{b^2}\right)(\cos\omega)(\sin\omega) = 2(4+d)$$

comparing the $(1-\alpha_1)\alpha_2$-terms of 5. and 1.

$$\Rightarrow \quad 2\left(\frac{1}{a^2}+\frac{1}{b^2}-\frac{2}{b^2}\right)(\cos\omega)(\sin\omega) = 2(4+d)$$

adding a zero-valued term inside the first bracketed term

$$\Rightarrow \quad 2\left(9+d^2-\frac{2}{b^2}\right)(\cos\omega)(\sin\omega) = 2(4+d) \qquad \text{Claim 7}$$

$$\Rightarrow \quad (\cos\omega)(\sin\omega) = \frac{4+d}{9+d^2-\frac{2}{b^2}} \qquad \text{rearranging terms}$$

$$\Rightarrow \quad (\cos\omega)^2(\sin\omega)^2 = \frac{(4+d)^2}{(9+d^2-\frac{2}{b^2})^2}$$

squaring both sides

$$\Rightarrow \quad \frac{5(4+d^2)b^4-(9+d^2)b^2+1}{(9+d^2)^2b^4-4(9+d^2)b^2+4} = \frac{(4+d)^2}{(9+d^2-\frac{2}{b^2})^2}$$

Claim 8

$$\Rightarrow \quad \frac{5(4+d^2)-\frac{9+d^2}{b^2}+\frac{1}{b^4}}{(9+d^2)^2-\frac{4(9+d^2)}{b^2}+\frac{4}{b^2}} - \frac{(4+d)^2}{(9+d^2-\frac{2}{b^2})^2} = 0\,,$$

reducing the first fraction by b^4 and rearranging terms

as desired.

11. Find R code on the book homepage.

A.2 Solutions for ▶ Chap. 2

Solutions for ▶ Sect. 2.2

Solution 2.1 We prove the five claims in turn.

1. The first claim follows readily from the properties of minima.

   Indeed, we find

$$\begin{aligned}\min_{\boldsymbol{\alpha}'\in\mathbb{R}^{p+1}} \|\boldsymbol{y}-X'\boldsymbol{\alpha}'\|_2^2 &= \min_{\alpha_{p+1}\in\mathbb{R}}\min_{\boldsymbol{\alpha}\in\mathbb{R}^p}\|\boldsymbol{y}-X\boldsymbol{\alpha}-\alpha\boldsymbol{x}\|_2^2 && X'=(X,\boldsymbol{x})\\ &\le \min_{\boldsymbol{\alpha}\in\mathbb{R}^p}\|\boldsymbol{y}-X\boldsymbol{\alpha}\|_2^2\,, && \text{consider } \alpha_{p+1}=0\end{aligned}$$

   as desired.

2. The proof of this claim consists of simple but slightly tedious derivations.

   Note first that the proof is complete if we can find a vector $\boldsymbol{\alpha}'\in\mathbb{R}^{p+1}$ such that

$$\|\boldsymbol{y}-X'\boldsymbol{\alpha}'\|_2^2 < \min_{\boldsymbol{\alpha}\in\mathbb{R}^p}\|\boldsymbol{y}-X\boldsymbol{\alpha}\|_2^2\,.$$

   To this end, we define $\boldsymbol{\alpha}' := (\widehat{\boldsymbol{\beta}}_{\mathrm{ls}}{}^\top, \alpha_{p+1})^\top$ with $\alpha_{p+1}\in\mathbb{R}$ specified later. Now,

$$\begin{aligned}&\|\boldsymbol{y}-X'\boldsymbol{\alpha}'\|_2^2-\min_{\boldsymbol{\alpha}\in\mathbb{R}^p}\|\boldsymbol{y}-X\boldsymbol{\alpha}\|_2^2\\ &= \|\boldsymbol{y}-X'\boldsymbol{\alpha}'\|_2^2-\|\boldsymbol{y}-X\widehat{\boldsymbol{\beta}}_{\mathrm{ls}}\|_2^2 && \text{definition of } \widehat{\boldsymbol{\beta}}_{\mathrm{ls}}\end{aligned}$$

$$
\begin{aligned}
&= \|\boldsymbol{y} - X\widehat{\boldsymbol{\beta}}_{\text{ls}} - \alpha_{p+1}\boldsymbol{x}\|_2^2 - \|\boldsymbol{y} - X\widehat{\boldsymbol{\beta}}_{\text{ls}}\|_2^2 \\
&\qquad\qquad \text{substituting } X' = (X, \boldsymbol{x}) \text{ and } \boldsymbol{\alpha}' = (\widehat{\boldsymbol{\beta}}_{\text{ls}}{}^\top, \alpha_{p+1})^\top \\
&= \|\boldsymbol{y} - X\widehat{\boldsymbol{\beta}}_{\text{ls}}\|_2^2 - 2\langle \boldsymbol{y} - X\widehat{\boldsymbol{\beta}}_{\text{ls}},\, \alpha_{p+1}\boldsymbol{x}\rangle \\
&\quad + \|\alpha_{p+1}\boldsymbol{x}\|_2^2 - \|\boldsymbol{y} - X\widehat{\boldsymbol{\beta}}_{\text{ls}}\|_2^2 \qquad \text{expanding the first term} \\
&= -2\alpha_{p+1}\langle \boldsymbol{y} - X\widehat{\boldsymbol{\beta}}_{\text{ls}},\, \boldsymbol{x}\rangle + (\alpha_{p+1})^2\|\boldsymbol{x}\|_2^2\,. \\
&\qquad\qquad \text{consolidating terms and using} \\
&\qquad\qquad \text{the linearity/absolute homogeneity} \\
&\qquad\qquad \text{of inner products/norms}
\end{aligned}
$$

In view of the stated condition $\langle \boldsymbol{y} - X\widehat{\boldsymbol{\beta}}_{\text{ls}},\, \boldsymbol{x}\rangle \neq 0$, it must hold that $\boldsymbol{x} \neq \boldsymbol{0}_n$. Therefore, we can massage the display further into

$$
\begin{aligned}
&\|\boldsymbol{y} - X'\boldsymbol{\alpha}'\|_2^2 - \min_{\boldsymbol{\alpha}\in\mathbb{R}^p} \|\boldsymbol{y} - X\boldsymbol{\alpha}\|_2^2 \\
&\quad = \|\boldsymbol{x}\|_2^2\left(\frac{\langle \boldsymbol{y} - X\widehat{\boldsymbol{\beta}}_{\text{ls}},\, \boldsymbol{x}\rangle}{\|\boldsymbol{x}\|_2^2} - \alpha_{p+1}\right)^2 - \frac{\left(\langle \boldsymbol{y} - X\widehat{\boldsymbol{\beta}}_{\text{ls}},\, \boldsymbol{x}\rangle\right)^2}{\|\boldsymbol{x}\|_2^2}\,.
\end{aligned}
$$

Setting $\alpha_{p+1} := \langle \boldsymbol{y} - X\widehat{\boldsymbol{\beta}}_{\text{ls}},\, \boldsymbol{x}\rangle / \|\boldsymbol{x}\|_2^2$, this yields

$$
\|\boldsymbol{y} - X'\boldsymbol{\alpha}'\|_2^2 - \min_{\boldsymbol{\alpha}\in\mathbb{R}^p} \|\boldsymbol{y} - X\boldsymbol{\alpha}\|_2^2 = -\frac{\left(\langle \boldsymbol{y} - X\widehat{\boldsymbol{\beta}}_{\text{ls}},\, \boldsymbol{x}\rangle\right)^2}{\|\boldsymbol{x}\|_2^2}\,,
$$

which implies—again in view of the stated condition $\langle \boldsymbol{y} - X\widehat{\boldsymbol{\beta}}_{\text{ls}},\, \boldsymbol{x}\rangle \neq 0$—that

$$
\|\boldsymbol{y} - X'\boldsymbol{\alpha}'\|_2^2 - \min_{\boldsymbol{\alpha}\in\mathbb{R}^p} \|\boldsymbol{y} - X\boldsymbol{\alpha}\|_2^2 < 0\,,
$$

and thus, rearranging,

$$
\|\boldsymbol{y} - X'\boldsymbol{\alpha}'\|_2^2 < \min_{\boldsymbol{\alpha}\in\mathbb{R}^p} \|\boldsymbol{y} - X\boldsymbol{\alpha}\|_2^2\,,
$$

as desired.

3. We establish a proof by contradiction.

   Consider a least-squares estimator of the form $(\widehat{\boldsymbol{\beta}}_{\text{ls}})' = ((\widehat{\boldsymbol{\beta}}_{\text{ls}})'_{-}{}^\top, 0)^\top$ for some $(\widehat{\boldsymbol{\beta}}_{\text{ls}})'_{-} \in \mathbb{R}^p$. It then holds that

$$
\min_{\boldsymbol{\alpha}'\in\mathbb{R}^{p+1}} \|\boldsymbol{y} - X'\boldsymbol{\alpha}'\|_2^2 = \|\boldsymbol{y} - X'(\widehat{\boldsymbol{\beta}}_{\text{ls}})'\|_2^2 \qquad \text{definition of } (\widehat{\boldsymbol{\beta}}_{\text{ls}})'
$$

$$= \|\boldsymbol{y} - X(\widehat{\boldsymbol{\beta}}_{\text{ls}})'_{-}\|_2^2$$

$(\widehat{\boldsymbol{\beta}}_{\text{ls}})'_{p+1} = 0$ by assumption; $X' = (X, \boldsymbol{x})$

$$\geq \min_{\boldsymbol{\alpha} \in \mathbb{R}^p} \|\boldsymbol{y} - X\boldsymbol{\alpha}\|_2^2 .$$

taking the minimum

This contradicts the strict inequality of 2. and thus proves the claim.

4. For proving this claim, we argue with linear dependence.

   Recall that if $\text{rank}[X] \geq n$, the columns of X form a basis for $\mathbb{R}^n$. Applied to the columns of $X' \in \mathbb{R}^{n \times (p+1)}$, this means that for every $\alpha_{p+1} \in \mathbb{R}$, there exists a $\boldsymbol{\gamma} \in \mathbb{R}^p$ such that $\alpha_{p+1}\boldsymbol{x} = X\boldsymbol{\gamma}$. We can use this in the following derivation:

$$\min_{\boldsymbol{\alpha}' \in \mathbb{R}^{p+1}} \|\boldsymbol{y} - X'\boldsymbol{\alpha}'\|_2^2$$

$$= \min_{\boldsymbol{\alpha} \in \mathbb{R}^p} \min_{\alpha_{p+1} \in \mathbb{R}} \|\boldsymbol{y} - X\boldsymbol{\alpha} - \alpha_{p+1}\boldsymbol{x}\|_2^2$$

properties of minima; $X' = (X, \boldsymbol{x})$

$$= \min_{\boldsymbol{\alpha} \in \mathbb{R}^p} \min_{\boldsymbol{\gamma} \in \mathbb{R}^p} \|\boldsymbol{y} - X\boldsymbol{\alpha} - X\boldsymbol{\gamma}\|_2^2$$ above insight: $\alpha_{p+1}\boldsymbol{x} = X\boldsymbol{\gamma}$

$$= \min_{\boldsymbol{\alpha} \in \mathbb{R}^p} \|\boldsymbol{y} - X\boldsymbol{\alpha}\|_2^2 ,$$ $\boldsymbol{\alpha}$ taking the role of $\boldsymbol{\alpha} + \boldsymbol{\gamma}$

   as desired.

5. We prove this by constructing and verifying a specific solution.

   Set $\boldsymbol{\gamma}' := (\widehat{\boldsymbol{\beta}}_{\text{ls}}{}^\top, 0)^\top + (\boldsymbol{\gamma}^\top, -\alpha_{p+1})^\top \in \mathbb{R}^p$, where $\alpha_{p+1} \in \mathbb{R} \setminus \{0\}$ and $\boldsymbol{\gamma} \in \mathbb{R}^p$ such that $\alpha_{p+1}\boldsymbol{x} = X\boldsymbol{\gamma}$ (cf. the proof of 4.). Then,

$$\|\boldsymbol{y} - X'\boldsymbol{\gamma}'\|_2^2$$

$$= \|\boldsymbol{y} - X\widehat{\boldsymbol{\beta}}_{\text{ls}} - X\boldsymbol{\gamma} + \alpha'_{p+1}\boldsymbol{x}\|_2^2$$ choice of $\boldsymbol{\gamma}'$; $X' = (X, \boldsymbol{x})$

$$= \|\boldsymbol{y} - X\widehat{\boldsymbol{\beta}}_{\text{ls}}\|_2^2$$ $\alpha_{p+1}\boldsymbol{x} = X\boldsymbol{\gamma}$ by construction

$$= \min_{\boldsymbol{\alpha} \in \mathbb{R}^p} \|\boldsymbol{y} - X\boldsymbol{\alpha}\|_2^2$$ definition of $\widehat{\boldsymbol{\beta}}_{\text{ls}}$

$$= \min_{\boldsymbol{\alpha}' \in \mathbb{R}^{p+1}} \|\boldsymbol{y} - X'\boldsymbol{\alpha}'\|_2^2 .$$ 4.

Hence, $(\widehat{\boldsymbol{\beta}}_{\mathrm{ls}})' := \boldsymbol{\gamma}'$ is a least-squares solution with a non-zero-valued last coordinate, as desired.

Solutions for ▶ Sect. 2.4

Solution 2.3 All proofs follow from the definitions in straightforward ways.

1. For all $\boldsymbol{a}, \boldsymbol{b} \in \mathbb{R}^p$, we find

$$\begin{aligned}
\overline{\hbar}[\boldsymbol{a}+\boldsymbol{b}] &= \sup\left\{\langle \boldsymbol{a}+\boldsymbol{b},\, \boldsymbol{c}\rangle \;:\; \boldsymbol{c}\in\mathbb{R}^p,\ \hbar[\boldsymbol{c}]\le 1\right\} && \text{definition of the dual function}\\
&= \sup\left\{\langle \boldsymbol{a},\, \boldsymbol{c}\rangle + \langle \boldsymbol{b},\, \boldsymbol{c}\rangle \;:\; \boldsymbol{c}\in\mathbb{R}^p,\ \hbar[\boldsymbol{c}]\le 1\right\} && \text{linearity of inner products}\\
&\le \sup\left\{\langle \boldsymbol{a},\, \boldsymbol{c}\rangle \;:\; \boldsymbol{c}\in\mathbb{R}^p,\ \hbar[\boldsymbol{c}]\le 1\right\}\\
&\quad + \sup\left\{\langle \boldsymbol{b},\, \boldsymbol{c}\rangle \;:\; \boldsymbol{c}\in\mathbb{R}^p,\ \hbar[\boldsymbol{c}]\le 1\right\} && \text{properties of suprema}\\
&= \overline{\hbar}[\boldsymbol{a}] + \overline{\hbar}[\boldsymbol{b}]\,, && \text{definition of the dual function}
\end{aligned}$$

as desired.

2. For all $a \in \mathbb{R}$ and $\boldsymbol{b} \in \mathbb{R}^p$, we find

$$\begin{aligned}
\overline{\hbar}[a\boldsymbol{b}] &= \sup\left\{\langle a\boldsymbol{b},\, \boldsymbol{c}\rangle \;:\; \boldsymbol{c}\in\mathbb{R}^p,\ \hbar[\boldsymbol{c}]\le 1\right\} && \text{definition of the dual function}\\
&= \sup\left\{\langle |a|\,\mathrm{sign}[a]\boldsymbol{b},\, \boldsymbol{c}\rangle \;:\; \boldsymbol{c}\in\mathbb{R}^p,\ \hbar[\boldsymbol{c}]\le 1\right\} && a = |a|\,\mathrm{sign}[a]\\
&= \sup\left\{|a|\langle \mathrm{sign}[a]\boldsymbol{b},\, \boldsymbol{c}\rangle \;:\; \boldsymbol{c}\in\mathbb{R}^p,\ \hbar[\boldsymbol{c}]\le 1\right\} && \text{linearity of inner products}\\
&= |a|\sup\left\{\langle \mathrm{sign}[a]\boldsymbol{b},\, \boldsymbol{c}\rangle \;:\; \boldsymbol{c}\in\mathbb{R}^p,\ \hbar[\boldsymbol{c}]\le 1\right\} && \text{properties of suprema}\\
&= |a|\overline{\hbar}\big[\mathrm{sign}[a]\boldsymbol{b}\big]\,, && \text{definition of the dual function}
\end{aligned}$$

as desired.

3. For all $a \in \mathbb{R}$ and $\boldsymbol{b} \in \mathbb{R}^p$, we find

$$\begin{aligned}
\overline{\hbar}[a\boldsymbol{b}] &= \sup\left\{\langle a\boldsymbol{b},\, \boldsymbol{c}\rangle \;:\; \boldsymbol{c}\in\mathbb{R}^p,\ \hbar[\boldsymbol{c}]\le 1\right\} && \text{definition of the dual function}\\
&= \sup\left\{\langle |a|\,\mathrm{sign}[a]\boldsymbol{b},\, \boldsymbol{c}\rangle \;:\; \boldsymbol{c}\in\mathbb{R}^p,\ \hbar[\boldsymbol{c}]\le 1\right\} && a = |a|\,\mathrm{sign}[a]
\end{aligned}$$

$$= \sup\left\{ |a|\langle \boldsymbol{b},\, \mathrm{sign}[a]\boldsymbol{c}\rangle \;:\; \boldsymbol{c} \in \mathbb{R}^p,\, \hbar[\boldsymbol{c}] \le 1 \right\}$$ linearity of inner products

$$= \sup\left\{ |a|\langle \boldsymbol{b},\, \boldsymbol{c}\rangle \;:\; \boldsymbol{c} \in \mathbb{R}^p,\, \hbar\big[\mathrm{sign}[a]\boldsymbol{c}\big] \le 1 \right\}$$ reparametrization: $\boldsymbol{c} \mapsto \mathrm{sign}[a]\boldsymbol{c}$

$$= \sup\left\{ |a|\langle \boldsymbol{b},\, \boldsymbol{c}\rangle \;:\; \boldsymbol{c} \in \mathbb{R}^p,\, \hbar\big[\boldsymbol{c}\big] \le 1 \right\}$$ assumed absolute homogeneity of $\hbar$; $|\mathrm{sign}[a]| = 1$

$$= |a| \sup\left\{ \langle \boldsymbol{b},\, \boldsymbol{c}\rangle \;:\; \boldsymbol{c} \in \mathbb{R}^p,\, \hbar[\boldsymbol{c}] \le 1 \right\}$$ properties of suprema

$$= |a|\overline{\hbar}\big[\boldsymbol{b}\big]\,,$$ definition of the dual function

as desired.

<u>Details:</u> It actually suffices that $\hbar$ is symmetric (verify that symmetry is a weaker assumption than absolute homogeneity).

4. For all $\boldsymbol{a} \in \mathbb{R}^p$, we find

$$\overline{\hbar}[\boldsymbol{a}] = \sup\left\{ \langle \boldsymbol{a},\, \boldsymbol{c}\rangle \;:\; \boldsymbol{c} \in \mathbb{R}^p,\, \hbar[\boldsymbol{c}] \le 1 \right\}$$ definition of the dual function

$$\ge \langle \boldsymbol{a},\, \boldsymbol{0}_p\rangle$$ $\hbar[\boldsymbol{0}_p] \le 1$ by assumption; set $\boldsymbol{c} = \boldsymbol{0}_p$

$$= 0\,,$$ linearity of inner products

as desired.

5. For all $\boldsymbol{a} \in \mathbb{R}^p$, we find

$$\overline{\hbar}[-\boldsymbol{a}] = \sup\left\{ \langle -\boldsymbol{a},\, \boldsymbol{c}\rangle \;:\; \boldsymbol{c} \in \mathbb{R}^p,\, \hbar[\boldsymbol{c}] \le 1 \right\}$$ definition of dual functions

$$= \sup\left\{ \langle \boldsymbol{a},\, -\boldsymbol{c}\rangle \;:\; \boldsymbol{c} \in \mathbb{R}^p,\, \hbar[\boldsymbol{c}] \le 1 \right\}$$ linearity of inner products

$$= \sup\left\{ \langle \boldsymbol{a},\, \boldsymbol{c}\rangle \;:\; \boldsymbol{c} \in \mathbb{R}^p,\, \hbar[-\boldsymbol{c}] \le 1 \right\}$$ reparametrization: $\boldsymbol{c} \mapsto -\boldsymbol{c}$

$$= \sup\left\{ \langle \boldsymbol{a},\, \boldsymbol{c}\rangle \;:\; \boldsymbol{c} \in \mathbb{R}^p,\, \hbar[\boldsymbol{c}] \le 1 \right\}$$ assumed symmetry of $\hbar$

$$= \overline{\hbar}[\boldsymbol{a}]\,,$$ definition of the dual function

as desired.

6. The triangle inequality and the absolute homogeneity follow from 1. and 3., respectively. The non-negativity follows from 4. Hence, what is left to show is the

definiteness: $\overline{\hbar}[\mathbf{0}_p] = 0$. This follows similarly as in the proofs above, noting that for every $\boldsymbol{a} \neq \mathbf{0}_p$ and every norm $\hbar$, it holds that $\boldsymbol{c} := \boldsymbol{a}/\hbar[\boldsymbol{a}]$ satisfies $\hbar[\boldsymbol{c}] = \hbar[\boldsymbol{a}/\hbar[\boldsymbol{a}]] = \hbar[\boldsymbol{a}]/\hbar[\boldsymbol{a}] = 1$:

$$\begin{aligned}\overline{\hbar}[\mathbf{0}_p] &= \sup\left\{\langle \mathbf{0}_p, \boldsymbol{c}\rangle : \boldsymbol{c} \in \mathbb{R}^p, \hbar[\boldsymbol{c}] \leq 1\right\} && \text{definition of dual functions}\\ &= \sup\left\{0 : \boldsymbol{c} \in \mathbb{R}^p, \hbar[\boldsymbol{c}] \leq 1\right\} && \text{linearity of inner products}\\ &= 0\,, && \text{above comment}\end{aligned}$$

as desired.
Details: The last fact $\overline{\hbar}[\mathbf{0}_p] = 0$ also follows from Theorem 2.4.1.

7. For all $\boldsymbol{a}, \boldsymbol{b} \in \mathbb{R}^p$ and $w \in (0, 1)$, we find

$$\begin{aligned}\overline{\hbar}\big[w\boldsymbol{a} + (1-w)\boldsymbol{b}\big] &\leq \overline{\hbar}\big[w\boldsymbol{a}\big] + \overline{\hbar}\big[(1-w)\boldsymbol{b}\big] && \text{Claim 1 (triangle inequality)}\\ &= |w|\overline{\hbar}\big[\operatorname{sign}[w]\boldsymbol{a}\big] + |1-w|\overline{\hbar}\big[\operatorname{sign}[1-w]\boldsymbol{b}\big] && \text{Claim 2 (absolute semi-homogeneity)}\\ &= w\overline{\hbar}[\boldsymbol{a}] + (1-w)\overline{\hbar}[\boldsymbol{b}]\,, && w \in (0,1) \text{, which implies } |w| = w,\ |1-w| = 1-w, \text{ and } \operatorname{sign}[w] = \operatorname{sign}[1-w] = 1\end{aligned}$$

as desired.

The same proof route applies to $w \in \{0, 1\}$, but for the sake of clarity we disentangle this case from the above one. For, say, $w = 0$ (the proof for $w = 1$ is very similar), we find

$$\begin{aligned}\overline{\hbar}\big[w\boldsymbol{a} + (1-w)\boldsymbol{b}\big] &= \overline{\hbar}\big[(1-w)\boldsymbol{b}\big] && w = 0\\ &= |1-w|\overline{\hbar}\big[\operatorname{sign}[1-w]\boldsymbol{b}\big] && \text{Claim 2 (absolute semi-homogeneity)}\\ &= (1-w)\overline{\hbar}[\boldsymbol{b}] && w = 0\\ &= w\overline{\hbar}[\boldsymbol{a}] + (1-w)\overline{\hbar}[\boldsymbol{b}]\,, && w = 0;\ 0 \cdot (\pm\infty) = 0 \text{ by our conventions on Page X}\end{aligned}$$

as desired.

8. and 9. Finding such examples is left to the reader.

Solutions for ▶ Sect. 2.5

Solution 2.5 We prove the claim by induction in k.

Induction basis: In the case $k = 1$, the assumption $a_1 + \cdots + a_k = 1$ specializes to $a_1 = 1$. Hence,

$$\begin{aligned} f\Big[\sum_{j=1}^{k} a_j \boldsymbol{b}^j\Big] &= f\big[a_1 \boldsymbol{b}^1\big] && k = 1 \\ &= a_1 \cdot f\big[\boldsymbol{b}^1\big] && a_1 = 1 \\ &= \sum_{j=1}^{k} a_j f\big[\boldsymbol{b}^j\big], && k = 1 \end{aligned}$$

which proves the claim for $k = 1$.

Induction step: Now, we establish the induction step $k \mapsto k+1$, that is, we show that if the claim is true for a $k \in \{1, 2, \ldots\}$, the claim is also true for $k + 1$.

In the case $a_{k+1} = 1$, the assumption $a_1, \ldots, a_{k+1} \in [0, 1]$ such that $a_1 + \cdots + a_{k+1} = 1$ implies $a_1 = \cdots = a_k = 0$. The proof of the induction step is then the same as the proof for the induction basis.

In the case $a_{k+1} < 1$, we observe

$$\begin{aligned} f\Big[\sum_{j=1}^{k+1} a_j \boldsymbol{b}^j\Big] &= f\Big[\sum_{j=1}^{k} a_j \boldsymbol{b}^j + a_{k+1} \boldsymbol{b}^{k+1}\Big] \\ &\qquad \text{splitting the sum into two parts} \\ &= f\Big[(1 - a_{k+1}) \sum_{j=1}^{k} \frac{a_j}{1 - a_{k+1}} \boldsymbol{b}^j + a_{k+1} \boldsymbol{b}^{k+1}\Big] \\ &\qquad a_{k+1} < 1 \text{ by assumption; linearity of sums} \\ &\le (1 - a_{k+1})\, f\Big[\sum_{j=1}^{k} \frac{a_j}{1 - a_{k+1}} \boldsymbol{b}^j\Big] + a_{k+1} f\big[\boldsymbol{b}^{k+1}\big]. \\ &\qquad \text{Definition 2.5.1 (convexity) applied with} \\ &\qquad w = 1 - a_{k+1},\ \boldsymbol{a} = \textstyle\sum_{j=1}^{k} a_j \boldsymbol{b}^j / (1 - a_{k+1}),\ \boldsymbol{b} = \boldsymbol{b}^{k+1} \end{aligned}$$

Now, $a_j/(1-a_{k+1}) \geq 0$ since $a_1, \ldots, a_{k+1} \geq 0$ and $a_1 + \cdots + a_{k+1} = 1$, and

$$\begin{aligned}\sum_{j=1}^{k} \frac{a_j}{1-a_{k+1}} &= \frac{1}{1-a_{k+1}} \sum_{j=1}^{k} a_j && \text{linearity of sums}\\ &= \frac{1}{1-a_{k+1}}(1-a_{k+1}) && a_1+\cdots+a_{k+1}=1 \text{ by assumption}\\ &= 1\,,\end{aligned}$$

(which then also implies that $a_j/(1-a_{k+1}) \leq 1$) so that we can use the induction argument to derive

$$f\Bigg[\sum_{j=1}^{k} \frac{a_j}{1-a_{k+1}} \boldsymbol{b}^j\Bigg] \leq \sum_{j=1}^{k} \frac{a_j}{1-a_{k+1}} f[\boldsymbol{b}^j]\,.$$

Thus, we conclude that

$$\begin{aligned}&f\Bigg[\sum_{j=1}^{k+1} a_j \boldsymbol{b}^j\Bigg]\\ &\leq (1-a_{k+1}) \sum_{j=1}^{k} \frac{a_j}{1-a_{k+1}} f[\boldsymbol{b}^j] + a_{k+1} f[\boldsymbol{b}^{k+1}] && \text{combining the above inequalities}\\ &= \sum_{j=1}^{k+1} a_j f[\boldsymbol{b}^j]\,, && \text{summarizing terms}\end{aligned}$$

as desired.

Solution 2.10 The proof is a straightforward reformulation of the lasso's KKT equation. We show this in three steps, as indicated by the layout of the exercise.

1. The first result follows almost directly from the KKT conditions (2.7).

   These conditions are in the lasso case

$$-2X^\top(\boldsymbol{y} - X\widehat{\boldsymbol{\beta}}_{\text{lasso}}) + r\widehat{\boldsymbol{\kappa}} = \boldsymbol{0}_p$$

for a vector $\widehat{\boldsymbol{\kappa}} \in \partial\|\widehat{\boldsymbol{\beta}}_{\text{lasso}}\|_1$. Rearranging the terms in the equality yields

$$2X^\top X\widehat{\boldsymbol{\beta}}_{\text{lasso}} = X^\top \boldsymbol{y} - r\widehat{\boldsymbol{\kappa}}$$

and dividing through by $2n$ then

$$\frac{X^\top X\widehat{\boldsymbol{\beta}}_{\text{lasso}}}{n} = \frac{X^\top \boldsymbol{y}}{2n} - \frac{r\widehat{\boldsymbol{\kappa}}}{2n}.$$

We can finally use $X^\top X = n\mathrm{I}_{p\times p}$ to derive

$$\widehat{\boldsymbol{\beta}}_{\text{lasso}} = \frac{X^\top \boldsymbol{y}}{n} - \frac{r\widehat{\boldsymbol{\kappa}}}{2n},$$

as desired.

2. The three implications can be derived from the equation in 1. through basic algebra. In fact, we only need to prove the ⇒'s, as the ⇐'s then follow logically.

   First implication: Assume that $|(X^\top \boldsymbol{y})_j| \le r/2$.

   We do a proof by contradiction. Assume first $(\widehat{\beta}_{\text{lasso}})_j > 0$. Then, the jth coordinate of 1. multiplied through by n gives

$$(X^\top \boldsymbol{y})_j - \frac{r\widehat{\kappa}_j}{2} > 0,$$

which can be reformulated as

$$(X^\top \boldsymbol{y})_j > \frac{r\widehat{\kappa}_j}{2}.$$

Hence, since $\widehat{\kappa}_j = 1$ for $(\widehat{\beta}_{\text{lasso}})_j > 0$ (see Example 2.5.2),

$$(X^\top \boldsymbol{y})_j > \frac{r}{2},$$

which implies (recall that $r \ge 0$)

$$\left|(X^\top \boldsymbol{y})_j\right| > \frac{r}{2},$$

contradicting our initial assumption.

   Similarly, if $(\widehat{\beta}_{\text{lasso}})_j < 0$, Claim 1 yields

$$(X^\top \boldsymbol{y})_j - \frac{r\widehat{\kappa}_j}{2} < 0,$$

which can be reformulated as

$$-(X^\top \boldsymbol{y})_j \;>\; -\frac{r\widehat{\kappa}_j}{2}\,.$$

Hence, since $\widehat{\kappa}_j = -1$ for $(\widehat{\beta}_{\text{lasso}})_j < 0$,

$$-(X^\top \boldsymbol{y})_j \;>\; \frac{r}{2}\,,$$

which implies

$$\left|(X^\top \boldsymbol{y})_j\right| \;>\; \frac{r}{2}\,,$$

contradicting our initial assumption.

Second implication: Assume that $(X^\top \boldsymbol{y})_j > r/2$. We then find

$$\begin{aligned}
(\widehat{\beta}_{\text{lasso}})_j &= \frac{(X^\top \boldsymbol{y})_j}{n} - \frac{r\widehat{\kappa}_j}{2n} && j\text{th coordinate of 1.}\\
&\geq \frac{(X^\top \boldsymbol{y})_j}{n} - \frac{r}{2n} && \widehat{\kappa}_j \leq 1 \text{ by Example 2.5.2}\\
&> 0\,, && (X^\top \boldsymbol{y})_j > r/2 \text{ by assumption}
\end{aligned}$$

as desired.

Third implication: Assume that $(X^\top \boldsymbol{y})_j < -r/2$. We then find

$$\begin{aligned}
(\widehat{\beta}_{\text{lasso}})_j &= \frac{(X^\top \boldsymbol{y})_j}{n} - \frac{r\widehat{\kappa}_j}{2n} && j\text{th coordinate of 1.}\\
&\leq \frac{(X^\top \boldsymbol{y})_j}{n} + \frac{r}{2n} && \widehat{\kappa}_j \geq -1 \text{ by Example 2.5.2}\\
&< 0\,, && (X^\top \boldsymbol{y})_j < -r/2 \text{ by assumption}
\end{aligned}$$

as desired.

3. The proof of this part uses 1. and 2. and the properties of the signum function and of the positive part.

   Note first that for $|(X^\top \boldsymbol{y})_j| \leq r/2$, the right-hand side of the desired equality is equal to zero, which is correct in view of the second implication of 2. We can thus assume $|(X^\top \boldsymbol{y})_j| > r/2$ in the following.

   If $(X^\top \boldsymbol{y})_j > r/2$, it holds that $\widehat{\kappa}_j = \text{sign}[(\widehat{\beta}_{\text{lasso}})_j] = 1$ through the second implication of Claim 2 and Example 2.5.2. Similarly, if $-(X^\top \boldsymbol{y})_j > r/2$, it holds that $\widehat{\kappa}_j = \text{sign}[(\widehat{\beta}_{\text{lasso}})_j] = -1$.

Hence,

$$
\begin{aligned}
(\widehat{\beta}_{\text{lasso}})_j &= \frac{(X^\top \boldsymbol{y})_j}{n} - \frac{r\widehat{\kappa}_j}{2n} && \text{again from 1.} \\
&= \begin{cases} \frac{|(X^\top \boldsymbol{y})_j|}{n} - \frac{r}{2n} & \text{if } (X^\top \boldsymbol{y})_j > r/2 \\ -\frac{|(X^\top \boldsymbol{y})_j|}{n} + \frac{r}{2n} & \text{if } -(X^\top \boldsymbol{y})_j > r/2 \end{cases} \\
& && \text{two preceding observations} \\
&= \text{sign}\left[(X^\top \boldsymbol{y})_j\right]\left(\frac{|(X^\top \boldsymbol{y})_j|}{n} - \frac{r}{2n}\right) \\
& && \text{definition of the sign function} \\
&= \text{sign}\left[(X^\top \boldsymbol{y})_j\right]\left(\frac{|(X^\top \boldsymbol{y})_j|}{n} - \frac{r}{2n}\right)_+, \\
& && |(X^\top \boldsymbol{y})_j| \geq r/2 \text{ by assumption}
\end{aligned}
$$

as desired.

Solution 2.11 We prove the five parts in order.

1. This equation is a simple reformulation of the lasso's KKT condition.

   Equation (2.7) states

$$
-2X^\top\big(\boldsymbol{y} - X\widehat{\boldsymbol{\beta}}_{\text{lasso}}[r]\big) + r\widehat{\boldsymbol{\kappa}} = \boldsymbol{0}_p
$$

   for a vector $\widehat{\boldsymbol{\kappa}} \in \boldsymbol{\partial}\|\widehat{\boldsymbol{\beta}}_{\text{lasso}}[r]\|_1$. Rearranging the terms yields

$$
2X^\top X\widehat{\boldsymbol{\beta}}_{\text{lasso}}[r] = 2X^\top \boldsymbol{y} - r\widehat{\boldsymbol{\kappa}},
$$

   and then multiplying both sides by $(X^\top X)^{-1}/2$

$$
\widehat{\boldsymbol{\beta}}_{\text{lasso}}[r] = \underbrace{(X^\top X)^{-1}X^\top \boldsymbol{y}}_{\widehat{\boldsymbol{\beta}}_{\text{ls}}} - \frac{r}{2}(X^\top X)^{-1}\widehat{\boldsymbol{\kappa}},
$$

   as desired.

2. This inequality follows readily from 1.

   Verify first that if $A \in \mathbb{R}^{p\times p}$ is a positive definite matrix with ordered eigenvalues $m_p \geq \cdots \geq m_1 > 0$, the ordered eigenvalues of A^{-1} are $1/m_1 \geq \cdots \geq 1/m_p > 0$, and it holds that $\|A^{-1}\boldsymbol{a}\|_2 \leq \|\boldsymbol{a}\|_2/m_1$.

We then find

$$\begin{aligned}
&\|X\widehat{\boldsymbol{\beta}}_{\text{lasso}}[r] - X\widehat{\boldsymbol{\beta}}_{\text{ls}}\|_2^2 \\
&= \|-\frac{r}{2}X(X^\top X)^{-1}\widehat{\boldsymbol{\kappa}}\|_2^2 && \text{by 1.} \\
&= \frac{r^2\|X(X^\top X)^{-1}\widehat{\boldsymbol{\kappa}}\|_2^2}{4} && \text{absolute homogeneity of norms} \\
&= \frac{r^2\big(X(X^\top X)^{-1}\widehat{\boldsymbol{\kappa}}\big)^\top X(X^\top X)^{-1}\widehat{\boldsymbol{\kappa}}}{4} && \text{definition of the } \ell_2\text{-norm} \\
&= \frac{r^2\widehat{\boldsymbol{\kappa}}^\top\big((X^\top X)^{-1}\big)^\top X^\top X(X^\top X)^{-1}\widehat{\boldsymbol{\kappa}}}{4} && \text{3. in Lemma B.2.1 (reversion of transposition)} \\
&= \frac{r^2\widehat{\boldsymbol{\kappa}}^\top\big((X^\top X)^{-1}\big)^\top\widehat{\boldsymbol{\kappa}}}{4} && \text{simplifying} \\
&= \frac{r^2\widehat{\boldsymbol{\kappa}}^\top(X^\top X)^{-1}\widehat{\boldsymbol{\kappa}}}{4} && \text{using 1. in Lemma B.2.6 and the fact that } X^\top X \text{ is symmetric} \\
&\le \frac{r^2\|\widehat{\boldsymbol{\kappa}}\|_2\|(X^\top X)^{-1}\widehat{\boldsymbol{\kappa}}\|_2}{4} && \text{Cauchy–Schwarz inequality–see Example 2.4.1} \\
&\le \frac{r^2\|\widehat{\boldsymbol{\kappa}}\|_2^2}{4m_1}\,. && \text{previous comments applied to } A = X^\top X
\end{aligned}$$

Now, recall that $|\widehat{\kappa}_j| \le 1$ since $\widehat{\boldsymbol{\kappa}} \in \partial\|\widehat{\boldsymbol{\beta}}_{\text{lasso}}[r]\|_1$ (see Exercise 2.5.2), so that the definition of the ℓ_2-norm and simple algebra yield

$$\|\widehat{\boldsymbol{\kappa}}\|_2^2 = \sum_{j=1}^{p}|\widehat{\kappa}_j|^2 \le \sum_{j=1}^{p} 1 = p\,.$$

This combined with the previous display then implies

$$\|X\widehat{\boldsymbol{\beta}}_{\text{lasso}}[r] - X\widehat{\boldsymbol{\beta}}_{\text{ls}}\|_2^2 \le \frac{r^2 p}{4m_1}\,,$$

as desired.

3. The claim follows again readily from the lasso's KKT conditions.

   Once more, recall that Eq. (2.7) states that $\widehat{\boldsymbol{\beta}}_{\text{lasso}}[r]$ is a solution of the lasso if and only if

$$-2X^\top\big(\boldsymbol{y} - X\widehat{\boldsymbol{\beta}}_{\text{lasso}}[r]\big) + r\widehat{\boldsymbol{\kappa}} = \mathbf{0}_p$$

   for a $\widehat{\boldsymbol{\kappa}} \in \partial\|\widehat{\boldsymbol{\beta}}_{\text{lasso}}[r]\|_1$. Setting $\widehat{\boldsymbol{\beta}}_{\text{lasso}}[r] = \mathbf{0}_p$ and rearranging yield that $\mathbf{0}_p$ is a solution if and only if

$$2X^\top\boldsymbol{y} = r\widehat{\boldsymbol{\kappa}}$$

   for a $\widehat{\boldsymbol{\kappa}} \in \partial\|\mathbf{0}_p\|_1$.

   Next, recall that $\widehat{\boldsymbol{\kappa}} \in \partial\|\mathbf{0}_p\|_1$ is equivalent to $\widehat{\kappa}_j \in [-1, 1]$ for all $j \in \{1, \ldots, p\}$—see Example 2.5.2. Consequently, formulated in terms of the individual coordinates of the vectors, $\mathbf{0}_p$ is a solution if and only if for all $j \in \{1, \ldots, p\}$, there is a $\widehat{\kappa}_j \in [-1, 1]$ such that

$$2(X^\top\boldsymbol{y})_j = r\widehat{\kappa}_j\,.$$

   The latter is true if and only if $2|(X^\top\boldsymbol{y})_j| \leq r$ for all $j \in \{1, \ldots, p\}$, that is, $2\|X^\top\boldsymbol{y}\|_\infty \leq r$, as desired.

4. For this question, we leverage the estimator's definition directly.

   Assume that $\mathbf{0}_p$ is a lasso solution, that is, $\mathbf{0}_p$ is a minimizer of the lasso's objective function. Then, the value of the lasso's objective function at any solution $\widehat{\boldsymbol{\beta}}_{\text{lasso}}[r] \in \mathbb{R}^p$ must equal the value at $\mathbf{0}_p$:

$$\|\boldsymbol{y}-X\widehat{\boldsymbol{\beta}}_{\text{lasso}}[r]\|_2^2+r\|\widehat{\boldsymbol{\beta}}_{\text{lasso}}[r]\|_1 = \|\boldsymbol{y} - X\mathbf{0}_p\|_2^2+r\|\mathbf{0}_p\|_1 = \|\boldsymbol{y}\|_2^2\,.$$

   Expanding the first term on the left-hand side of this equality yields

$$\|\boldsymbol{y}\|_2^2-2\langle\boldsymbol{y},\, X\widehat{\boldsymbol{\beta}}_{\text{lasso}}[r]\rangle+\|X\widehat{\boldsymbol{\beta}}_{\text{lasso}}[r]\|_2^2+r\|\widehat{\boldsymbol{\beta}}_{\text{lasso}}[r]\|_1 = \|\boldsymbol{y}\|_2^2$$

   and simplifying and rearranging then

$$\|X\widehat{\boldsymbol{\beta}}_{\text{lasso}}[r]\|_2^2 + r\|\widehat{\boldsymbol{\beta}}_{\text{lasso}}[r]\|_1 = 2\langle\boldsymbol{y},\, X\widehat{\boldsymbol{\beta}}_{\text{lasso}}[r]\rangle\,.$$

Using the properties of inner products, the Hölder inequality (2.6), and the fact that $r \geq \|X^\top \boldsymbol{y}\|_\infty$, we can bound the right-hand side of this equality according to

$$\begin{aligned}2\langle \boldsymbol{y},\, X\widehat{\boldsymbol{\beta}}_{\text{lasso}}[r]\rangle &= 2\langle X^\top \boldsymbol{y},\, \widehat{\boldsymbol{\beta}}_{\text{lasso}}[r]\rangle\\ &\leq 2\|X^\top \boldsymbol{y}\|_\infty \|\widehat{\boldsymbol{\beta}}_{\text{lasso}}[r]\|_1 \leq r\|\widehat{\boldsymbol{\beta}}_{\text{lasso}}[r]\|_1\,.\end{aligned}$$

Plugging this back into the foregoing display gives

$$\|X\widehat{\boldsymbol{\beta}}_{\text{lasso}}[r]\|_2^2 + r\|\widehat{\boldsymbol{\beta}}_{\text{lasso}}[r]\|_1 \leq r\|\widehat{\boldsymbol{\beta}}_{\text{lasso}}[r]\|_1$$

and, therefore,

$$\|X\widehat{\boldsymbol{\beta}}_{\text{lasso}}[r]\|_2^2 \leq 0\,,$$

which means that $X\widehat{\boldsymbol{\beta}}_{\text{lasso}}[r] = \mathbf{0}_n$ by the positive definiteness of norms.

We can plug this into the previously derived equality $\|X\widehat{\boldsymbol{\beta}}_{\text{lasso}}[r]\|_2^2 + r\|\widehat{\boldsymbol{\beta}}_{\text{lasso}}[r]\|_1 = 2\langle \boldsymbol{y},\, X\widehat{\boldsymbol{\beta}}_{\text{lasso}}[r]\rangle$ to find

$$r\|\widehat{\boldsymbol{\beta}}_{\text{lasso}}[r]\|_1 = 0$$

by the linearity of inner products. Since $r > 0$ by assumption, we can again use the positive definiteness of norms to derive from this equality that $\widehat{\boldsymbol{\beta}}_{\text{lasso}}[r] = \mathbf{0}_p$, as desired.

5. This is a simple algebra exercise.

   Observe first that the positive definiteness of norms yields

$$2\|X^\top \boldsymbol{y}\|_\infty = 0 \quad \Rightarrow \quad X^\top \boldsymbol{y} = \mathbf{0}_p\,.$$

Therefore, the lasso's objective function becomes

$$\begin{aligned}&\|\boldsymbol{y} - X\boldsymbol{\alpha}\|_2^2 + r\|\boldsymbol{\alpha}\|_1\\ &= \|\boldsymbol{y} - X\boldsymbol{\alpha}\|_2^2 && r = 0 \text{ by assumption}\\ &= \|\boldsymbol{y}\|_2^2 - 2\langle \boldsymbol{y},\, X\boldsymbol{\alpha}\rangle + \|X\boldsymbol{\alpha}\|_2^2 && \text{expanding the squared-norm}\\ &= \|\boldsymbol{y}\|_2^2 - 2\langle X^\top \boldsymbol{y},\, \boldsymbol{\alpha}\rangle + \|X\boldsymbol{\alpha}\|_2^2 && \text{properties of the inner product}\\ &= \|\boldsymbol{y}\|_2^2 - 2\langle \mathbf{0}_p,\, \boldsymbol{\alpha}\rangle + \|X\boldsymbol{\alpha}\|_2^2 && \text{previous display}\\ &= \|\boldsymbol{y}\|_2^2 + \|X\boldsymbol{\alpha}\|_2^2\,. && \text{linearity of the inner product}\end{aligned}$$

Hence, since $\|\boldsymbol{y}\|_2^2$ does not depend on $\boldsymbol{\alpha}$,

$$\begin{aligned}\operatorname*{arg\,min}_{\boldsymbol{\alpha}\in\mathbb{R}^p}\left\{\|\boldsymbol{y}-X\boldsymbol{\alpha}\|_2^2+r\|\boldsymbol{\alpha}\|_1\right\} &= \operatorname*{arg\,min}_{\boldsymbol{\alpha}\in\mathbb{R}^p}\|X\boldsymbol{\alpha}\|_2^2\\ &= \{\boldsymbol{\alpha}\in\mathbb{R}^p\,:\,X\boldsymbol{\alpha}=\boldsymbol{0}_n\}\,,\end{aligned}$$

as desired.

Alternatively, one could verify that the KKT conditions imply in our case (where $2X^\top\boldsymbol{y}=r\widehat{\boldsymbol{\kappa}}/2=\boldsymbol{0}_p$) that $X^\top X\widehat{\boldsymbol{\beta}}_{\text{lasso}}=\boldsymbol{0}_p$. Multiplying both sides of this equation by $\widehat{\boldsymbol{\beta}}_{\text{lasso}}$ yields $\|X\widehat{\boldsymbol{\beta}}_{\text{lasso}}\|_2^2=0$, from which the proof follows readily.

A.3 Solutions for ▶ Chap. 3

Solutions for ▶ Sect. 3.1

Solution 3.1 Refer to online resources such as Wikipedia.

Solutions for ▶ Sect. 3.3

Solution 3.2 We prove the six claims in order.

1. The proof of this claim is a simple algebra exercise.

   Consider two matrices $\Omega',\Omega''\in\mathcal{S}_d^+$ and a constant $w\in[0,1]$. We have to show that $w\Omega'+(1-w)\Omega''\in\mathcal{S}_d^+$.

   The symmetry of the matrix in question is proved as follows:

$$\begin{aligned}&\left(w\Omega'+(1-w)\Omega''\right)^\top\\ &= w\Omega'^\top+(1-w)\Omega''^\top \qquad \text{2. in Lemma B.2.1 (linearity of transposition)}\\ &= w\Omega'+(1-w)\Omega''\,, \qquad \Omega',\Omega''\text{ are symmetric by assumption}\end{aligned}$$

   as desired.

The positive definiteness of the matrix is proved as follows: for every $\boldsymbol{b} \in \mathbb{R}^d \setminus \{\boldsymbol{0}_d\}$,

$$\begin{aligned}
&\boldsymbol{b}^\top\big(w\Omega' + (1-w)\Omega''\big)\boldsymbol{b} \\
&= w\boldsymbol{b}^\top\Omega'\boldsymbol{b} + (1-w)\boldsymbol{b}^\top\Omega''\boldsymbol{b} && \text{linearity of matrix–vector multiplications} \\
&> 0\,, && \Omega', \Omega'' \text{ positive definite by assumption; } w, 1-w \geq 0 \text{ by assumption}
\end{aligned}$$

as desired.

This concludes the proof of Claim 1.

2. This claim follows directly from the linearity of matrix multiplications and of the trace function.

   Indeed, these linearity properties applied in sequence yield for all $\Omega', \Omega'' \in \mathbb{R}^{d\times d}$ and $w \in [0, 1]$ that

$$\begin{aligned}
\operatorname{trace}\big[A\big(w\Omega' + (1-w)\Omega''\big)\big] &= \operatorname{trace}\big[wA\Omega' + (1-w)A\Omega''\big] \\
&= w\operatorname{trace}[A\Omega'] + (1-w)\operatorname{trace}[A\Omega'']\,,
\end{aligned}$$

   which implies the desired claim.

3. This proof is again a simple algebra exercise.

   According to Lemma B.2.11 (singular value decomposition), there are orthogonal matrices $U, V \in \mathbb{R}^{d\times d}$ and a diagonal matrix $D \in \mathbb{R}^{d\times d}$ with diagonal elements and the singular values $m_1, \ldots, m_d$ of A such that (i) $A = UDV^\top$.

   Moreover, it holds by Lemma B.2.8 (determinant of orthogonal matrices) and 2. in Lemma B.2.3 (basic properties of determinants) that (ii) $|\det[U]| = |\det[V^\top]| = 1$.

   We then find

$$\begin{aligned}
|\det[A]| &= |\det[UDV^\top]| && A = UDV^\top \text{ by (i)} \\
&= |\det[U]\det[D]\det[V^\top]| && \text{1. in Lemma B.2.3 (multiplicativity of the determinant) applied twice} \\
&= |\det[D]| && |\det[U]| = |\det[V^\top]| = 1 \text{ by (ii)}
\end{aligned}$$

$$= \left|\prod_{j=1}^{d} D_{jj}\right| \qquad \text{3. in Lemma B.2.3}$$

$$= \prod_{j=1}^{d} m_j\,, \qquad \text{diag}\, D_{jj} = m_j > 0 \text{ by the second part of Lemma B.2.11}$$

as stated in the first claim.

The second claim follows similarly—see Lemmas B.2.9 and B.2.10.

4. This follows from 3. and the strict concavity of the logarithm. The detailed derivations are extensive nevertheless; therefore, we separate them into five steps.

Step 1: We first show that

$$\det\left[\Omega + tA\right] \;=\; \det[\Omega] \cdot \det\left[\mathrm{I}_{d\times d} + t\Omega^{-\frac{1}{2}}A\Omega^{-\frac{1}{2}}\right].$$

We only need there the fact that $\Omega \in \mathcal{S}_d^+$: the factor t and the matrix A can be arbitrary.

The matrix Ω is symmetric and positive definite by assumption. Then, by 1. in Lemma B.2.5, it is also invertible. Hence, Ω has an invertible square-root $\Omega^{\frac{1}{2}}$ in the sense of Corollary B.2.1, and (using also the linearity of matrix–matrix and scalar–matrix multiplications) we can write

$$\Omega + tA \;=\; \Omega^{\frac{1}{2}}(\mathrm{I}_{d\times d} + t\Omega^{-\frac{1}{2}}A\Omega^{-\frac{1}{2}})\Omega^{\frac{1}{2}}\,.$$

This allows us to derive

$$\begin{aligned}
&\det\left[\Omega + tA\right] \\
&= \det\left[\Omega^{\frac{1}{2}}(\mathrm{I}_{d\times d} + t\Omega^{-\frac{1}{2}}A\Omega^{-\frac{1}{2}})\Omega^{\frac{1}{2}}\right] && \text{previous display} \\
&= \det[\Omega^{\frac{1}{2}}] \cdot \det\left[\mathrm{I}_{d\times d} + t\Omega^{-\frac{1}{2}}A\Omega^{-\frac{1}{2}}\right] \cdot \det[\Omega^{\frac{1}{2}}] && \text{1. in Lemma B.2.3 (multiplicativity of the determinant) applied twice} \\
&= \det[\Omega^{\frac{1}{2}}\Omega^{\frac{1}{2}}] \cdot \det\left[\mathrm{I}_{d\times d} + t\Omega^{-\frac{1}{2}}A\Omega^{-\frac{1}{2}}\right] && \text{1. in Lemma B.2.3 to combine first and third factor} \\
&= \det[\Omega] \cdot \det\left[\mathrm{I}_{d\times d} + t\Omega^{-\frac{1}{2}}A\Omega^{-\frac{1}{2}}\right], && \text{Corollary B.2.1}
\end{aligned}$$

as desired.

Step 2: We now show that $\mathrm{I}_{d\times d} + t\Omega^{-\frac{1}{2}}A\Omega^{-\frac{1}{2}}$ is symmetric and positive definite.

The symmetry (see Definition B.2.1) follows from a short calculation:

$$\begin{aligned}
&\big(\mathrm{I}_{d\times d} + t\Omega^{-\frac{1}{2}}A\Omega^{-\frac{1}{2}}\big)^\top \\
&= (\mathrm{I}_{d\times d})^\top + t\big(\Omega^{-\frac{1}{2}}A\Omega^{-\frac{1}{2}}\big)^\top \\
&\qquad\qquad \text{2. in Lemma B.2.1 (linearity of transposition)} \\
&= \mathrm{I}_{d\times d} + t(\Omega^{-\frac{1}{2}})^\top A^\top (\Omega^{-\frac{1}{2}})^\top \\
&\qquad\qquad (\mathrm{I}_{d\times d})^\top = \mathrm{I}_{d\times d}\text{; 3. in Lemma B.2.1 (reversion of transposition) applied twice} \\
&= \mathrm{I}_{d\times d} + t\Omega^{-\frac{1}{2}}A\Omega^{-\frac{1}{2}}\,. \\
&\qquad\qquad \Omega^{-\frac{1}{2}} \text{ is symmetric by Corollary B.2.1 and 2. of Lemma B.2.6; } A \text{ symmetric by assumption}
\end{aligned}$$

Also the positive definiteness follows readily: Consider $\boldsymbol{b} \in \mathbb{R}^d \setminus \{\boldsymbol{0}_d\}$. Then, since $\Omega^{\frac{1}{2}}$ is invertible by Corollary B.2.1, there is a $\boldsymbol{c} \in \mathbb{R}^d \setminus \{\boldsymbol{0}_d\}$ such that $\boldsymbol{b} = \Omega^{\frac{1}{2}}\boldsymbol{c}$ (namely $\boldsymbol{c} = \Omega^{-\frac{1}{2}}\boldsymbol{b}$), and we find

$$\begin{aligned}
&\boldsymbol{b}^\top\big(\mathrm{I}_{d\times d} + t\Omega^{-\frac{1}{2}}A\Omega^{-\frac{1}{2}}\big)\boldsymbol{b} \\
&= (\Omega^{\frac{1}{2}}\boldsymbol{c})^\top\big(\mathrm{I}_{d\times d} + t\Omega^{-\frac{1}{2}}A\Omega^{-\frac{1}{2}}\big)\Omega^{\frac{1}{2}}\boldsymbol{c} \\
&\qquad\qquad \boldsymbol{b} = \Omega^{\frac{1}{2}}\boldsymbol{c} \text{ by definition} \\
&= \boldsymbol{c}^\top(\Omega^{\frac{1}{2}})^\top\big(\mathrm{I}_{d\times d} + t\Omega^{-\frac{1}{2}}A\Omega^{-\frac{1}{2}}\big)\Omega^{\frac{1}{2}}\boldsymbol{c} \\
&\qquad\qquad \text{3. in Lemma B.2.1 (reversion of transposition)} \\
&= \boldsymbol{c}^\top\Omega^{\frac{1}{2}}\big(\mathrm{I}_{d\times d} + t\Omega^{-\frac{1}{2}}A\Omega^{-\frac{1}{2}}\big)\Omega^{\frac{1}{2}}\boldsymbol{c} \\
&\qquad\qquad \Omega^{\frac{1}{2}} \text{ is symmetric by Corollary B.2.1} \\
&= \boldsymbol{c}^\top\big(\Omega + tA\big)\boldsymbol{c} \\
&\qquad\qquad \text{linearity of matrix–matrix/scalar–matrix multiplications} \\
&> 0\,, \qquad\qquad \Omega + tA \text{ positive definite by assumption}
\end{aligned}$$

as desired.

Step 3: We now show that

$$-\log\det\big[\Omega + tA\big] \;=\; -\log\det[\Omega] - \sum_{j=1}^{d}\log[m_j]\,,$$

where $m_1, \ldots, m_d > 0$ are the eigenvalues of $\mathrm{I}_{d\times d} + t\Omega^{-\frac{1}{2}}A\Omega^{-\frac{1}{2}}$.

Since $\Omega, \Omega + tA \in \mathcal{S}_d^+$ by assumption, and $\mathrm{I}_{d\times d} + t\Omega^{-\frac{1}{2}}A\Omega^{-\frac{1}{2}} \in \mathcal{S}_d^+$ by Step 2, Lemma B.2.4 implies that the determinants of all three matrices are strictly positive, and we can therefore take (negative) logarithms in the result of Step 1:

$$
\begin{aligned}
&- \log\det\big[\Omega + tA\big] \\
&= -\log\big[\det[\Omega]\cdot\det[\mathrm{I}_{d\times d} + t\Omega^{-\frac{1}{2}}A\Omega^{-\frac{1}{2}}]\big] && \text{Step 1} \\
&= -\log\det[\Omega] - \log\det[\mathrm{I}_{d\times d} + t\Omega^{-\frac{1}{2}}A\Omega^{-\frac{1}{2}}]\,. \\
&\qquad\qquad\text{rules for the logarithm: } \log[ab] = \log[a] + \log[b]
\end{aligned}
$$

Now, since $\mathrm{I}_{d\times d}+t\Omega^{-\frac{1}{2}}A\Omega^{-\frac{1}{2}}$ is symmetric and positive definite according to Step 2, we find in view of Claim 3 of the exercise that

$$
\begin{aligned}
-\log\det\big[\Omega + tA\big] &= -\log\det[\Omega] - \log\Big[\prod_{j=1}^{d} m_j\Big] \\
&= -\log\det[\Omega] - \sum_{j=1}^{d}\log[m_j]\,,
\end{aligned}
$$

where $m_1, \ldots, m_d > 0$ are the eigenvalues of $\mathrm{I}_{d\times d} + t\Omega^{-\frac{1}{2}}A\Omega^{-\frac{1}{2}}$, and where we have used again the rules for the logarithm. This is the desired identity.

Step 4: We now compute the eigenvalues $m_1, \ldots, m_d$ of $\mathrm{I}_{d\times d} + t\Omega^{-\frac{1}{2}}A\Omega^{-\frac{1}{2}}$:

$$
m_j = 1 + t\widetilde{m}_j \qquad \text{for all } j \in \{1, \ldots, d\}\,,
$$

where $\widetilde{m}_1, \ldots, \widetilde{m}_d$ are the eigenvalues of $\Omega^{-\frac{1}{2}}A\Omega^{-\frac{1}{2}}$.

One can show similarly as in Step 2 that $\Omega^{-\frac{1}{2}}A\Omega^{-\frac{1}{2}}$ is symmetric. Hence, according to the spectral decomposition in Lemma B.2.9, it admits a basis of eigenvectors $\boldsymbol{q}_1, \ldots, \boldsymbol{q}_d \in \mathbb{R}^d$ with eigenvalues $\widetilde{m}_1, \ldots, \widetilde{m}_d$. By Definition B.2.7 of eigenvectors and eigenvalues and the linearity of matrix multiplications,

$$
(\mathrm{I}_{d\times d} + t\Omega^{-\frac{1}{2}}A\Omega^{-\frac{1}{2}})\boldsymbol{q}_j = (1 + t\widetilde{m}_j)\boldsymbol{q}_j\,.
$$

This means that $\boldsymbol{q}_j$ is also an eigenvector of $\mathrm{I}_{d\times d} + t\Omega^{-\frac{1}{2}}A\Omega^{-\frac{1}{2}}$ with eigenvalue $1+t\widetilde{m}_j$. Hence, $\boldsymbol{q}_1, \ldots, \boldsymbol{q}_d \in \mathbb{R}^d$ is a basis of eigenvectors of that matrix with eigenvalues $1+t\widetilde{m}_1, \ldots, 1+t\widetilde{m}_d$. The desired statement then follows from this.

Step 5: We finally show that the function

$$t \mapsto -\log\det[\Omega + tA]$$

is strictly convex on $[0, \tilde{t}]$.

In view of Steps 3 and 4, we need to show strict convexity of

$$t \mapsto -\log\det[\Omega] - \sum_{j=1}^{d} \log[1 + t\widetilde{m}_j]$$

on $[0, \tilde{t}]$, where $\widetilde{m}_1, \ldots, \widetilde{m}_d$ are the eigenvalues of $\Omega^{-\frac{1}{2}}A\Omega^{-\frac{1}{2}}$.

The first term is constant in t and, therefore, convex. Let us then look at the remaining functions

$$t \mapsto -\log[1 + t\widetilde{m}_j] \qquad \text{for all } j \in \{1, \ldots, d\}.$$

Taking derivatives, we find

$$\frac{\partial^2}{\partial t^2}\left(-\log[1+t\widetilde{m}_j]\right) = \frac{\partial}{\partial t}\left(-\frac{\widetilde{m}_j}{1 + t\widetilde{m}_j}\right) = \frac{(\widetilde{m}_j)^2}{(1 + t\widetilde{m}_j)^2}.$$

The right-hand side is strictly positive (for $\widetilde{m}_j \neq 0$) or at least non-negative (for $\widetilde{m}_j = 0$). This implies that the function in question is strictly convex (for $\widetilde{m}_j \neq 0$) or at least convex (for $\widetilde{m}_j = 0$)—we omit the details here.

Verify that $A \neq \mathbf{0}_{d\times d}$ implies that $\widetilde{m}_j \neq 0$ for at least one $j \in \{1, \ldots, d\}$. This means that the function in question is a sum of one or more convex functions and at least one strictly convex function, and one can show similarly as in Lemma 2.5.1 (where the domain is $\mathbb{R}^d$ rather than an interval) that such a function is strictly convex. This concludes the proof.

Details: The assumed positive definiteness of $\Omega + tA$ ensures that $1 + t\widetilde{m}_j > 0$, but $\widetilde{m}_j$ itself can be negative.

5. We need to show that for all $w \in (0, 1)$ and $\Omega', \Omega'' \in \mathcal{S}_d^+$ with $\Omega' \neq \Omega''$, it holds that

$$\begin{aligned} &- \log\det\left[w\Omega' + (1-w)\Omega''\right] \\ &\qquad < \; -w\log\det[\Omega'] - (1-w)\log\det[\Omega'']\,. \end{aligned}$$

We do this via Claim 4.

Fix two matrices $\Omega', \Omega'' \in \mathcal{S}_d^+$, $\Omega' \neq \Omega''$. It then holds that $\Omega := \Omega'' \in \mathcal{S}_d^+$ and that $A := \Omega' - \Omega'' \in \mathbb{R}^{d\times d}\setminus\{\mathbf{0}_{d\times d}\}$ is symmetric. Further, it holds that $\Omega+tA$ is symmetric and positive definite for every $t \in [0, \tilde{t}]$ with $\tilde{t} := 1$. According to Claim 4, this implies that $t \mapsto -\log\det[\Omega+tA]$ is strictly convex on $[0, \tilde{t}]$; hence, by the definition of strict convexity (use the statement in the exercise with $p = 1$), it holds for every $w \in (0, 1)$ and $t', t'' \in [0, \tilde{t}]$ with $t' \neq t''$ that

$$\begin{aligned} &- \log\det\left[\Omega + (wt' + (1-w)t'')A\right] \\ &< \; -w\log\det\left[\Omega+t'A\right] - (1-w)\log\det\left[\Omega+t''A\right]. \end{aligned}$$

Recalling that $\Omega = \Omega''$ and $A = \Omega' - \Omega''$ and setting $t' = 1$ and $t'' = 0$ give

$$\begin{aligned} &- \log\det\left[\Omega'' + (w\cdot 1 + (1-w)\cdot 0)(\Omega' - \Omega'')\right] \\ &< \; -w\log\det\left[\Omega'' + 1\cdot(\Omega' - \Omega'')\right] \\ &\qquad\qquad - (1-w)\log\det\left[\Omega'' + 0\cdot(\Omega' - \Omega'')\right]. \end{aligned}$$

Consolidating both sides yields

$$\begin{aligned} &- \log\det\left[w\Omega' + (1-w)\Omega''\right] \\ &< \; -w\log\det[\Omega'] - (1-w)\log\det[\Omega'']\,, \end{aligned}$$

as desired.

6. This claim follows directly from 2., 5., and Lemma 2.5.1, which states that the sum of a convex function and a strictly convex function is again a strictly convex function.

Solution 3.3 We prove the five claims in order.

1. The proof of the first claim is based on the linearity of the trace function.

By the definition of the trace, we find

$$\text{trace}[A\Omega] = \sum_{j=1}^{d} (A\Omega)_{jj} = \sum_{j=1}^{d}\sum_{i=1}^{d} A_{ji}\Omega_{ij}\,.$$

Therefore, taking derivatives yields for all $i,j \in \{1,\dots,d\}$

$$\frac{\partial}{\partial\Omega_{ij}}\text{trace}[A\Omega] = A_{ji} = (A^\top)_{ij}\,,$$

which is in matrix form

$$\frac{\partial}{\partial\Omega}\text{trace}[A\Omega] = A^\top\,,$$

as desired.

2. For this proof, we use the Laplace expansion of determinants in Lemma B.2.13: denoting the cofactor matrix of Ω by C, we find for all $i,j \in \{1,\dots,d\}$ that

$$\begin{aligned}
\frac{\partial}{\partial\Omega_{ij}}\log\bigl[\det[\Omega]\bigr] &= \frac{1}{\det[\Omega]}\frac{\partial}{\partial\Omega_{ij}}\det[\Omega] \\
&\qquad \text{chain rule; } \tfrac{d}{da}\log[a] = 1/a \\
&= \frac{1}{\det[\Omega]}\frac{\partial}{\partial\Omega_{ij}}\sum_{k=1}^{d} C_{kj}\Omega_{kj} \\
&\qquad \text{Lemma B.2.13 (Laplace expansion of determinants)} \\
&= \frac{C_{ij}}{\det[\Omega]} \qquad \text{sum rule and} \\
&\qquad \text{(i) in Lemma B.2.12 (properties of cofactor matrices)} \\
&= \bigl((\Omega^{-1})^\top\bigr)_{ij}\,, \\
&\qquad \text{(ii) in Lemma B.2.12 (properties of cofactor matrices)}
\end{aligned}$$

which can be written in the desired matrix form.

3. This part follows readily from the hint, the KKT conditions, and Claims 1 and 2 above.

   Exercise 3.2 ensures that the objective function is strictly convex. Hence, if a minimizer exists, it must be unique.

To check the existence and the form of the minimizer, we just need to set derivatives to zero (KKT conditions):

$$\frac{\partial}{\partial\Omega}\Big|_{\Omega=\widehat{\Theta}}\big(\text{trace}[A\Omega]-\log\big[\det[\Omega]\big]\big) = \mathbf{0}_{d\times d}$$
KKT conditions for $\widehat{\Theta}$

$$\Rightarrow \quad A^\top - (\widehat{\Theta}^{-1})^\top = \mathbf{0}_{d\times d}$$
sum rule and 1. and 2.

$$\Rightarrow \quad \widehat{\Theta} = A^{-1}\,.$$
A and $\widehat{\Theta}$ are invertible by assumption

This shows that the minimizer indeed exists and is equal to A^{-1}, as desired.

4. For this part, we use the fact that sets that live in spaces that are of a dimension smaller than the ambient spaces' dimension have Gauss measure equal to 0.

First, symmetry is straightforward:

$$\Big(\frac{1}{n}\sum_{i=1}^{n} z_i z_i^\top\Big)^\top = \frac{1}{n}\sum_{i=1}^{n}\big(z_i z_i^\top\big)^\top$$
2. in Lemma B.2.1 (linearity of transposition)

$$= \frac{1}{n}\sum_{i=1}^{n} z_i z_i^\top\,, \qquad (AB)^\top = B^\top A^\top$$

as desired.

For the invertibility, consider first the case $d = 1$. Then,

$$\mathbb{P}\Big\{\frac{1}{n}\sum_{i=1}^{n} z_i z_i^\top \text{ not invertible}\Big\}$$

$$= \mathbb{P}\Big\{\frac{1}{n}\sum_{i=1}^{n}(z^i)^2 = 0\Big\} \qquad d = 1 \text{ by assumption}$$

$$= \mathbb{P}\big\{z^i = 0\ \forall i \in \{1,\ldots,d\}\big\}$$
all summands are non-negative

$$\leq \mathbb{P}\{z^1 = 0\}$$

probability functions are increasing: $\mathbb{P}\{\mathscr{A}\} \leq \mathbb{P}\{\mathscr{A}'\}$ if $\mathscr{A} \subset \mathscr{A}'$

$$= 0\,,$$

affine subspaces with codimension larger or equal to one are nullsets of Gauss distributions

as desired.

Consider now the case $d > 1$. Take the first k outcomes $z_1, \ldots, z_k$, $k \in \{1, \ldots, d-1\}$. These vectors span an affine subspace of dimension at most k, which makes a nullset with respect to any (non-degenerate) Gauss distribution on the $\mathbb{R}^d$. Hence, z_{k+1} is linear independent of the first k outcomes with probability 1. Since unions of finitely many nullsets are still nullsets, we conclude by induction that the first $z_1, \ldots, z_d$ form a basis of the $\mathbb{R}^d$ with probability 1.

Now,

$$\mathbb{P}\left\{\frac{1}{n}\sum_{i=1}^{n} z_i z_i^\top \text{ not invertible}\right\}$$

$$= \mathbb{P}\left\{\min_{\boldsymbol{a}\in\mathbb{R}^d\setminus\{\boldsymbol{0}_d\}} \boldsymbol{a}^\top\Big(\frac{1}{n}\sum_{i=1}^{n} z_i z_i^\top\Big)\boldsymbol{a} = 0\right\}$$

A invertible $\Leftrightarrow \boldsymbol{a}^\top A\boldsymbol{a} \neq 0$ for all $\boldsymbol{a} \neq \boldsymbol{0}$

$$= \mathbb{P}\left\{\min_{\boldsymbol{a}\in\mathbb{R}^d\setminus\{\boldsymbol{0}_d\}} \frac{1}{n}\sum_{i=1}^{n} \boldsymbol{a}^\top z_i z_i^\top \boldsymbol{a} = 0\right\}$$

linearity of sums

$$= \mathbb{P}\left\{\min_{\boldsymbol{a}\in\mathbb{R}^d\setminus\{\boldsymbol{0}_d\}} \frac{1}{n}\sum_{i=1}^{n} (\boldsymbol{a}^\top z_i)^2 = 0\right\}$$

symmetry of inner products

$$= \mathbb{P}\big\{\exists \boldsymbol{a} \in \mathbb{R}^d \setminus \{\boldsymbol{0}_d\} \,:\, \boldsymbol{a}^\top z_i = 0\ \forall i \in \{1, \ldots, n\}\big\}$$

all summands are non-negative

$$= \mathbb{P}\big\{\exists \boldsymbol{a} \in \mathbb{R}^d \setminus \{\boldsymbol{0}_d\} \,:\, \boldsymbol{a} \perp z_i = 0\ \forall i \in \{1, \ldots, n\}\big\}$$

reformulation

$$\leq \mathbb{P}\big\{\exists \boldsymbol{a} \in \mathbb{R}^d \setminus \{\boldsymbol{0}_d\} \,:\, \boldsymbol{a} \perp z_i = 0\ \forall i \in \{1, \ldots, d\}\big\}$$

$n \geq d$ by assumption and $\mathbb{P}\{\mathscr{A}\} \leq \mathbb{P}\{\mathscr{A}'\}$ if $\mathscr{A} \subset \mathscr{A}'$

$$\leq \mathbb{P}\{z^1, \ldots, z^d \text{ is not a basis of the } \mathbb{R}^d\}$$

by definition, bases span the entire ambient space

$$= 0\,,$$

above insights

as desired.

Details: The fact that affine subspaces with codimension larger or equal to one have Gauss measure zero can be proved as follows (an affine subspace that has dimension s has codimension $d - s$ with respect to the $\mathbb{R}^d$): Consider an affine subspace $\mathscr{A}$ of dimension k in $\mathbb{R}^d$, $k < d$. There is a rotation R such that for every element $\boldsymbol{a} \in R\mathscr{A}$, it holds that $a_d = 0$. Denoting the Lebesgue measure on $\mathbb{R}^d$ by $\mathbb{P}$, we then find

$$
\begin{aligned}
\mathbb{P}\mathscr{A} &= \mathbb{P}R\mathscr{A} && \text{the Lebesgue measure on } \mathbb{R}^d \\
& && \text{is rotation invariant (we omit that proof)} \\
&\leq \mathbb{P}\{\boldsymbol{a} \in \mathbb{R}^d \;:\; a_d = 0\} && \\
& && \text{definition of the rotation } R;\ \mathbb{P}\{\mathscr{A}\} \leq \mathbb{P}\{\mathscr{A}'\} \text{ if } \mathscr{A} \subset \mathscr{A}' \\
&= \mathbb{P}\bigcup_{i=1}^{\infty}\big\{\boldsymbol{a} \in \mathbb{R}^d \;:\; a_1, \ldots, a_{d-1} \in [-i, i], a_d = 0\big\} && \\
& && \text{reformulation of the event} \\
&= \lim_{i\to\infty} \mathbb{P}\big\{\boldsymbol{a} \in \mathbb{R}^d \;:\; a_1, \ldots, a_{d-1} \in [-i, i], a_d = 0\big\} && \\
& && \text{measures are countably additive} \\
&= \lim_{i\to\infty} \big([-i, i]^{d-1} \cdot 0\big) && \text{definition of the} \\
& && \text{Lebesgue measure in Dudley (2002, Theorem 3.2.6} \\
& && \text{on p. 98 and Chapter 4.4 on pp. 134ff)} \\
&= 0\,. && \text{taking the limit}
\end{aligned}
$$

(Note that one cannot take boxes $\{\boldsymbol{a} \in \mathbb{R}^d : |a_d| \leq 1/i\}$ instead, because then the stated definition of the Lebesgue measure does not apply.) Since the Lebesgue measure dominates all (non-degenerate) Gauss distributions, this proves that affine subspaces of dimension at most $d - 1$ are Gauss nullsets in $\mathbb{R}^d$.

5. In view of the formulation of the maximum likelihood estimator on Page 88, this claim follows directly from 3. and 4. when taking $A = \sum_{i=1}^{n} z_i z_i^\top/n$.

Solutions for ▶ Sect. 3.4

Solution 3.4 In essence, we reformulate basic properties of the least-squares solutions.

1. The proof of the first claim is a reorganization of the least-squares' KKT condition.

   From the least-squares definition

$$\widehat{\boldsymbol{\beta}}^j \in \underset{\boldsymbol{\alpha}\in\mathbb{R}^{d-1}}{\arg\min} \|\boldsymbol{y}_j - X_{-j}\boldsymbol{\alpha}\|_2^2 ,$$

we find by setting derivatives to zero (KKT conditions) that

$$\frac{\partial}{\partial\boldsymbol{\alpha}}\Big|_{\boldsymbol{\alpha}=\widehat{\boldsymbol{\beta}}^j} \|\boldsymbol{y}_j - X_{-j}\boldsymbol{\alpha}\|_2^2 = \mathbf{0}_{d-1} \qquad \text{KKT conditions}$$

$$\Rightarrow \quad -2(X_{-j})^\top(\boldsymbol{y}_j - X_{-j}\widehat{\boldsymbol{\beta}}^j) = \mathbf{0}_{d-1} \qquad \text{computing the derivative}$$

$$\Rightarrow \quad -2\left((\boldsymbol{z}_1)_{\{j\}^\complement}, \cdots, (\boldsymbol{z}_n)_{\{j\}^\complement}\right)\left(\begin{pmatrix}(\boldsymbol{z}_1)_j\\ \vdots \\ (\boldsymbol{z}_n)_j\end{pmatrix} - \begin{pmatrix}((\boldsymbol{z}_1)_{\{j\}^\complement})^\top\\ \vdots \\ ((\boldsymbol{z}_n)_{\{j\}^\complement})^\top\end{pmatrix}\cdot\widehat{\boldsymbol{\beta}}^j\right)$$

$$= \mathbf{0}_{d-1} \qquad \text{definition of the } \boldsymbol{y}_j\text{'s and } X_{-j}\text{'s}$$

$$\Rightarrow \quad -2\left((\boldsymbol{z}_1)_{\{j\}^\complement}, \cdots, (\boldsymbol{z}_n)_{\{j\}^\complement}\right)\left(-\begin{pmatrix}(\boldsymbol{z}_1)^\top\\ \vdots \\ (\boldsymbol{z}_n)^\top\end{pmatrix}\cdot\underline{\widehat{\boldsymbol{\beta}}^j}\right) = \mathbf{0}_{d-1}$$

$$(\underline{\widehat{\boldsymbol{\beta}}^j})_j = -1 \text{ by definition}$$

$$\Rightarrow \quad \frac{1}{n}\left((\boldsymbol{z}_1)_{\{j\}^\complement}, \cdots, (\boldsymbol{z}_n)_{\{j\}^\complement}\right)\begin{pmatrix}(\boldsymbol{z}_1)^\top\\ \vdots \\ (\boldsymbol{z}_n)^\top\end{pmatrix}\cdot\underline{\widehat{\boldsymbol{\beta}}^j} = \mathbf{0}_{d-1}\,.$$

$$\text{consolidating and dividing both sides by } 2n$$

Now, we find for all $k, l \in \{1, \ldots, d\}, k \neq j$,

$$\frac{1}{n}\left(\left((\boldsymbol{z}_1)_{\{j\}^\complement}, \cdots, (\boldsymbol{z}_n)_{\{j\}^\complement}\right)\begin{pmatrix}(\boldsymbol{z}_1)^\top\\ \vdots \\ (\boldsymbol{z}_n)^\top\end{pmatrix}\right)_{kl}$$

$$= \frac{1}{n}\sum_{i=1}^n (\boldsymbol{z}_i)_k(\boldsymbol{z}_i)_l$$

$$\text{computing the matrix–matrix multiplication}$$

$$= \left(\frac{1}{n}\sum_{i=1}^n \boldsymbol{z}_i\boldsymbol{z}_i^\top\right)_{kl}.$$

$$\text{rewriting in terms of the observation vectors}$$

Combining this with the foregoing display yields the desired claim.

2. This is a straightforward calculation.

We find

$$\|\boldsymbol{y}_j - X_{-j}\widehat{\boldsymbol{\beta}}^j\|_2^2 = \langle \boldsymbol{y}_j - X_{-j}\widehat{\boldsymbol{\beta}}^j, \boldsymbol{y}_j - X_{-j}\widehat{\boldsymbol{\beta}}^j \rangle$$

definition of the ℓ_2-norm

$$= \langle \boldsymbol{y}_j, \boldsymbol{y}_j - X_{-j}\widehat{\boldsymbol{\beta}}^j \rangle - \langle X_{-j}\widehat{\boldsymbol{\beta}}^j, \boldsymbol{y}_j - X_{-j}\widehat{\boldsymbol{\beta}}^j \rangle$$

linearity of the inner product

$$= \langle \boldsymbol{y}_j, \boldsymbol{y}_j - X_{-j}\widehat{\boldsymbol{\beta}}^j \rangle - \langle \frac{\widehat{\boldsymbol{\beta}}^j}{2}, 2(X_{-j})^\top (\boldsymbol{y}_j - X_{-j}\widehat{\boldsymbol{\beta}}^j) \rangle$$

linearity of inner product; property (B.1) of transposition

$$= \langle \boldsymbol{y}_j, \boldsymbol{y}_j - X_{-j}\widehat{\boldsymbol{\beta}}^j \rangle - \langle \frac{\widehat{\boldsymbol{\beta}}^j}{2}, \mathbf{0}_{d-1} \rangle$$

$2(X_{-j})^\top (\boldsymbol{y}_j - X_{-j}\widehat{\boldsymbol{\beta}}^j) = \mathbf{0}_{d-1}$ by the KKT conditions for the least-squares—see 1. above

$$= \langle \boldsymbol{y}_j, \boldsymbol{y}_j - X_{-j}\widehat{\boldsymbol{\beta}}^j \rangle$$

linearity of the inner product

$$= \sum_{i=1}^n (\boldsymbol{y}_i)_j \Big((\boldsymbol{y}_i)_j - \sum_{k \neq j} (\boldsymbol{y}_i)_k (\underline{\widehat{\boldsymbol{\beta}}^j})_k \Big)$$

definition of the $\boldsymbol{y}_j$'s, X_{-j}'s, and $\underline{\widehat{\boldsymbol{\beta}}^j}$'s

$$= \sum_{i=1}^n (\boldsymbol{y}_i)_j \Big(-\sum_{k=1}^d (\boldsymbol{y}_i)_k (\underline{\widehat{\boldsymbol{\beta}}^j})_k \Big)$$

$(\underline{\widehat{\boldsymbol{\beta}}^j})_j = -1$ by definition

$$= -n \sum_{k=1}^d \Big(\frac{1}{n} \sum_{i=1}^n (\boldsymbol{y}_i)_j (\boldsymbol{y}_i)_k \Big) (\underline{\widehat{\boldsymbol{\beta}}^j})_k$$

linearity of sums

$$= -n\sum_{k=1}^{d}\left(\frac{1}{n}\sum_{i=1}^{n}z_i z_i^\top\right)_{jk}(\underline{\widehat{\beta}}^j)_k$$

as above

$$= -n\left(\frac{1}{n}\sum_{i=1}^{n}z_i z_i^\top\right)_{j\{1,\ldots,d\}}\underline{\widehat{\beta}}^j\,.$$

formulating in terms of matrix–vector multiplications

Dividing both sides by $-n$ yields the desired result.

3. We plug the results from above into the definition of the neighborhood selection estimator.

   The two claims above can be combined into

$$\left(\frac{1}{n}\sum_{i=1}^{n}z_i z_i^\top\right)\underline{\widehat{\beta}}^j = -\frac{\|y_j - X_{-j}\widehat{\beta}^j\|_2^2}{n}e_j\,,$$

where $e_j \in \mathbb{R}^d$ is the jth standard unit vector: $(e_j)_k = 1$ if $k = j$ and $(e_j)_k = 0$ otherwise. By assumption, we can invert the empirical covariance matrix, so that the equation can be written as

$$\underline{\widehat{\beta}}^j = -\frac{\|y_j - X_{-j}\widehat{\beta}^j\|_2^2}{n}\left(\frac{1}{n}\sum_{i=1}^{n}z_i z_i^\top\right)^{-1}e_j\,.$$

With this in mind, we find for all $k, l \in \{1, \ldots, d\}$ that

$$(\widehat{\Theta}_{\text{ns}})_{kl} = -\frac{\frac{n}{\|y_k - X_{-k}\widehat{\beta}^k\|_2^2}(\underline{\widehat{\beta}}^k)_l + \frac{n}{\|y_l - X_{-l}\widehat{\beta}^l\|_2^2}(\underline{\widehat{\beta}}^l)_k}{2}$$

Definition (3.6)

$$= \frac{\left(\left(\frac{1}{n}\sum_{i=1}^{n}z_i z_i^\top\right)^{-1}e_k\right)_l + \left(\left(\frac{1}{n}\sum_{i=1}^{n}z_i z_i^\top\right)^{-1}e_l\right)_k}{2}$$

preceding display

$$= \frac{\left(\left(\frac{1}{n}\sum_{i=1}^{n}z_i z_i^\top\right)^{-1}\right)_{lk} + \left(\left(\frac{1}{n}\sum_{i=1}^{n}z_i z_i^\top\right)^{-1}\right)_{kl}}{2}$$

e_k, e_l are the kth and lth unit vectors, respectively

$$= \left(\left(\frac{1}{n}\sum_{i=1}^{n}z_i z_i^\top\right)^{-1}\right)_{kl}\,,$$

the empirical covariance matrix (and, therefore, also its inverse—see 2. in Lemma B.2.6) is symmetric

as desired.

A.4 Solutions for ▶ Chap. 4

Solutions for ▶ Sect. 4.2

Solution 4.2 The proof relies only on Properties (i) and (ii).
Our first observation is that

$$
\begin{aligned}
\mathbb{P}\Big\{\bigcup_{j=1}^{k}\mathscr{A}_j\Big\} &= \mathbb{P}\Big\{\bigcup_{j=1}^{k}\Big(\mathscr{A}_j\setminus\bigcup_{i=1}^{j-1}\mathscr{A}_i\Big)\Big\} && \text{verify that } \cup_{j=1}^{k}\mathscr{A}_j=\cup_{j=1}^{k}(\mathscr{A}_j\setminus\cup_{i=1}^{j-1}\mathscr{A}_i), \text{ where we set } \cup_{i=1}^{0}\mathscr{A}_i:=\varnothing\\
&= \mathbb{P}\Big\{\mathscr{A}_k\setminus\bigcup_{i=1}^{k-1}\mathscr{A}_i\Big\}+\mathbb{P}\Big\{\bigcup_{j=1}^{k-1}\Big(\mathscr{A}_j\setminus\bigcup_{i=1}^{j-1}\mathscr{A}_i\Big)\Big\} && \text{the events } \mathscr{A}_k\setminus\cup_{i=1}^{k-1}\mathscr{A}_i \text{ and } \cup_{j=1}^{k-1}(\mathscr{A}_j\setminus\cup_{i=1}^{k-1}\mathscr{A}_i) \text{ are mutually disjoint; Property (i)}\\
&= \ldots = \sum_{j=1}^{k}\mathbb{P}\Big\{\mathscr{A}_j\setminus\bigcup_{i=1}^{j-1}\mathscr{A}_i\Big\}. && \text{Property (i) applied } k-2 \text{ more times in a similar fashion}
\end{aligned}
$$

Our second observation is that for all $j\in\{1,\ldots,k\}$,

$$
\begin{aligned}
&\mathbb{P}\{\mathscr{A}_j\}\\
&= \mathbb{P}\Big\{\Big(\mathscr{A}_j\setminus\bigcup_{i=1}^{j-1}\mathscr{A}_i\Big)\cup\Big(\mathscr{A}_j\cap\bigcup_{i=1}^{j-1}\mathscr{A}_i\Big)\Big\} && \mathscr{A}=(\mathscr{A}\setminus\mathscr{B})\cup(\mathscr{A}\cap\mathscr{B}) \text{ for all two sets } \mathscr{A},\mathscr{B}\\
&= \mathbb{P}\Big\{\mathscr{A}_j\setminus\bigcup_{i=1}^{j-1}\mathscr{A}_i\Big\}+\mathbb{P}\Big\{\mathscr{A}_j\cap\bigcup_{i=1}^{j-1}\mathscr{A}_i\Big\} && \text{the events } \mathscr{A}_j\setminus\cup_{i=1}^{j-1}\mathscr{A}_i \text{ and } \mathscr{A}_j\cap\cup_{i=1}^{j-1}\mathscr{A}_i \text{ are disjoint; Property (i)}\\
&\geq \mathbb{P}\Big\{\mathscr{A}_j\setminus\bigcup_{i=1}^{j-1}\mathscr{A}_i\Big\}. && \text{Property (ii)}
\end{aligned}
$$

Combining the two observations yields the desired inequality.

Solution 4.3 We exploit the symmetry properties of the Gauss density.

We find

$$
\begin{aligned}
\mathbb{P}\{|z| \geq a\} &= \int \mathbb{1}\{|z| \geq a\} \frac{1}{\sqrt{2\pi}} e^{-\frac{z^2}{2}} dz \\
&\qquad \text{specific form of Gauss densities} \\
&= \int_{-\infty}^{-a} \frac{1}{\sqrt{2\pi}} e^{-\frac{z^2}{2}} dz + \int_{a}^{\infty} \frac{1}{\sqrt{2\pi}} e^{-\frac{z^2}{2}} dz \\
&\qquad \text{linearity of integrals} \\
&= \int_{a}^{\infty} \frac{1}{\sqrt{2\pi}} e^{-\frac{z^2}{2}} dz + \int_{a}^{\infty} \frac{1}{\sqrt{2\pi}} e^{-\frac{z^2}{2}} dz \\
&\qquad z \mapsto -z \text{ in the first term} \\
&= 2\int_{a}^{\infty} \frac{1}{\sqrt{2\pi}} e^{-\frac{z^2}{2}} dz \qquad \text{consolidating} \\
&= 2\int_{0}^{\infty} \frac{1}{\sqrt{2\pi}} e^{-\frac{(z+a)^2}{2}} dz \qquad z \mapsto z+a \\
&= 2\int_{0}^{\infty} \frac{1}{\sqrt{2\pi}} e^{-\frac{z^2}{2}} e^{-za} e^{-\frac{a^2}{2}} dz \\
&\qquad \text{expanding the exponent} \\
&\leq 2\int_{0}^{\infty} \frac{1}{\sqrt{2\pi}} e^{-\frac{z^2}{2}} e^{-\frac{a^2}{2}} dz \\
&\qquad e^{-za} \leq 1 \text{ since } z, a \geq 0; \text{ monotonicity of integrals} \\
&= 2e^{-\frac{a^2}{2}} \int_{0}^{\infty} \frac{1}{\sqrt{2\pi}} e^{-\frac{z^2}{2}} dz \\
&\qquad \text{linearity of integrals} \\
&= e^{-\frac{a^2}{2}} \int_{-\infty}^{\infty} \frac{1}{\sqrt{2\pi}} e^{-\frac{z^2}{2}} dz \\
&\qquad \text{symmetry of the integrand exploited similarly as above} \\
&= e^{-\frac{a^2}{2}}, \qquad \text{densities integrate to one}
\end{aligned}
$$

as desired.

Details: Using the Cramér–Chernoff method instead of our rudimentary approach yields the slightly looser bound $\mathbb{P}\{z \geq a\} \leq e^{-\frac{a^2}{2}}$ from Boucheron et al. (2013, Section 2.2 on pp. 21ff).

Solutions for ▶ Sect. 4.3

Solution 4.5 We use Plots α–δ:

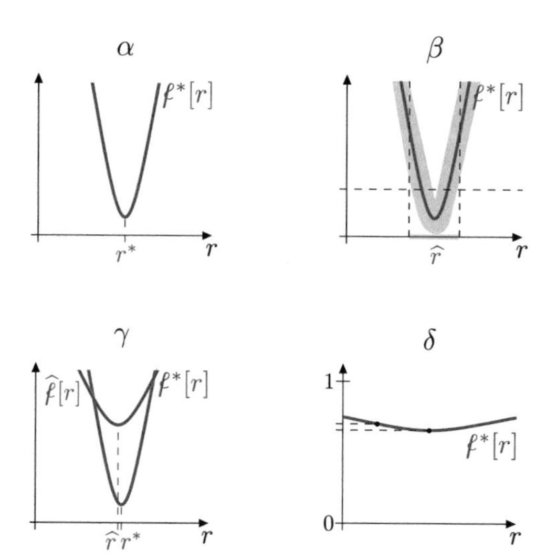

1. By definition (4.1), the optimal tuning parameter r^* is the minimizer of the prediction error $\mathscr{f}^*$: see Plot α. In the depicted case, it seems that $\mathscr{f}^*$ is continuous; then, by definition of continuity, it holds that: for every $\delta > 0$ there is a $\varepsilon > 0$ such that $|\mathscr{f}^*[r] - \mathscr{f}^*[r^*]| < \delta$ for all r with $|r - r^*| < \varepsilon$.
2. The fact that the values $\widehat{\mathscr{f}}[r]$ are in the red shaded area for all $r \in \mathcal{R}$ implies that $\widehat{\mathscr{f}}[r^*]$ is below the black, dashed, horizontal line in Plot β. Now, the estimated tuning parameter $\widehat{r}$ is the minimizer of the estimated prediction errors $\widehat{\mathscr{f}}$ by definition (4.2), which implies that $\widehat{\mathscr{f}}[\widehat{r}] \leq \widehat{\mathscr{f}}[r^*]$. Using again that $\widehat{\mathscr{f}}$ is in the red shaded area, we find that the tuning parameters for which $\widehat{\mathscr{f}}[r]$ can be below the black line are limited to the blue shaded area in Plot β.

   This is a common pattern: typically, the better the estimate of the prediction error, the closer the corresponding estimate for the tuning parameter is to the optimal one.
3. We mark the tuning parameters according to (4.1) and (4.2): see Plot γ. Even though $\widehat{\mathscr{f}}$ is not a good estimator of $\mathscr{f}^*$ (for example, $\widehat{\mathscr{f}}[r^*] \gg \mathscr{f}^*[r^*]$), the corresponding tuning parameter $\widehat{r}$ is close to r^*.

4. The curve ℓ^* is relatively flat (see the scaling of the y-axis), so that *all* tuning parameters $r \in \mathcal{R}$ entail nearly the same prediction error: see Plot γ. In particular, we do *not* require $\widehat{r} \approx r^*$ for $\ell^*[\widehat{r}] \approx \ell^*[r^*]$.

Solution 4.6 It is not suited: Recall that cross-validation uses $\boldsymbol{y}$ as an empirical counterpart of $X\boldsymbol{\beta}$. The regression vector $\boldsymbol{\beta}$ does not have such a straightforward counterpart.

A.5 Solutions for ▶ Chap. 5

Solutions for ▶ Sect. 5.1

Solution 5.1 The proofs are short calculations.

1. The proof of the first claim invokes basics of conditional expectations.

   We first find by Durrett (2010, Theorem 5.1.7 on p. 228) that

$$\mathbb{E}[\boldsymbol{u}|X] = \mathbf{0}_p \quad \Rightarrow \quad \mathbb{E}[X^\top \boldsymbol{u}|X] = \mathbf{0}_p\,.$$

   Then,

$$\begin{aligned}
&\mathbb{E}[X^\top(\boldsymbol{y} - X\boldsymbol{\beta})] \\
&= \mathbb{E}[X^\top \boldsymbol{u}] && \text{linear model: } \boldsymbol{y} = X\boldsymbol{\beta} + \boldsymbol{u} \\
&= \mathbb{E}\big[\mathbb{E}[X^\top \boldsymbol{u} \mid X]\big] && \mathbb{E}[X^\top \boldsymbol{u}] = \mathbb{E}[\mathbb{E}[X^\top \boldsymbol{u} \mid X]] \text{ by the law of iterated expectations} \\
&= \mathbb{E}\big[\mathbf{0}_p\big] && \text{above display} \\
&= \mathbf{0}_p\,, && \text{linearity of expectations}
\end{aligned}$$

   as desired.

2. This claim follows directly from comparing the definition of the Z-estimator in the claim and from the formulation of the least-squares estimator at the end of Example 5.1.1: the equations differ only in a constant ($\tilde{\mathfrak{z}}_Z = -\mathfrak{z}_Z/2$), which means that the two definitions of the estimators are equivalent.

Solution 5.2 We give one example for each of the two parts of the exercise. The examples assume $p = d$.

1. For $M_{\mathfrak{z}Z} = \mathbf{0}_{p\times p}$, the generalized Newton–Raphson algorithm always stays at its starting point $\widehat{\boldsymbol{\beta}}^0$—see Display (5.3)— which might not be a least-squares solution.
2. For $M_{\mathfrak{z}Z} = \mathrm{I}_{p\times p}$ (rather than $M_{\mathfrak{z}Z} = \mathrm{I}_{p\times p}/2$), the generalized Newton–Raphson algorithm does not necessarily converge: similarly as in the first display of Example 5.1.3, we can derive

$$\widehat{\boldsymbol{\beta}}^{i+1} = 2M_{\mathfrak{z}Z}X^\top \boldsymbol{y} + \left(\mathrm{I}_{p\times p} - 2M_{\mathfrak{z}Z}X^\top X\right)\widehat{\boldsymbol{\beta}}^i$$
$$= 2X^\top \boldsymbol{y} - \widehat{\boldsymbol{\beta}}^i\,,$$

so that

$$\widehat{\boldsymbol{\beta}}^1 = 2X^\top \boldsymbol{y} - \widehat{\boldsymbol{\beta}}^0\,,$$
$$\widehat{\boldsymbol{\beta}}^2 = 2X^\top \boldsymbol{y} - \widehat{\boldsymbol{\beta}}^1 = 2X^\top \boldsymbol{y} - (2X^\top \boldsymbol{y} - \widehat{\boldsymbol{\beta}}^0) = \widehat{\boldsymbol{\beta}}^0\,,$$
$$\widehat{\boldsymbol{\beta}}^3 = 2X^\top \boldsymbol{y} - \widehat{\boldsymbol{\beta}}^2 = 2X^\top \boldsymbol{y} - \widehat{\boldsymbol{\beta}}^0\,,$$
$$\widehat{\boldsymbol{\beta}}^4 = 2X^\top \boldsymbol{y} - \widehat{\boldsymbol{\beta}}^3 = 2X^\top \boldsymbol{y} - (2X^\top \boldsymbol{y} - \widehat{\boldsymbol{\beta}}^0) = \widehat{\boldsymbol{\beta}}^0\,,$$
$$\vdots$$

This means that for the stated choice of surrogate inverse, the algorithm only converges if $\widehat{\boldsymbol{\beta}}^0 = X^\top \boldsymbol{y}$.

Solutions for ▶ Sect. 5.2

Solution 5.3 The proofs of 1. and 2. are simple reformulations of the KKT conditions. The third part follows from the fact that $r = 0$ in the case of the least-squares estimator.

1. This indeed follows almost directly from the stated KKT conditions.

   The terms of the KKT conditions can be rearranged to

$$r\widehat{\boldsymbol{\kappa}} = 2X^\top(\boldsymbol{y} - X\widehat{\boldsymbol{\beta}})\,,$$

which yields after multiplying through by $M_{\mathfrak{z}Z}$ that

$$rM_{\mathfrak{z}Z}\widehat{\boldsymbol{\kappa}} = 2M_{\mathfrak{z}Z}X^\top(\boldsymbol{y} - X\widehat{\boldsymbol{\beta}})\,.$$

Using this and the linearity of matrix–vector multiplications then gives

$$\begin{aligned}\widehat{\boldsymbol{\beta}} + rM_{\jmath_Z}\widehat{\boldsymbol{\kappa}} &= \widehat{\boldsymbol{\beta}} + 2M_{\jmath_Z}X^\top(\boldsymbol{y} - X\widehat{\boldsymbol{\beta}}) \\ &= 2M_{\jmath_Z}X^\top\boldsymbol{y} + \big(\mathrm{I}_{p\times p} - 2M_{\jmath_Z}X^\top X\big)\widehat{\boldsymbol{\beta}}\,,\end{aligned}$$

as desired.

2. This is a further reformulation of the equality in 1.
   We find

$$\begin{aligned}
\widehat{\boldsymbol{\beta}} + rM_{\jmath_Z}\widehat{\boldsymbol{\kappa}} &= 2M_{\jmath_Z}X^\top\boldsymbol{y} \\
&\quad + \big(\mathrm{I}_{p\times p} - 2M_{\jmath_Z}X^\top X\big)\widehat{\boldsymbol{\beta}} && \text{Claim 1} \\
\Leftrightarrow\quad \widehat{\boldsymbol{\beta}} + rM_{\jmath_Z}\widehat{\boldsymbol{\kappa}} &= 2M_{\jmath_Z}X^\top(X\boldsymbol{\beta} + \boldsymbol{u}) \\
&\quad + \big(\mathrm{I}_{p\times p} - 2M_{\jmath_Z}X^\top X\big)\widehat{\boldsymbol{\beta}} \\
& \text{linear model: } \boldsymbol{y} = X\boldsymbol{\beta} + \boldsymbol{u} \\
\Leftrightarrow\quad \widehat{\boldsymbol{\beta}} - \boldsymbol{\beta} &= -rM_{\jmath_Z}\widehat{\boldsymbol{\kappa}} + 2M_{\jmath_Z}X^\top\boldsymbol{u} \\
&\quad + \big(2M_{\jmath_Z}X^\top X - \mathrm{I}_{p\times p}\big)(\boldsymbol{\beta} - \widehat{\boldsymbol{\beta}}) \\
& \text{linearity of matrix–vector multiplications and rearranging terms} \\
\Leftrightarrow\quad \mathbb{E}[\widehat{\boldsymbol{\beta}} - \boldsymbol{\beta}] &= -\mathbb{E}[rM_{\jmath_Z}\widehat{\boldsymbol{\kappa}}] + 2\mathbb{E}[M_{\jmath_Z}X^\top\boldsymbol{u}] \\
&\quad + \mathbb{E}\big[\big(2M_{\jmath_Z}X^\top X - \mathrm{I}_{p\times p}\big)(\boldsymbol{\beta} - \widehat{\boldsymbol{\beta}})\big]\,. \\
& \text{taking expectations on both sides; linearity of expectations}
\end{aligned}$$

Now, by the assumed symmetry of $M_{\jmath_Z}X^\top\boldsymbol{u}$ and by the linearity of expectations,

$$\begin{aligned}2\mathbb{E}[M_{\jmath_Z}X^\top\boldsymbol{u}] &= \mathbb{E}[M_{\jmath_Z}X^\top\boldsymbol{u}] + \mathbb{E}[-M_{\jmath_Z}X^\top\boldsymbol{u}] \\ &= \mathbb{E}[M_{\jmath_Z}X^\top\boldsymbol{u}] - \mathbb{E}[M_{\jmath_Z}X^\top\boldsymbol{u}] = \mathbf{0}_p\,,\end{aligned}$$

and $\mathbb{E}[(2M_{\jmath_Z}X^\top X - \mathrm{I}_{p\times p})(\boldsymbol{\beta} - \widehat{\boldsymbol{\beta}})] \approx \mathbf{0}_p$ by assumption. Plugging these two observations in the above display yields

$$\mathbb{E}[\widehat{\boldsymbol{\beta}} - \boldsymbol{\beta}] \approx -\mathbb{E}[rM_{\jmath_Z}\widehat{\boldsymbol{\kappa}}]\,,$$

as desired.

3. The least-squares estimator corresponds to $r = 0$. Hence, $rM_{\jmath_Z}\widehat{\boldsymbol{\kappa}} = \mathbf{0}_p$, which implies that the Newton–Raphson update $\widehat{\boldsymbol{\beta}}_{\mathrm{ls}} \mapsto \widehat{\boldsymbol{\beta}}_{\mathrm{ls}} + rM_{\jmath_Z}\widehat{\boldsymbol{\kappa}} = \widehat{\boldsymbol{\beta}}_{\mathrm{ls}}$ leaves *any*

least-squares solution unchanged *irrespective* of $M_{\mathfrak{z}Z}$. This generalizes the observations in Examples 5.1.2 and 5.1.3 that the *specific* least-squares solutions $\widehat{\boldsymbol{\beta}}_{\mathrm{ls}} = (X^\top X)^{-1}X^\top \boldsymbol{y}$ and $\widehat{\boldsymbol{\beta}}_{\mathrm{ls}} = (X^\top X)^{+}X^\top \boldsymbol{y}$, respectively, remain unchanged under the (generalized) Newton–Raphson algorithm with the *specific* choices $M_{\mathfrak{z}Z} = (X^\top X)^{-1}/2$ and $M_{\mathfrak{z}Z} = (X^\top X)^{+}/2$, respectively.

The fact that $rM_{\mathfrak{z}Z}\widehat{\boldsymbol{\kappa}} = \mathbf{0}_p$ also implies by linearity of expectations that under the conditions of 2., it holds that $\mathbb{E}[\widehat{\boldsymbol{\beta}} - \boldsymbol{\beta}] = \mathbf{0}_p$ (which is commensurate with the results of 2.), that is, the least-squares estimator is unbiased.

Solution 5.4 The proof relies on the properties of standard Gauss random variables.

1. The proof of this equality is a simple calculation based on Property (i).

   By assumption on $\boldsymbol{u}$, it holds that $u_1/\sigma, \ldots, u_n/\sigma$ are independent standard Gauss random variables. Thus,

$$
\begin{aligned}
&\mathbb{E}\|\boldsymbol{u}\|_2^2\\
&= \mathbb{E}\sum_{i=1}^{n} u_i^2 && \text{writing out the squared } \ell_2\text{-norm}\\
&= \sigma^2 \sum_{i=1}^{n} \mathbb{E}\big[(u_i/\sigma)^2\big] && \text{linearity of expectations and sums}\\
&= n\sigma^2 \mathbb{E}\big[(u_1/\sigma)^2\big] && u_1/\sigma, \ldots, u_n/\sigma \text{ are all identically distributed (previous comment)}\\
&= n\sigma^2, && z := u_1/\sigma \text{ is standard Gauss (previous comment); Property (i)}
\end{aligned}
$$

   as desired.

2. This proof is again straightforward but slightly more tedious.

   We find

$$
\begin{aligned}
&\mathbb{E}\Big[\big(\|\boldsymbol{u}\|_2^2 - n\sigma^2\big)^2\Big]\\
&= \mathbb{E}\Bigg[\bigg(\sum_{i=1}^{n} u_i^2 - n\sigma^2\bigg)^2\Bigg] && \text{writing out } \|\boldsymbol{u}\|_2^2
\end{aligned}
$$

$$
\begin{aligned}
&= \mathbb{E}\Bigg[\Bigg(\sum_{i=1}^{n}(u_i^2-\sigma^2)\Bigg)^2\Bigg] && \text{summarizing terms}\\
&= \mathbb{E}\Bigg[\sum_{i,j=1}^{n}(u_i^2-\sigma^2)(u_j^2-\sigma^2)\Bigg] && \text{multiplying out the square}\\
&= \sum_{i,j=1}^{n}\mathbb{E}\big[(u_i^2-\sigma^2)(u_j^2-\sigma^2)\big] && \text{linearity of expectations}\\
&= \sum_{\substack{i,j=1\\ i\neq j}}^{n}\mathbb{E}\big[(u_i^2-\sigma^2)(u_j^2-\sigma^2)\big]+\sum_{i=1}^{n}\mathbb{E}\big[(u_i^2-\sigma^2)^2\big]\\
& && \text{linearity of sums}\\
&= \sum_{\substack{i,j=1\\ i\neq j}}^{n}\mathbb{E}\big[u_i^2-\sigma^2\big]\mathbb{E}\big[u_j^2-\sigma^2\big]+\sum_{i=1}^{n}\mathbb{E}\big[(u_i^2-\sigma^2)^2\big]\\
& && u_i, u_j \text{ independent for } i\neq j\text{—cf. the proof of Claim 1}\\
&= \sigma^4\sum_{\substack{i,j=1\\ i\neq j}}^{n}\big(\mathbb{E}\big[(u_i/\sigma)^2\big]-1\big)\big(\mathbb{E}\big[(u_j/\sigma)^2\big]-1\big)\\
&\quad+\sum_{i=1}^{n}\mathbb{E}\big[(u_i^2-\sigma^2)^2\big] && \text{linearity of expectations and sums}\\
&= \sum_{i=1}^{n}\mathbb{E}\big[(u_i^2-\sigma^2)^2\big]\\
& && \mathbb{E}[(u_i/\sigma)^2]=1 \text{ by Property (i)—recall that}\\
& && z:=u_i/\sigma \text{ is standard Gauss-distributed}\\
&= \sum_{i=1}^{n}\mathbb{E}\big[u_i^4-2\sigma^2u_i^2+\sigma^4\big] && \text{expanding the square}\\
&= \sigma^4\sum_{i=1}^{n}\big(\mathbb{E}\big[(u_i/\sigma)^4\big]-2\mathbb{E}\big[(u_i/\sigma)^2\big]+1\big)\\
& && \text{linearity of expectations and sums}\\
&= \sigma^4\sum_{i=1}^{n}\big(3-2+1\big) && \text{Properties (ii) and (i)}\\
&= 2n\sigma^4\,, && \text{consolidating}
\end{aligned}
$$

as desired.

3. This proof is based on the Markov inequality.

   For every constant $t \in (0, 1)$, it holds that

$$\mathbb{P}\left\{ \frac{\|\boldsymbol{u}\|_2}{\sqrt{n}} \notin [\sqrt{1-t}\,\sigma, \sqrt{1+t}\,\sigma] \right\}$$

$$= \mathbb{P}\left\{ \frac{\|\boldsymbol{u}\|_2^2}{n} \notin [(1-t)\sigma^2, (1+t)\sigma^2] \right\}$$

$a_1 \leq a_2 \leq a_3 \Leftrightarrow a_1^2 \leq a_2^2 \leq a_3^2$ for all $a_1, a_2, a_3 \in [0, \infty)$

$$= \mathbb{P}\left\{ \frac{\|\boldsymbol{u}\|_2^2}{n} - \sigma^2 \notin [-t\sigma^2, t\sigma^2] \right\}$$

$a_1 \leq a_2 \leq a_3 \Leftrightarrow a_1 - b \leq a_2 - b \leq a_3 - b$ for all $a_1, a_2, a_3, b \in \mathbb{R}$

$$= \mathbb{P}\left\{ \left(\frac{\|\boldsymbol{u}\|_2^2}{n} - \sigma^2 \right)^2 > t^2\sigma^4 \right\}$$

$-a_1 \leq a_2 \leq a_1 \Leftrightarrow a_2^2 \leq a_1^2$ for all $a_1 \in [0, \infty)$, $a_2 \in \mathbb{R}$

$$\leq \mathbb{P}\left\{ \left(\frac{\|\boldsymbol{u}\|_2^2}{n} - \sigma^2 \right)^2 \geq t^2\sigma^4 \right\} \qquad \mathbb{P}\{\mathscr{A}\} \leq \mathbb{P}\{\mathscr{B}\} \text{ for } \mathscr{A} \subset \mathscr{B}$$

$$\leq \frac{\mathbb{E}\left[\left(\frac{\|\boldsymbol{u}\|_2^2}{n} - \sigma^2\right)^2\right]}{t^2\sigma^4}$$

Markov inequality applied to $x = (\|\boldsymbol{u}\|_2^2/n - \sigma^2)^2$ and $a = t^2\sigma^4$

$$\leq \frac{\mathbb{E}\left[\left(\|\boldsymbol{u}\|_2^2 - n\sigma^2\right)^2\right]}{n^2t^2\sigma^4} \qquad \text{linearity of expectations}$$

$$\leq \frac{2n\sigma^4}{n^2t^2\sigma^4} \qquad \text{Claim 2}$$

$$\leq \frac{2}{nt^2}, \qquad \text{consolidating}$$

   as desired.

4. This proof is a consequence of Claim 3.

   By the monotonicity of probabilities ($\mathbb{P}\{\mathscr{A}\} \leq \mathbb{P}\{\mathscr{B}\}$ for $\mathscr{A} \subset \mathscr{B}$), it holds that $\mathbb{P}\{|\|\boldsymbol{u}\|_2|/\sqrt{n} - \sigma \geq b\}$ is non-increasing in b: for all $b, b' \in (0, \infty)$, $b \leq b'$, it holds that

$$\mathbb{P}\left\{ \left| \frac{\|\boldsymbol{u}\|_2}{\sqrt{n}} - \sigma \right| \geq b \right\} \geq \mathbb{P}\left\{ \left| \frac{\|\boldsymbol{u}\|_2}{\sqrt{n}} - \sigma \right| \geq b' \right\}.$$

This means that if the claim is proved for a given b, it is automatically proved also for all larger b'; in particular, we can assume that $b \in (0, \sigma)$ in the following.

Given such a b, set $t := 1 - (1 - b/\sigma)^2$. In view of $b \in (0, \sigma)$, it holds that $t \in (0, 1)$, $\sqrt{1-t} = 1 - b/\sigma$, and

$$
\begin{aligned}
&\sqrt{1+t}\\
&= \sqrt{1 + 1 - (1 - b/\sigma)^2} && t = 1 - (1 - b/\sigma)^2 \text{ by definition}\\
&= \sqrt{1 + 1 - 1 + 2b/\sigma - (b/\sigma)^2} && \text{expanding the square}\\
&= \sqrt{1 + 2b/\sigma - (b/\sigma)^2} && \text{consolidating}\\
&\le \sqrt{1 + 2b/\sigma + (b/\sigma)^2} && \text{adding } 2(b/\sigma)^2 \ge 0 \text{ under the square}\\
&= \sqrt{(1 + b/\sigma)^2} && \text{binomial formula}\\
&= 1 + b/\sigma\,. && \text{taking the square-root}
\end{aligned}
$$

Using these properties of t, we finally find

$$
\begin{aligned}
&\lim_{n\to\infty} \mathbb{P}\left\{\left|\frac{\|\boldsymbol{u}\|_2}{\sqrt{n}} - \sigma\right| \ \ge\ b\right\}\\
&= \lim_{n\to\infty} \mathbb{P}\left\{\frac{\|\boldsymbol{u}\|_2}{\sqrt{n}} \notin [\sigma - b, \sigma + b]\right\}\\
&\qquad |a_1 - a_2| \ge a_3 \Leftrightarrow a_1 \notin [a_2 - a_3, a_2 + a_3] \text{ for } a_1, a_2, a_3 \in [0, \infty)\\
&= \lim_{n\to\infty} \mathbb{P}\left\{\frac{\|\boldsymbol{u}\|_2}{\sqrt{n}} \notin [(1 - b/\sigma)\sigma, (1 + b/\sigma)\sigma]\right\}\\
&\qquad \text{factoring out } \sigma \text{ in the interval description}\\
&\le \lim_{n\to\infty} \mathbb{P}\left\{\frac{\|\boldsymbol{u}\|_2}{\sqrt{n}} \notin [\sqrt{1-t}\,\sigma, \sqrt{1+t}\,\sigma]\right\}\\
&\qquad \text{above properties of } t;\ \mathbb{P}\{\mathscr{A}\} \le \mathbb{P}\{\mathscr{B}\} \text{ for } \mathscr{A} \subset \mathscr{B}\\
&\le \lim_{n\to\infty} \frac{2}{nt^2} \qquad \text{Claim 3}\\
&= 0\,, \qquad \text{taking the limit in } n
\end{aligned}
$$

as desired.

A.6 Solutions for ▶ Chap. 6

Solutions for ▶ Sect. 6.2

Solution 6.1 Claim 1 follows directly from Lemma 6.2.2 by noting that for the identity link function, $g'[a] = 1$ for all $a \in \mathbb{R}$ (so that especially $g'\big[\|y - X\widehat{\beta}\|_2^2\big] = 1$).

The first inequality of Claim 2 follows directly from Lemma 6.2.1 by setting $\boldsymbol{\alpha} = \boldsymbol{\beta}$; the second inequality of Claim 2 is derived exactly as the inequality in Lemma 6.2.2 except for setting $\boldsymbol{\alpha} = \boldsymbol{\beta}$ and taking the limit $a \to 0$ in the end.

Solutions for ▶ Sect. 6.4

Solution 6.4 All proofs center around Definition 6.4.1.

1. Swapping $\mathcal{S}$ and $\mathcal{S}^{\complement}$ just means swapping $h_{\mathcal{S}}$ and $h_{\mathcal{S}^{\complement}}$—see Definition 6.4.1.
2. Set $k := 1$ and $\mathcal{A}_1 := \{1, \dots, p\}$.
3. For $\mathcal{S} = \varnothing$ or $\mathcal{S} = \{1, \dots, p\}$, the edr function—just as any other non-negative function—is clearly decomposable: set $h_{\mathcal{S}}[\boldsymbol{a}_{\mathcal{S}}] := 0$, $h_{\mathcal{S}^{\complement}}[\boldsymbol{a}_{\mathcal{S}^{\complement}}] := \|\boldsymbol{a}_{\mathcal{S}^{\complement}}\|_2$ and $h_{\mathcal{S}}[\boldsymbol{a}_{\mathcal{S}}] := \|\boldsymbol{a}_{\mathcal{S}}\|_2$, $h_{\mathcal{S}^{\complement}}[\boldsymbol{a}_{\mathcal{S}^{\complement}}] := 0$, respectively.

   For other $\mathcal{S}$, instead, the edr function is not decomposable: If it were, then it must hold that $h_{\mathcal{S}}[\boldsymbol{a}_{\mathcal{S}}] = \|\boldsymbol{a}_{\mathcal{S}}\|_2$ and $h_{\mathcal{S}^{\complement}}[\boldsymbol{a}_{\mathcal{S}^{\complement}}] = \|\boldsymbol{a}_{\mathcal{S}^{\complement}}\|_2$ (consider $\boldsymbol{a}_{\mathcal{S}}$ variable, $\boldsymbol{a}_{\mathcal{S}^{\complement}} = \boldsymbol{0}_{|\mathcal{S}^{\complement}|}$ fixed and $\boldsymbol{a}_{\mathcal{S}^{\complement}}$ variable, $\boldsymbol{a}_{\mathcal{S}} = \boldsymbol{0}_{|\mathcal{S}|}$ fixed, respectively). But then $h[\boldsymbol{a}] = \|\boldsymbol{a}\|_2$ and $h_{\mathcal{S}}[\boldsymbol{a}_{\mathcal{S}}] + h_{\mathcal{S}^{\complement}}[\boldsymbol{a}_{\mathcal{S}^{\complement}}] = \|\boldsymbol{a}_{\mathcal{S}}\|_2 + \|\boldsymbol{a}_{\mathcal{S}^{\complement}}\|_2$ are different for many $\boldsymbol{a} \in \mathbb{R}^p$, which contradicts the decomposability.

   In contrast, the ridge estimator's squared ℓ_2-norm can be written for every $\mathcal{S}$ as

   $$\|\boldsymbol{a}\|_2^2 = \sum_{j=1}^{p}(a_j)^2 = \sum_{j\in\mathcal{S}}(a_j)^2 + \sum_{j\in\mathcal{S}^{\complement}}(a_j)^2 = \|\boldsymbol{a}_{\mathcal{S}}\|_2^2 + \|\boldsymbol{a}_{\mathcal{S}^{\complement}}\|_2^2\,,$$

   which makes it decomposable with subfunctions $h_{\mathcal{S}} : \boldsymbol{a}_{\mathcal{S}} \mapsto \|\boldsymbol{a}_{\mathcal{S}}\|_2^2$ and $h_{\mathcal{S}^{\complement}} : \boldsymbol{a}_{\mathcal{S}^{\complement}} \mapsto \|\boldsymbol{a}_{\mathcal{S}^{\complement}}\|_2^2$.
4. Set $k := p$ and $\mathcal{A}_j := \{j\}$.
5. Set $h_{\mathcal{S}}[\boldsymbol{a}_{\mathcal{S}}] := \|\boldsymbol{a}_{\mathcal{S}}\|_1$ and $h_{\mathcal{S}^{\complement}}[\boldsymbol{a}_{\mathcal{S}^{\complement}}] := \|\boldsymbol{a}_{\mathcal{S}^{\complement}}\|_1$ and recall that $\|\boldsymbol{a}\|_1 = \|\boldsymbol{a}_{\mathcal{S}}\|_1 + \|\boldsymbol{a}_{\mathcal{S}^{\complement}}\|_1$ by the definition of the ℓ_1-norms.

6. One can prove this claim along the lines of the proof of 3. In particular, by the same arguments as above, the subfunctions of an $\mathcal{S}$-decomposable group-lasso prior $\hbar$ must be

$$\hbar_{\mathcal{S}} \;:\; \boldsymbol{a}_{\mathcal{S}} \;\mapsto\; \sum_{j=1}^{k} \|\boldsymbol{a}_{\mathcal{A}_j \cap \mathcal{S}}\|_2 \quad \text{and}$$

$$\hbar_{\mathcal{S}^{\complement}} \;:\; \boldsymbol{a}_{\mathcal{S}^{\complement}} \;\mapsto\; \sum_{j=1}^{k} \|\boldsymbol{a}_{\mathcal{A}_j \cap \mathcal{S}^{\complement}}\|_2 \,.$$

The equality $\hbar[\boldsymbol{a}] = \hbar_{\mathcal{S}}[\boldsymbol{a}_{\mathcal{S}}] + \hbar_{\mathcal{S}^{\complement}}[\boldsymbol{a}_{\mathcal{S}^{\complement}}]$, that is,

$$\sum_{j=1}^{k} \|\boldsymbol{a}_{\mathcal{A}_j}\|_2 = \sum_{j=1}^{k} \big(\|\boldsymbol{a}_{\mathcal{A}_j \cap \mathcal{S}}\|_2 + \|\boldsymbol{a}_{\mathcal{A}_j \cap \mathcal{S}^{\complement}}\|_2\big)\,,$$

then holds if and only if either $\mathcal{A}_j \subset \mathcal{S}$ or $\mathcal{A}_j \subset \mathcal{S}^{\complement}$.

Solution 6.5 We prove the four statements in order.

1. The algebra in this proof is slightly tedious, but the educational result justifies the effort:

$$\min_{\boldsymbol{\delta}\in\mathscr{C}} \frac{\|X\boldsymbol{\delta}\|_2^2}{n\|\boldsymbol{\delta}\|_1^2} = \min_{\boldsymbol{\delta}\in\mathscr{C}} \frac{\|X_{\{1,2\}}\boldsymbol{\delta}_{\{1,2\}}\|_2^2 + \|X_{\{3,4\}}\boldsymbol{\delta}_{\{3,4\}}\|_2^2}{n\big(\|\boldsymbol{\delta}_{\{1,2\}}\|_1 + \|\boldsymbol{\delta}_{\{3,4\}}\|_1\big)^2}$$

assumed form of $X/\sqrt{n}$;
decomposability of the ℓ_2^2- and ℓ_1-functions

$$= \min_{\boldsymbol{\delta}_{\{1,2\}}\in\mathbb{R}^2} \min_{\substack{\boldsymbol{\delta}_{\{3,4\}}\in\mathbb{R}^2\\ \boldsymbol{\delta}\in\mathscr{C}}} \frac{\|X_{\{1,2\}}\boldsymbol{\delta}_{\{1,2\}}\|_2^2 + \|X_{\{3,4\}}\boldsymbol{\delta}_{\{3,4\}}\|_2^2}{n\big(\|\boldsymbol{\delta}_{\{1,2\}}\|_1 + \|\boldsymbol{\delta}_{\{3,4\}}\|_1\big)^2}$$

separating the minimum into two parts

$$= \min_{\boldsymbol{\delta}_{\{1,2\}}\in\mathbb{R}^2} \min_{\substack{\boldsymbol{\delta}_{\{3,4\}}\in\mathbb{R}^2\\ \boldsymbol{\delta}\in\mathscr{C}}} \frac{\|X_{\{1,2\}}\boldsymbol{\delta}_{\{1,2\}}\|_2^2}{n\big(\|\boldsymbol{\delta}_{\{1,2\}}\|_1 + \|\boldsymbol{\delta}_{\{3,4\}}\|_1\big)^2}$$

take $\delta_3 = -\delta_4$ for every fixed $\|\boldsymbol{\delta}_{\{3,4\}}\|_1$;
verify that $\boldsymbol{\delta}$ with such $\boldsymbol{\delta}_{\{3,4\}}$ exist in $\mathscr{C}$ for every $\boldsymbol{\delta}_{\{1,2\}}$

$$= \min_{\boldsymbol{\delta}_{\{1,2\}}\in\mathbb{R}^2} \min_{\substack{\boldsymbol{\delta}_{\{3,4\}}\in\mathbb{R}^2\\ \boldsymbol{\delta}\in\mathscr{C}}} \frac{(\delta_1 + \delta_2/2)^2 + 3\delta_2^2/4}{\big(\|\boldsymbol{\delta}_{\{1,2\}}\|_1 + \|\boldsymbol{\delta}_{\{3,4\}}\|_1\big)^2}$$

specific form of $X/\sqrt{n}$

$$= \min_{\delta_{\{3,4\}}\in\mathbb{R}^2} \min_{\substack{\delta_{\{1,2\}}\in\mathbb{R}^2\\ \delta\in\mathscr{C}}} \frac{\delta_1^2+\delta_2^2+\delta_1\delta_2}{\left(\|\boldsymbol{\delta}_{\{1,2\}}\|_1+\|\boldsymbol{\delta}_{\{3,4\}}\|_1\right)^2}$$

expanding the square; interchanging the minima

$$= \min_{\delta_{\{3,4\}}\in\mathbb{R}^2} \min_{\substack{\delta_{\{1,2\}}\in\mathbb{R}^2\\ \delta\in\mathscr{C}}} \frac{\delta_1^2+\delta_2^2-|\delta_1||\delta_2|}{\left(\|\boldsymbol{\delta}_{\{1,2\}}\|_1+\|\boldsymbol{\delta}_{\{3,4\}}\|_1\right)^2}$$

take δ_1, δ_2 with different signs for all fixed $\delta_1^2+\delta_2^2$ and $\|\boldsymbol{\delta}_{\{1,2\}}\|_1$;
verify that $\boldsymbol{\delta}$ with such $\boldsymbol{\delta}_{\{1,2\}}$ exist in $\mathscr{C}$ for every $\boldsymbol{\delta}_{\{3,4\}}$

$$= \min_{\delta_{\{3,4\}}\in\mathbb{R}^2} \min_{\substack{\delta_{\{1,2\}}\in\mathbb{R}^2\\ \delta\in\mathscr{C}}} \frac{\left(|\delta_1|+|\delta_2|\right)^2-3|\delta_1||\delta_2|}{\left(\|\boldsymbol{\delta}_{\{1,2\}}\|_1+\|\boldsymbol{\delta}_{\{3,4\}}\|_1\right)^2}$$

rearranging terms

$$= \min_{\delta_{\{3,4\}}\in\mathbb{R}^2} \min_{\substack{\delta_{\{1,2\}}\in\mathbb{R}^2\\ \delta\in\mathscr{C}}} \frac{\left(|\delta_1|+|\delta_2|\right)^2-3\left(|\delta_1|+|\delta_2|-|\delta_2|\right)|\delta_2|}{\left(\|\boldsymbol{\delta}_{\{1,2\}}\|_1+\|\boldsymbol{\delta}_{\{3,4\}}\|_1\right)^2}$$

adding a zero-valued term

$$= \min_{\delta_{\{3,4\}}\in\mathbb{R}^2} \min_{\substack{\delta_{\{1,2\}}\in\mathbb{R}^2\\ \delta\in\mathscr{C}}} \frac{\|\boldsymbol{\delta}_{\{1,2\}}\|_1{}^2-3(\|\boldsymbol{\delta}_{\{1,2\}}\|_1-|\delta_2|)|\delta_2|}{\left(\|\boldsymbol{\delta}_{\{1,2\}}\|_1+\|\boldsymbol{\delta}_{\{3,4\}}\|_1\right)^2}$$

definition of the ℓ_1-norm

$$= \min_{\delta_{\{3,4\}}\in\mathbb{R}^2} \min_{\substack{\delta_{\{1,2\}}\in\mathbb{R}^2\\ \delta\in\mathscr{C}}} \frac{3|\delta_2|^2-3\|\boldsymbol{\delta}_{\{1,2\}}\|_1|\delta_2|+\|\boldsymbol{\delta}_{\{1,2\}}\|_1{}^2}{\left(\|\boldsymbol{\delta}_{\{1,2\}}\|_1+\|\boldsymbol{\delta}_{\{3,4\}}\|_1\right)^2}$$

multiplying out the bracket in the denominator
and rearranging terms

$$= \min_{\delta_{\{3,4\}}\in\mathbb{R}^2} \min_{\substack{\delta_{\{1,2\}}\in\mathbb{R}^2\\ \delta\in\mathscr{C}}} \frac{3\left(|\delta_2|-\|\boldsymbol{\delta}_{\{1,2\}}\|_1/2\right)^2+\|\boldsymbol{\delta}_{\{1,2\}}\|_1{}^2/4}{\left(\|\boldsymbol{\delta}_{\{1,2\}}\|_1+\|\boldsymbol{\delta}_{\{3,4\}}\|_1\right)^2}$$

rearranging terms further

$$= \min_{\delta_{\{3,4\}}\in\mathbb{R}^2} \min_{\substack{\delta_{\{1,2\}}\in\mathbb{R}^2\\ \delta\in\mathscr{C}}} \frac{\|\boldsymbol{\delta}_{\{1,2\}}\|_1{}^2/4}{\left(\|\boldsymbol{\delta}_{\{1,2\}}\|_1+\|\boldsymbol{\delta}_{\{3,4\}}\|_1\right)^2}$$

take $\delta_2 = -\delta_1$ for given $\|\boldsymbol{\delta}_{\{1,2\}}\|_1$;
verify that $\boldsymbol{\delta}$ with such $\boldsymbol{\delta}_{\{1,2\}}$ exist in $\mathscr{C}$ for every $\boldsymbol{\delta}_{\{3,4\}}$

$$= \min_{\delta\in\mathscr{C}} \frac{\|\boldsymbol{\delta}_{\{1,2\}}\|_1{}^2}{4\|\boldsymbol{\delta}\|_1^2},$$

simplifying and using the decomposability of the ℓ_1-norm

as desired.

Details: Since $\mathcal{S} \neq \varnothing$, it holds that $\mathcal{C} \neq \varnothing$. However, for example, the set $\{\boldsymbol{\delta}_{\{1,2\}} \in \mathbb{R}^2 : \boldsymbol{\delta} \in \mathcal{C}\}$ can well be empty for given $\boldsymbol{\delta}_{\{3,4\}}$. This means that above (and similarly below), we take minima over empty sets. As a convention, we have set those minima to infinity: $\min_{\boldsymbol{a}\in\varnothing} \not{f}[\boldsymbol{a}] := \infty$ for every function $\not{f}$—see Page IX. One can check that this is commensurate with our proof.

2. Again, the proof is a somewhat tedious exercise in linear algebra.

   We first observe that

$$\begin{aligned}
\min_{\boldsymbol{\delta}\in\mathcal{C}} \frac{\|X\boldsymbol{\delta}\|_2^2}{n\|\boldsymbol{\delta}\|_1^2} &= \min_{\boldsymbol{\delta}\in\mathcal{C}} \frac{\|\boldsymbol{\delta}_{\{1,2\}}\|_1^2}{4\|\boldsymbol{\delta}\|_1^2} && \text{Claim 1}\\
&= \min_{\boldsymbol{\delta}\in\mathcal{C}} \frac{\|\boldsymbol{\delta}_{\{1,2\}}\|_1^2}{4\big(\|\boldsymbol{\delta}_{\{1,2\}}\|_1 + \|\boldsymbol{\delta}_{\{3,4\}}\|_1\big)^2} && \text{decomposability of the } \ell_1\text{-norm}\\
&= \min_{\boldsymbol{\delta}_{\{1,2\}}\in\mathbb{R}^2} \min_{\substack{\boldsymbol{\delta}_{\{3,4\}}\in\mathbb{R}^2\\ \boldsymbol{\delta}\in\mathcal{C}}} \frac{\|\boldsymbol{\delta}_{\{1,2\}}\|_1^2}{4\big(\|\boldsymbol{\delta}_{\{1,2\}}\|_1 + \|\boldsymbol{\delta}_{\{3,4\}}\|_1\big)^2}\,. && \text{separating the minimum into two parts}
\end{aligned}$$

We assume now $\mathcal{S} = \{1\}$ (the case $\mathcal{S} = \{2\}$ can be studied similarly). Then, since $\|\boldsymbol{\delta}_{\mathcal{S}^\complement}\|_1 \leq (v+1)\|\boldsymbol{\delta}_{\mathcal{S}}\|_1/(v-1)$ for $\boldsymbol{\delta} \in \mathcal{C}$, it holds for all $\boldsymbol{\delta} \in \mathcal{C}$ that $(v+1)|\delta_1| \geq (v-1)(|\delta_2| + \|\boldsymbol{\delta}_{\{3,4\}}\|_1)$. Since $\|\boldsymbol{\delta}_{\{3,4\}}\|_1 \geq 0$, it is sufficient to consider the outer minimum over $\boldsymbol{\delta}_{\{1,2\}} \in \mathbb{R}^2$ such that (i) $(v+1)|\delta_1| \geq (v-1)|\delta_2|$. Next, by similar reasons and since $\mathbf{0}_4 \notin \mathcal{C}$ by definition, it is sufficient to consider (ii) $\delta_1 \neq 0$. Moreover, $\|\boldsymbol{\delta}_{\mathcal{S}^\complement}\|_1 \leq (v+1)\|\boldsymbol{\delta}_{\mathcal{S}}\|_1/(v-1)$ for $\boldsymbol{\delta} \in \mathcal{C}$ together with $\mathcal{S} = \{1\}$ imply that $\|\boldsymbol{\delta}_{\{3,4\}}\|_1 \leq (v+1)|\delta_1|/(v-1) - |\delta_2|$. With the restrictions (i) and (ii) on $\boldsymbol{\delta}_{\{1,2\}}$, the inner minimum in the last line of the display above is always over a non-empty set, and the minimum is attained if $\|\boldsymbol{\delta}_{\{3,4\}}\|_1$ is maximally large; therefore, it is sufficient to consider the inner minimum over $\boldsymbol{\delta}$ such that (iii) $\|\boldsymbol{\delta}_{\{3,4\}}\|_1 = (v+1)|\delta_1|/(v-1) - |\delta_2|$. Plugging (i)–(iii) into the above display and reformulating yields

$$\min_{\boldsymbol{\delta}\in\mathscr{C}} \frac{\|X\boldsymbol{\delta}\|_2^2}{n\|\boldsymbol{\delta}\|_1^2}$$

$$= \min_{\substack{\boldsymbol{\delta}_{\{1,2\}}\in\mathbb{R}^2\\(v+1)|\delta_1|\geq(v-1)|\delta_2|\\\delta_1\neq 0}} \frac{\|\boldsymbol{\delta}_{\{1,2\}}\|_1^2}{4\bigl(\|\boldsymbol{\delta}_{\{1,2\}}\|_1+(v+1)|\delta_1|/(v-1)-|\delta_2|\bigr)^2}$$

(i), (ii), and (iii)

$$= \min_{\substack{\boldsymbol{\delta}_{\{1,2\}}\in\mathbb{R}^2\\(v+1)|\delta_1|\geq(v-1)|\delta_2|\\\delta_1\neq 0}} \frac{\bigl(|\delta_1|+|\delta_2|\bigr)^2}{4\bigl(2v|\delta_1|/(v-1)\bigr)^2}$$

definition of the ℓ_1-norm

$$= \min_{\delta_1\in\mathbb{R}\setminus\{0\}} \min_{\substack{\delta_2\in\mathbb{R}\\(v+1)|\delta_1|\geq(v-1)|\delta_2|}} \frac{\bigl(|\delta_1|+|\delta_2|\bigr)^2}{4\bigl(2v|\delta_1|/(v-1)\bigr)^2}$$

separating the minimum into two parts

$$= \min_{\delta_1\in\mathbb{R}\setminus\{0\}} \frac{|\delta_1|^2}{4\bigl(2v|\delta_1|/(v-1)\bigr)^2} \qquad \text{setting } \delta_2=0$$

$$= \frac{(v-1)^2}{16v^2}\,, \qquad \text{simplifying}$$

as desired.

3. Similarly as above,

$$\min_{\boldsymbol{\delta}\in\mathscr{C}} \frac{\|X\boldsymbol{\delta}\|_2^2}{\|\boldsymbol{\delta}\|_1^2}$$

$$= \min_{\boldsymbol{\delta}\in\mathscr{C}} \frac{\|\boldsymbol{\delta}_{\{1,2\}}\|_1^2}{4\|\boldsymbol{\delta}\|_1^2} \qquad \text{Claim 1}$$

$$= \min_{\boldsymbol{\delta}\in\mathscr{C}} \frac{\|\boldsymbol{\delta}_{\{1,2\}}\|_1^2}{4\bigl(\|\boldsymbol{\delta}_{\{1,2\}}\|_1+\|\boldsymbol{\delta}_{\{3,4\}}\|_1\bigr)^2}$$

decomposability of the ℓ_1-norm

$$= \min_{\boldsymbol{\delta}_{\{1,2\}}\in\mathbb{R}^2} \min_{\substack{\boldsymbol{\delta}_{\{3,4\}}\in\mathbb{R}^2\\\boldsymbol{\delta}\in\mathscr{C}}} \frac{\|\boldsymbol{\delta}_{\{1,2\}}\|_1^2}{4\bigl(\|\boldsymbol{\delta}_{\{1,2\}}\|_1+\|\boldsymbol{\delta}_{\{3,4\}}\|_1\bigr)^2}$$

separating the minimum into two parts

$$= \min_{\boldsymbol{\delta}_{\{1,2\}}\in\mathbb{R}^2\setminus\{\mathbf{0}_2\}} \frac{\|\boldsymbol{\delta}_{\{1,2\}}\|_1^2}{4\bigl(\|\boldsymbol{\delta}_{\{1,2\}}\|_1+(v+1)\|\boldsymbol{\delta}_{\{1,2\}}\|_1/(v-1)\bigr)^2}$$

same argument as in 2. above

$$= \min_{\boldsymbol{\delta}_{\{1,2\}} \in \mathbb{R}^2 \setminus \{\mathbf{0}_2\}} \frac{1}{4\bigl(1+(v+1)/(v-1)\bigr)^2}$$
dividing through by $\|\boldsymbol{\delta}_{\{1,2\}}\|_1^2$

$$= \frac{(v-1)^2}{16v^2}\,,$$
simplifying

as desired.

4. We approach this again via 1. Since the argument of the minimum of 1.'s right-hand side is non-negative for all $\boldsymbol{\delta}$, it suffices to show that there is a $\boldsymbol{\delta} \in \mathscr{C}$ such that (i) $\|\boldsymbol{\delta}_{\{1,2\}}\|_1^2 = 0$ and (ii) $4\|\boldsymbol{\delta}\|_1^2 > 0$.
   For this, we assume without loss of generality that $\{3\} \subset \mathcal{S}$ and define $\boldsymbol{\delta} := (0, 0, 1, 0)^\top$. Then, $\|\boldsymbol{\delta}_{\mathcal{S}^\complement}\|_1 = 0 \le (v+1)/(v-1) = (v+1)\|\boldsymbol{\delta}_{\mathcal{S}}\|_1/(v-1)$, that is, $\boldsymbol{\delta} \in \mathscr{C}$, and one can also check that (i) and (ii) are indeed satisfied.
   Details: Alternatively, one can start directly from 1.'s left-hand side and take $\boldsymbol{\delta} := (0, 0, 1, -1)^\top$.

A.7 Solutions for ▶ Chap. 7

Solutions for ▶ Sect. 7.2

Solution 7.1 We prove the two statements in order.

1. The proof of the first inequality is based on the Hölder inequality; the proof of the second inequality is just basic algebra.
   First inequality: If $k < l < \infty$, we find for every $\boldsymbol{c} \in \mathbb{R}^p$,

$$\|\boldsymbol{c}\|_k^k = \sum_{j=1}^{p} |c_j|^k$$
definition of the ℓ_q-norm

$$= \sum_{j=1}^{p} \bigl(|c_j|^k \cdot 1\bigr)$$
multiplying with a one-valued factor

$$= \langle \boldsymbol{a}, \boldsymbol{b} \rangle$$
where $\boldsymbol{a} := (|c_1|^k, \ldots, |c_p|^k)^\top$ and $\boldsymbol{b} := (1, \ldots, 1)^\top$

$$\le \|\boldsymbol{a}\|_{l/k}\|\boldsymbol{b}\|_{1/(1-k/l)}$$
Hölder inequality (2.6) applied with $l \leftrightarrow l/k$ and $m \leftrightarrow 1/(1-k/l)$

$$= \Big(\sum_{j=1}^{p}\big||c_j|^k\big|^{l/k}\Big)^{k/l}\Big(\sum_{j=1}^{p}|1|^{1/(1-k/l)}\Big)^{1-k/l}$$

definition of the ℓ_q-norm; definition of $\boldsymbol{a}$ and $\boldsymbol{b}$

$$= \Big(\sum_{j=1}^{p}|c_j|^l\Big)^{k/l} p^{1-k/l} \qquad \text{simplifying}$$

$$= p^{1-k/l}\|\boldsymbol{c}\|_l^k \,. \qquad \text{definition of the } \ell_q\text{-norm; rearranging}$$

Taking the kth root on both sides yields

$$\|\boldsymbol{c}\|_k \;\le\; p^{1/k-1/l}\|\boldsymbol{c}\|_l \,,$$

which proves the first inequality.

If $k < l = \infty$, we find for every $\boldsymbol{c} \in \mathbb{R}^p$,

$$\|\boldsymbol{c}\|_k^k = \sum_{j=1}^{p}|c_j|^k \qquad \text{definition of the } \ell_q\text{-norm}$$

$$\le \sum_{j=1}^{p}\Big(\max_{j\in\{1,\dots,p\}}\{|c_j|\}\Big)^k$$

monotonicity of sum and exponentiation

$$= p\cdot\Big(\max_{j\in\{1,\dots,p\}}\{|c_j|\}\Big)^k \qquad \text{evaluating the sum}$$

$$= p^{1-k/l}\|\boldsymbol{c}\|_l^k \,, \qquad k/\infty = 0 \text{ by the conventions on Pages X; definition of the } \ell_q\text{-norm}$$

which—again after taking the kth root—proves the first inequality.

Second inequality: If $l \le k < \infty$, we first find that for each $\boldsymbol{c} \in \mathbb{R}^p$, it holds by the definition of the ℓ_q-norm that

$$|c_j| = \big(|c_j|^l\big)^{1/l} \;\le\; \Big(\sum_{i=1}^{p}|c_i|^l\Big)^{1/l} \;=\; \|\boldsymbol{c}\|_l \,.$$

We then use this to find for each $\boldsymbol{c} \in \mathbb{R}^p \setminus \{\boldsymbol{0}_p\}$ (the case $\boldsymbol{c} = \boldsymbol{0}_p$ follows from the linearity of norms)

$$\|\boldsymbol{c}\|_k^k = \|\boldsymbol{c}\|_l^k \cdot \|\boldsymbol{c}/\|\boldsymbol{c}\|_l\|_k^k \qquad \text{scalability of norms; } \boldsymbol{c} \neq \boldsymbol{0}_p$$

$$
\begin{aligned}
&= \|\boldsymbol{c}\|_l^k \cdot \sum_{j=1}^{p} \bigl(|c_j|/\|\boldsymbol{c}\|_l\bigr)^k && \text{definition of the } \ell_q\text{-norm}\\
&\le \|\boldsymbol{c}\|_l^k \cdot \sum_{j=1}^{p} \bigl(|c_j|/\|\boldsymbol{c}\|_l\bigr)^l && |c_j|/\|\boldsymbol{c}\|_l \le 1 \text{ by above; } k \ge l\\
&= \|\boldsymbol{c}\|_l^k \cdot \Bigl(\sum_{j=1}^{p} |c_j|^l\Bigr)/\|\boldsymbol{c}\|_l^l\\
& && \text{linearity of sums and exponentiation rules}\\
&= \|\boldsymbol{c}\|_l^k \cdot \|\boldsymbol{c}\|_l^l/\|\boldsymbol{c}\|_l^l && \text{definition of the } \ell_q\text{-norm}\\
&= \|\boldsymbol{c}\|_l^k\,. && \text{consolidating}
\end{aligned}
$$

Taking the kth root on both sides yields

$$\|\boldsymbol{c}\|_k \;\le\; \|\boldsymbol{c}\|_l\,,$$

which proves the second inequality.

The case $l = k = \infty$ should be obvious. If $l < k = \infty$, it holds for every $\boldsymbol{c} \in \mathbb{R}^p$,

$$
\begin{aligned}
\|\boldsymbol{c}\|_k &= \max_{j\in\{1,\dots,p\}} |c_j|\\
& && k = \infty \text{ by assumption; definition of the } \ell_q\text{-norm}\\
&= \Bigl(\max_{j\in\{1,\dots,p\}} |c_j|^l\Bigr)^{1/l} && \text{monotonicity of the maximum}\\
&\le \Bigl(\sum_{j=1}^{p} |c_j|^l\Bigr)^{1/l} && \text{sum of non-negative terms}\\
&= \|\boldsymbol{c}\|_l\,, && \text{definition of the } \ell_q\text{-norm}
\end{aligned}
$$

which proves the second inequality.

2. The conclusion follows directly from combining the second inequality of 1. (with $k = q$ and $l = 1$) and the last bound in Example 7.2.1.

Solutions for ▶ Sect. 7.3

Solution 7.3 The proof is a short exercise in convex analysis and linear algebra.

Recall first that the dual of the ℓ_1-norm is the corresponding ℓ_∞-norm (see 3. in Exercise 2.2); specifically, $\overline{\hbar}_{\mathcal{S}^\complement}[\boldsymbol{b}] = \|\boldsymbol{b}\|_\infty$ for $\boldsymbol{b} \in \mathbb{R}^{p-s}$. Recall second that $\|\boldsymbol{a}\|_\infty \le 1$ for all $\boldsymbol{a} \in \partial\hbar_{\mathcal{S}}[\widehat{\boldsymbol{\gamma}}_{\mathcal{S}}] = \partial\|\widehat{\boldsymbol{\gamma}}_{\mathcal{S}}\|_1$ (see Example 2.5.2). Using these two facts and the Hölder inequality, we find for all $\boldsymbol{a} \in \partial\hbar_{\mathcal{S}}[\widehat{\boldsymbol{\gamma}}_{\mathcal{S}}]$

$$\begin{aligned}
&\overline{\hbar}_{\mathcal{S}^\complement}\big[X_{\mathcal{S}^\complement}{}^\top X_{\mathcal{S}}(X_{\mathcal{S}}{}^\top X_{\mathcal{S}})^{-1}\boldsymbol{a}\big]\\
&= \|X_{\mathcal{S}^\complement}{}^\top X_{\mathcal{S}}(X_{\mathcal{S}}{}^\top X_{\mathcal{S}})^{-1}\boldsymbol{a}\|_\infty && \text{first fact above}\\
&= \max_{j\in\mathcal{S}^\complement} |\boldsymbol{x}_j{}^\top X_{\mathcal{S}}(X_{\mathcal{S}}{}^\top X_{\mathcal{S}})^{-1}\boldsymbol{a}|\\
& && \text{definition of the } \ell_\infty\text{-norm; } X = (\boldsymbol{x}_1,\dots,\boldsymbol{x}_p)\\
&= \max_{j\in\mathcal{S}^\complement} |\big(X_{\mathcal{S}}(X_{\mathcal{S}}{}^\top X_{\mathcal{S}})^{-1}\boldsymbol{a}\big)^\top \boldsymbol{x}_j| && \boldsymbol{b}^\top\boldsymbol{c} = \boldsymbol{c}^\top\boldsymbol{b} \text{ for all } \boldsymbol{b},\boldsymbol{c}\in\mathbb{R}^n\\
&= \max_{j\in\mathcal{S}^\complement} |\boldsymbol{a}^\top (X_{\mathcal{S}}{}^\top X_{\mathcal{S}})^{-1} X_{\mathcal{S}}{}^\top \boldsymbol{x}_j|\\
& && \text{3. in Lemma B.2.1 (reversion of transposition)}\\
&\le \max_{j\in\mathcal{S}^\complement} \|\boldsymbol{a}\|_\infty \|(X_{\mathcal{S}}{}^\top X_{\mathcal{S}})^{-1} X_{\mathcal{S}}{}^\top \boldsymbol{x}_j\|_1 && \text{Hölder inequality (2.6)}\\
&\le \max_{j\in\mathcal{S}^\complement} \|(X_{\mathcal{S}}{}^\top X_{\mathcal{S}})^{-1} X_{\mathcal{S}}{}^\top \boldsymbol{x}_j\|_1\,, && \text{second fact above}
\end{aligned}$$

as desired.

Solution 7.4 We tackle the three questions in order.

1. This follows from the properties of strictly convex functions.

   The restricted least-squares function $\boldsymbol{a} \mapsto \|\boldsymbol{y} - X_{\mathcal{S}}\boldsymbol{a}\|_2^2$ is strictly convex if $X_{\mathcal{S}}{}^\top X_{\mathcal{S}}$ is invertible (see 2. in Exercise 1.4), and the ℓ_1-prior function is convex (see Example 2.5.1); therefore, the restricted lasso problem in Definition 7.3.1 is strictly convex (see Lemma 2.5.1). Since strictly convex functions have unique minima (see 4. in Exercise 1.4), $\widehat{\boldsymbol{\gamma}}_{\mathcal{S}}$ is unique, as desired.
2. We show this with a simple example.

   Consider a design $X = (\boldsymbol{x}, \boldsymbol{x}) \in \mathbb{R}^{n\times 2}$ for an $\boldsymbol{x} \in \mathbb{R}^n$ with $\|\boldsymbol{x}\|_2^2 = n$ and $\text{sign}[\boldsymbol{x}^\top\boldsymbol{y}] = 1$, a lasso estimator with $r \in (0, 2\boldsymbol{x}^\top\boldsymbol{y})$, and the set $\mathcal{S} = \{1\}$. The lasso problem restricted to $\mathcal{S}$ is then orthogonal: $X_{\mathcal{S}}{}^\top X_{\mathcal{S}} = \boldsymbol{x}^\top\boldsymbol{x} = n = n\mathrm{I}_{1\times 1}$. (And in particular, the restricted Gram matrix $X_{\mathcal{S}}{}^\top X_{\mathcal{S}}$ is invertible.) Hence, in view of

Exercise 2.10, the unique solution of the restricted lasso problem is $\widehat{\gamma}_{\mathcal{S}} = \boldsymbol{x}^\top \boldsymbol{y}/n - r/(2n) > 0$.

Combining this observation with *(Dual 1)* yields

$$\begin{aligned}
\widehat{\nu}_{\mathcal{S}} &= 2\boldsymbol{x}^\top\Big(\boldsymbol{y} - \big(\boldsymbol{x}^\top \boldsymbol{y}/n - r/(2n)\big)\boldsymbol{x}\Big)/r \\
&\qquad\qquad \text{plugging the restricted lasso solution into } (\textit{Dual } 1) \\
&= 2\boldsymbol{x}^\top \boldsymbol{y}/r - 2\boldsymbol{x}^\top \boldsymbol{y}/r \cdot \boldsymbol{x}^\top \boldsymbol{x}/n + \boldsymbol{x}^\top \boldsymbol{x}/n \qquad \text{expanding} \\
&= 1\,, \qquad \boldsymbol{x}^\top \boldsymbol{x} = n;\ \text{consolidating}
\end{aligned}$$

and similarly, using *(Dual 2)* yields $\widehat{\nu}_{\mathcal{S}^\complement} = 1$. Hence, comparing to Example 2.5.2, we find that $\widehat{\boldsymbol{\nu}} = (\widehat{\nu}_{\mathcal{S}}, \widehat{\nu}_{\mathcal{S}^\complement})^\top \in \boldsymbol{\partial}\|\widehat{\boldsymbol{\gamma}}\|_1$, and then comparing to Example 2.5.3, we find that $\widehat{\boldsymbol{\gamma}}$ is a solution of the full lasso problem. In other words, the primal-dual construction was successful.

Details: The irrepresentability condition in Assumption 7.3.1 is not satisfied, though: since $\widehat{\gamma}_{\mathcal{S}} > 0$, it holds that $a := 1 \in \partial\|\widehat{\gamma}_{\mathcal{S}}\|_1$, and therefore,

$$\|X_{\mathcal{S}^\complement}{}^\top X_{\mathcal{S}}(X_{\mathcal{S}}{}^\top X_{\mathcal{S}})^{-1} a\|_\infty = \|n \cdot (1/n) \cdot 1\|_\infty = 1\,.$$

On the other hand, one can check readily that $(0, \widehat{\gamma}_{\mathcal{S}})^\top$ is yet another solution of the full lasso problem, which means that the primal vector $\widehat{\boldsymbol{\gamma}}$ is not the unique solution of the full problem.

3. This proof is a bit more challenging. However, it is still mainly based on convexity arguments.

We first observe that a sufficient condition for the claim to hold is $\operatorname{supp}[\widehat{\boldsymbol{\beta}}_{\text{lasso}}] \subset \mathcal{S}$ for all lasso solutions

$$\widehat{\boldsymbol{\beta}}_{\text{lasso}} \in \operatorname*{arg\,min}_{\boldsymbol{\alpha} \in \mathbb{R}^p} \big\{ \|\boldsymbol{y} - X\boldsymbol{\alpha}\|_2^2 + r\|\boldsymbol{\alpha}\|_1 \big\}\,.$$

Indeed, if $\operatorname{supp}[\widehat{\boldsymbol{\beta}}_{\text{lasso}}] \subset \mathcal{S}$, we can write $\widehat{\boldsymbol{\beta}} = (\widehat{\boldsymbol{\gamma}}_{\mathcal{S}}{}^\top, \boldsymbol{0}_{p-s}{}^\top)^\top$ with $\widehat{\boldsymbol{\gamma}}_{\mathcal{S}}$ unique as discussed in Claim 1.

We then proceed in five steps.

Step 1: We show that the primal-dual construction was successful, which implies that $\widehat{\boldsymbol{\nu}} \in \boldsymbol{\partial}\|\widehat{\boldsymbol{\gamma}}\|_1$ and

$$\|\boldsymbol{y} - X\widehat{\boldsymbol{\beta}}_{\text{lasso}}\|_2^2 + r\|\widehat{\boldsymbol{\beta}}_{\text{lasso}}\|_1 = \|\boldsymbol{y} - X\widehat{\boldsymbol{\gamma}}\|_2^2 + r\|\widehat{\boldsymbol{\gamma}}\|_1$$

for every lasso solution $\widehat{\boldsymbol{\beta}}_{\text{lasso}}$.

The fact (i) $\widehat{\boldsymbol{v}}_{\mathcal{S}} \in \partial\|\widehat{\boldsymbol{\gamma}}_{\mathcal{S}}\|_1$ follows as in the proof of Lemma 7.3.1 (use $r \in (0, \infty)$); the fact (ii) $\widehat{\boldsymbol{v}}_{\mathcal{S}^\complement} \in \partial\|\widehat{\boldsymbol{\gamma}}_{\mathcal{S}^\complement}\|_1$ follows from the dual feasibility condition $\|\widehat{\boldsymbol{v}}_{\mathcal{S}^\complement}\|_\infty \leq 1$ that is implied by the stipulated strict dual feasibility condition $\|\widehat{\boldsymbol{v}}_{\mathcal{S}^\complement}\|_\infty < 1$ and from *(Primal 2)* (which ensures $\widehat{\boldsymbol{\gamma}}_{\mathcal{S}^\complement} = \mathbf{0}_{p-s}$) and Example 2.5.2 (which states that $\partial\|\mathbf{0}_{p-s}\|_1 = \{\boldsymbol{b} \in \mathbb{R}^{p-s} : \|\boldsymbol{b}\|_\infty \leq 1\}$). In view of Example 2.5.3, these two facts ensure that the primal-dual construction was successful, which is expressed by the two statements.

Step 2: We now rearrange the equality of Step 1 to

$$
\begin{aligned}
&r\|\widehat{\boldsymbol{\beta}}_{\text{lasso}}\|_1 - r\langle\widehat{\boldsymbol{v}}, \widehat{\boldsymbol{\beta}}_{\text{lasso}}\rangle \\
&\quad = \|\boldsymbol{y} - X\widehat{\boldsymbol{\gamma}}\|_2^2 + \langle -2X^\top(\boldsymbol{y} - X\widehat{\boldsymbol{\gamma}}), \widehat{\boldsymbol{\beta}}_{\text{lasso}} - \widehat{\boldsymbol{\gamma}}\rangle - \|\boldsymbol{y} - X\widehat{\boldsymbol{\beta}}_{\text{lasso}}\|_2^2 .
\end{aligned}
$$

The quantities on the right-hand side will be upper-bounded by zero in Step 3; the quantities on the left-hand side will then be analyzed further in Steps 4 and 5.

Since $\widehat{\boldsymbol{v}} \in \partial\|\widehat{\boldsymbol{\gamma}}\|_1$ according to Step 1, Example 2.5.2 yields for all $j \in \{1, \ldots, p\}$

$$
\widehat{v}_j\widehat{\gamma}_j = \begin{cases} \operatorname{sign}[\widehat{\gamma}_j]\widehat{\gamma}_j = |\widehat{\gamma}_j| & \text{if } j \in \operatorname{supp}[\widehat{\boldsymbol{\gamma}}]; \\ \widehat{v}_j \cdot 0 = 0 = |\widehat{\gamma}_j| & \text{if } j \notin \operatorname{supp}[\widehat{\boldsymbol{\gamma}}]. \end{cases}
$$

Hence, $\|\widehat{\boldsymbol{\gamma}}\|_1 = \sum_{j=1}^p |\widehat{\gamma}_j| = \sum_{j=1}^p \widehat{v}_j\widehat{\gamma}_j = \langle\widehat{\boldsymbol{v}}, \widehat{\boldsymbol{\gamma}}\rangle$.

Plugging this observation into the equality derived in Step 1 gives

$$
\|\boldsymbol{y} - X\widehat{\boldsymbol{\beta}}_{\text{lasso}}\|_2^2 + r\|\widehat{\boldsymbol{\beta}}_{\text{lasso}}\|_1 = \|\boldsymbol{y} - X\widehat{\boldsymbol{\gamma}}\|_2^2 + r\langle\widehat{\boldsymbol{v}}, \widehat{\boldsymbol{\gamma}}\rangle .
$$

We then subtract $r\langle\widehat{\boldsymbol{v}}, \widehat{\boldsymbol{\beta}}_{\text{lasso}}\rangle$ from both sides and use the linearity of the inner product to obtain

$$
\begin{aligned}
&\|\boldsymbol{y} - X\widehat{\boldsymbol{\beta}}_{\text{lasso}}\|_2^2 + r\|\widehat{\boldsymbol{\beta}}_{\text{lasso}}\|_1 - r\langle\widehat{\boldsymbol{v}}, \widehat{\boldsymbol{\beta}}_{\text{lasso}}\rangle \\
&\qquad\qquad = \|\boldsymbol{y} - X\widehat{\boldsymbol{\gamma}}\|_2^2 + \langle r\widehat{\boldsymbol{v}}, \widehat{\boldsymbol{\gamma}} - \widehat{\boldsymbol{\beta}}_{\text{lasso}}\rangle .
\end{aligned}
$$

(Primal 2) and *(Dual 1&2)* taken together yield $r\widehat{\boldsymbol{v}} = 2X^\top(\boldsymbol{y} - X\widehat{\boldsymbol{\gamma}})$, so that we can further deduce from the prenultimate display that

$$
\begin{aligned}
&\|\boldsymbol{y} - X\widehat{\boldsymbol{\beta}}_{\text{lasso}}\|_2^2 + r\|\widehat{\boldsymbol{\beta}}_{\text{lasso}}\|_1 - r\langle\widehat{\boldsymbol{v}}, \widehat{\boldsymbol{\beta}}_{\text{lasso}}\rangle \\
&\qquad = \|\boldsymbol{y} - X\widehat{\boldsymbol{\gamma}}\|_2^2 + \langle 2X^\top(\boldsymbol{y} - X\widehat{\boldsymbol{\gamma}}), \widehat{\boldsymbol{\gamma}} - \widehat{\boldsymbol{\beta}}_{\text{lasso}}\rangle .
\end{aligned}
$$

Rearranging finally yields

$$
\begin{aligned}
&r\|\widehat{\boldsymbol{\beta}}_{\text{lasso}}\|_1 - r\langle \widehat{\boldsymbol{v}}, \widehat{\boldsymbol{\beta}}_{\text{lasso}}\rangle \\
&= \|\boldsymbol{y} - X\widehat{\boldsymbol{\gamma}}\|_2^2 + \langle -2X^\top(\boldsymbol{y} - X\widehat{\boldsymbol{\gamma}}), \widehat{\boldsymbol{\beta}}_{\text{lasso}} - \widehat{\boldsymbol{\gamma}}\rangle - \|\boldsymbol{y} - X\widehat{\boldsymbol{\beta}}_{\text{lasso}}\|_2^2,
\end{aligned}
$$

as desired.

Step 3: We now show that the equality from Step 2 entails the inequality

$$\|\widehat{\boldsymbol{\beta}}_{\text{lasso}}\|_1 \leq \langle \widehat{\boldsymbol{v}}, \widehat{\boldsymbol{\beta}}_{\text{lasso}}\rangle .$$

This inequality will allow us in Step 4 to bring the focus on the index set of irrelevant predictors.

Introducing the function $f : \boldsymbol{a} \mapsto \|\boldsymbol{y} - X\boldsymbol{a}\|_2^2$ permits us to write the right-hand side of the equality from Step 2 as

$$f[\widehat{\boldsymbol{\gamma}}] + \langle \nabla f[\widehat{\boldsymbol{\gamma}}], \widehat{\boldsymbol{\beta}}_{\text{lasso}} - \widehat{\boldsymbol{\gamma}}\rangle - f[\widehat{\boldsymbol{\beta}}_{\text{lasso}}] .$$

Since f is convex according to 1. in Exercise 1.4, it also holds that (see Definition 2.5.2 and Lemma 2.5.2)

$$f[\widehat{\boldsymbol{\beta}}_{\text{lasso}}] \geq f[\widehat{\boldsymbol{\gamma}}] + \langle \nabla f[\widehat{\boldsymbol{\gamma}}], \widehat{\boldsymbol{\beta}}_{\text{lasso}} - \widehat{\boldsymbol{\gamma}}\rangle ,$$

or equivalently,

$$f[\widehat{\boldsymbol{\gamma}}] + \langle \nabla f[\widehat{\boldsymbol{\gamma}}], \widehat{\boldsymbol{\beta}}_{\text{lasso}} - \widehat{\boldsymbol{\gamma}}\rangle - f[\widehat{\boldsymbol{\beta}}_{\text{lasso}}] \leq 0 .$$

Plugging this back into the equality from Step 2 gives

$$r\|\widehat{\boldsymbol{\beta}}_{\text{lasso}}\|_1 - r\langle \widehat{\boldsymbol{v}}, \widehat{\boldsymbol{\beta}}_{\text{lasso}}\rangle \leq 0 ,$$

which is—since $r \in (0, \infty)$ by assumption—equivalent to

$$\|\widehat{\boldsymbol{\beta}}_{\text{lasso}}\|_1 \leq \langle \widehat{\boldsymbol{v}}, \widehat{\boldsymbol{\beta}}_{\text{lasso}}\rangle ,$$

as desired.

Step 4: We now deduce from Step 3 that

$$\|(\widehat{\boldsymbol{\beta}}_{\text{lasso}})_{\mathcal{S}^\complement}\|_1 \leq \langle \widehat{\boldsymbol{v}}_{\mathcal{S}^\complement}, (\widehat{\boldsymbol{\beta}}_{\text{lasso}})_{\mathcal{S}^\complement}\rangle .$$

This inequality is the basis for analyzing in the final Step 5 the components of $\widehat{\boldsymbol{\beta}}_{\text{lasso}}$ that correspond to irrelevant predictors.

Since the primal-dual witness construction was successful according to Step 1, Example 2.5.3 implies $\|\widehat{\boldsymbol{v}}\|_\infty \leq 1$. Using this and the Hölder inequality gives

$$\begin{aligned}
&\langle \widehat{\boldsymbol{v}}, \widehat{\boldsymbol{\beta}}_{\text{lasso}} \rangle \\
&= \langle \widehat{\boldsymbol{v}}_{\mathcal{S}}, (\widehat{\boldsymbol{\beta}}_{\text{lasso}})_{\mathcal{S}} \rangle + \langle \widehat{\boldsymbol{v}}_{\mathcal{S}^\complement}, (\widehat{\boldsymbol{\beta}}_{\text{lasso}})_{\mathcal{S}^\complement} \rangle \\
&\qquad \text{decomposability of the inner product} \\
&\leq \|\widehat{\boldsymbol{v}}_{\mathcal{S}}\|_\infty \|(\widehat{\boldsymbol{\beta}}_{\text{lasso}})_{\mathcal{S}}\|_1 + \langle \widehat{\boldsymbol{v}}_{\mathcal{S}^\complement}, (\widehat{\boldsymbol{\beta}}_{\text{lasso}})_{\mathcal{S}^\complement} \rangle \\
&\qquad \text{Hölder inequality (2.6) applied to the first term} \\
&\leq \|(\widehat{\boldsymbol{\beta}}_{\text{lasso}})_{\mathcal{S}}\|_1 + \langle \widehat{\boldsymbol{v}}_{\mathcal{S}^\complement}, (\widehat{\boldsymbol{\beta}}_{\text{lasso}})_{\mathcal{S}^\complement} \rangle\,, \\
&\qquad \|\widehat{\boldsymbol{v}}\|_\infty \leq 1 \text{ as mentioned above}
\end{aligned}$$

so that together with Step 3

$$\begin{aligned}
&\|(\widehat{\boldsymbol{\beta}}_{\text{lasso}})_{\mathcal{S}^\complement}\|_1 \\
&= \|\widehat{\boldsymbol{\beta}}_{\text{lasso}}\|_1 - \|(\widehat{\boldsymbol{\beta}}_{\text{lasso}})_{\mathcal{S}}\|_1 \quad \text{decomposability of the } \ell_1\text{-norm} \\
&\leq \langle \widehat{\boldsymbol{v}}, \widehat{\boldsymbol{\beta}}_{\text{lasso}} \rangle - \|(\widehat{\boldsymbol{\beta}}_{\text{lasso}})_{\mathcal{S}}\|_1 \\
&\qquad \|\widehat{\boldsymbol{\beta}}_{\text{lasso}}\|_1 \leq \langle \widehat{\boldsymbol{v}}, \widehat{\boldsymbol{\beta}}_{\text{lasso}} \rangle \text{ by Step 3} \\
&\leq \|(\widehat{\boldsymbol{\beta}}_{\text{lasso}})_{\mathcal{S}}\|_1 + \langle \widehat{\boldsymbol{v}}_{\mathcal{S}^\complement}, (\widehat{\boldsymbol{\beta}}_{\text{lasso}})_{\mathcal{S}^\complement} \rangle - \|(\widehat{\boldsymbol{\beta}}_{\text{lasso}})_{\mathcal{S}}\|_1 \\
&\qquad \langle \widehat{\boldsymbol{v}}, \widehat{\boldsymbol{\beta}}_{\text{lasso}} \rangle \leq \|(\widehat{\boldsymbol{\beta}}_{\text{lasso}})_{\mathcal{S}}\|_1 + \langle \widehat{\boldsymbol{v}}_{\mathcal{S}^\complement}, (\widehat{\boldsymbol{\beta}}_{\text{lasso}})_{\mathcal{S}^\complement} \rangle \\
&\qquad \text{by the foregoing display} \\
&\leq \langle \widehat{\boldsymbol{v}}_{\mathcal{S}^\complement}, (\widehat{\boldsymbol{\beta}}_{\text{lasso}})_{\mathcal{S}^\complement} \rangle\,, \qquad \text{consolidating}
\end{aligned}$$

as desired.

Step 5: We finally derive from Step 4 that

$$\text{supp}[\widehat{\boldsymbol{\beta}}_{\text{lasso}}] \subset \mathcal{S}\,.$$

This inclusion implies Claim 3 as explained at the beginning.

This final step is the only part where the *strict* dual feasibility condition $\|\widehat{\boldsymbol{v}}_{\mathcal{S}^\complement}\|_\infty = \max_{j \in \mathcal{S}^\complement} |(\widehat{\boldsymbol{v}}_{\mathcal{S}^\complement})_j| < 1$ is invoked. It entails for all $j \in \mathcal{S}^\complement$

$$\widehat{v}_j \cdot (\widehat{\beta}_{\text{lasso}})_j \begin{cases} < |(\widehat{\beta}_{\text{lasso}})_j| & \text{if } j \in \text{supp}[\widehat{\boldsymbol{\beta}}_{\text{lasso}}]\,; \\ = 0 = |(\widehat{\beta}_{\text{lasso}})_j| & \text{if } j \notin \text{supp}[\widehat{\boldsymbol{\beta}}_{\text{lasso}}]\,. \end{cases}$$

Consequently, if $\operatorname{supp}[\widehat{\boldsymbol{\beta}}_{\text{lasso}}] \not\subset \mathcal{S}$, that is, $\mathcal{S}^{\complement} \cap \operatorname{supp}[\widehat{\boldsymbol{\beta}}_{\text{lasso}}] \neq \varnothing$, then

$$
\begin{aligned}
&\langle \widehat{\boldsymbol{v}}_{\mathcal{S}^{\complement}}, (\widehat{\boldsymbol{\beta}}_{\text{lasso}})_{\mathcal{S}^{\complement}} \rangle \\
&= \sum_{j \in \mathcal{S}^{\complement}} \widehat{v}_j \cdot (\widehat{\beta}_{\text{lasso}})_j \qquad \text{definition of the standard inner product} \\
&< \sum_{j \in \mathcal{S}^{\complement}} |(\widehat{\beta}_{\text{lasso}})_j| \\
&\qquad \text{previous display and assumption } \operatorname{supp}[\widehat{\boldsymbol{\beta}}_{\text{lasso}}] \not\subset \mathcal{S} \\
&= \|(\widehat{\boldsymbol{\beta}}_{\text{lasso}})_{\mathcal{S}^{\complement}}\|_1 \,, \qquad \text{definition of the } \ell_1\text{-norm}
\end{aligned}
$$

which contradicts the result of Step 4. Hence, $\operatorname{supp}[\widehat{\boldsymbol{\beta}}_{\text{lasso}}] \subset \mathcal{S}$, as desired.

This concludes the proof of Claim 3.

B Mathematical Background

B.1 Analysis

Lemma B.1.1

Generalized Triangle Inequalities For all $a, b \in \mathbb{R}$ and $c \in [1, \infty)$, it holds that

$$|a+b|^c \le 2^{c-1}|a|^c + 2^{c-1}|b|^c .$$

This inequality directly implies, for example, the fact that for all $\boldsymbol{a}, \boldsymbol{b} \in \mathbb{R}^p$

$$\|\boldsymbol{a}+\boldsymbol{b}\|_2^2 \le 2\|\boldsymbol{a}\|_2^2 + 2\|\boldsymbol{b}\|_2^2 .$$

Similarly, for all $a, b \in [0, \infty)$ and $c \in (0, 1]$, it holds that

$$(a+b)^c \le a^c + b^c .$$

The case $c = 1$ corresponds to the standard triangle inequality.

Proof of Lemma B.1.1 We start with the case $a, b \in \mathbb{R}$, $c \in [1, \infty)$. For $c = 1$, the stated inequality is just the standard triangle inequality; we can thus assume $c > 1$ in the following. Observe then the fact that the function

$$\begin{aligned} (0, \infty) &\to (0, \infty) \\ z &\mapsto z^c \end{aligned}$$

is convex; indeed, the function is infinitely many times differentiable with second derivative $c(c-1)z^{c-2} > 0$. Hence, recalling Definition 2.5.1 (convex functions), we find that

$$\begin{aligned} &|a+b|^c \\ &\le \big||a| + |b|\big|^c && \text{properties of the absolute value} \\ &= 2^c \left|\frac{|a|}{2} + \frac{|b|}{2}\right|^c \end{aligned}$$

absolute value is absolutely homogeneous (see Page IX)

$$\leq 2^c\Big(\frac{1}{2}||a||^c + \frac{1}{2}||b||^c\Big) \qquad \text{above-derived convexity}$$
$$= 2^{c-1}|a|^c + 2^{c-1}|b|^c\,, \qquad \text{simplification}$$

as desired.

We then look at the case $a, b \in [0, \infty)$, $c \in (0, 1]$. One can check readily the fact that the stated inequality holds for $a + b = 0$, so that we can assume $a + b > 0$ in the following. We then get

$$\begin{aligned}
1 &= \frac{a+b}{a+b} && \text{basic algebra}\\
&= \frac{a}{a+b} + \frac{b}{a+b} && \text{separating the fraction into two parts}\\
&\leq \Big(\frac{a}{a+b}\Big)^c + \Big(\frac{b}{a+b}\Big)^c\,, && a, b \leq a + b;\ c \leq 1
\end{aligned}$$

which can be brought in the desired form by multiplying all terms with $(a + b)^c$. □

Lemma B.1.2

Decomposition of the Squared ℓ_2-norm For all $\boldsymbol{a}, \boldsymbol{b} \in \mathbb{R}^p$, it holds that

$$\|\boldsymbol{a} + \boldsymbol{b}\|_2^2 = \|\boldsymbol{a}\|_2^2 + 2\langle \boldsymbol{a}, \boldsymbol{b}\rangle + \|\boldsymbol{b}\|_2^2\,.$$

Proof of Lemma B.1.2 The proof is a simple application of the definitions of the ℓ_2-norm on Page IX and the standard inner product on Page X:

$$\begin{aligned}
\|\boldsymbol{a} + \boldsymbol{b}\|_2^2 &= \sum_{j=1}^{p}(a_j + b_j)^2 = \sum_{j=1}^{p}\big(a_j^2 + 2a_jb_j + b_j^2\big)\\
&= \sum_{j=1}^{p} a_j^2 + 2\sum_{j=1}^{p} a_jb_j + \sum_{j=1}^{p} b_j^2 = \|\boldsymbol{a}\|_2^2 + 2\langle \boldsymbol{a}, \boldsymbol{b}\rangle + \|\boldsymbol{b}\|_2^2\,.
\end{aligned}$$

□

Lemma B.1.3

Decomposition of the Inner Product For all $\boldsymbol{a}, \boldsymbol{b} \in \mathbb{R}^p$ and $c \in (0, \infty)$, it holds that

$$-\frac{\|\boldsymbol{a}\|_2^2}{c} - \frac{c\|\boldsymbol{b}\|_2^2}{4} \leq \langle \boldsymbol{a}, \boldsymbol{b} \rangle \leq \frac{\|\boldsymbol{a}\|_2^2}{c} + \frac{c\|\boldsymbol{b}\|_2^2}{4},$$

and similarly, for every $d > 0$,

$$-\frac{\|\boldsymbol{a}\|_2^2}{c} - \frac{d^2 c\|\boldsymbol{b}\|_2^2}{4} \leq d\langle \boldsymbol{a}, \boldsymbol{b} \rangle \leq \frac{\|\boldsymbol{a}\|_2^2}{c} + \frac{d^2 c\|\boldsymbol{b}\|_2^2}{4}.$$

Proof of Lemma B.1.3 We derive

$$\begin{aligned}
0 &\leq \|\sqrt{2/c}\,\boldsymbol{a} - \sqrt{c/2}\,\boldsymbol{b}\|_2^2 && \text{non-negativity of norms}\\
&= \sum_{j=1}^{p} \left(\sqrt{2/c}\,a_j - \sqrt{c/2}\,\boldsymbol{b}_j\right)^2 && \text{definition of } \ell_2\text{-norm}\\
&= \sum_{j=1}^{p} \left(2/c \cdot a_j^2 + c/2 \cdot \boldsymbol{b}_j^2 - 2a_j\boldsymbol{b}_j\right) && \text{expanding}\\
&= 2/c \cdot \|\boldsymbol{a}\|_2^2 + c/2 \cdot \|\boldsymbol{b}\|_2^2 - 2\langle \boldsymbol{a}, \boldsymbol{b} \rangle\,. && \text{definition of the } \ell_2\text{-norm and of the standard inner product}
\end{aligned}$$

Rearranging then yields

$$\langle \boldsymbol{a}, \boldsymbol{b} \rangle \leq \frac{\|\boldsymbol{a}\|_2^2}{c} + \frac{c\|\boldsymbol{b}\|_2^2}{4}$$

as desired for the first part.

For the second part, we find for all $c, c', d \in (0, \infty)$, $c' = dc$,

$$\begin{aligned}
d\langle \boldsymbol{a}, \boldsymbol{b} \rangle &\leq d\left(\frac{\|\boldsymbol{a}\|_2^2}{c'} + \frac{c'\|\boldsymbol{b}\|_2^2}{4}\right) && \text{first part applied to } c'\\
&\leq \frac{\|\boldsymbol{a}\|_2^2}{c} + \frac{d^2 c\|\boldsymbol{b}\|_2^2}{4}, && c' = dc \text{ by assumption}
\end{aligned}$$

as desired.

The right-hand inequalities finally follow from setting $\boldsymbol{a} \to -\boldsymbol{a}$. □

B.2 Matrix Algebra

In this section, we review matrices and their properties. Example matrices that can accompany the below discussions are in ■ Table B.1.

Basic Definitions

Matrices over the real values generalize single numbers to rectangular arrays of numbers. Specifically, a matrix $A \in \mathbb{R}^{n \times p}$ is an array that consists of n rows and p columns, which amounts to $n \cdot p$ numbers in total. We call these individual numbers the *elements* of the matrix and denote them by A_{ij}, where $i \in \{1, \ldots, n\}$ identifies the row and $j \in \{1, \ldots, p\}$ the column:

$$A = \begin{pmatrix} A_{11} & \cdots & A_{1p} \\ \vdots & \ddots & \vdots \\ A_{n1} & \cdots & A_{np} \end{pmatrix}.$$

For example, the last matrix in the first line of ■ Table B.1 has three rows and two columns with a total of six entries, and $A_{22} = 1$ while $A_{32} = 0$. Special cases of matrices are numbers $A = a \in \mathbb{R}^{1 \times 1} = \mathbb{R}$ and (column) vectors $A = \boldsymbol{a} \in \mathbb{R}^{p \times 1} = \mathbb{R}^p$.

Addition and multiplication generalize from numbers to matrices as follows: The *sum of two matrices* $A, B \in \mathbb{R}^{n \times p}$ is the matrix $A + B \in \mathbb{R}^{n \times p}$ with elements $(A + B)_{ij} = A_{ij} + B_{ij}$ for all $i \in \{1, \ldots, n\}, j \in \{1, \ldots, p\}$. The difference of two matrices $A, B \in \mathbb{R}^{n \times p}$ is then $A - B := A + (-B)$, where $-B \in \mathbb{R}^{p \times p}$ is defined through $(-B)_{ij} := -B_{ij}$. Observe that the two matrices must have the same dimensions. The *product of two matrices* $A \in \mathbb{R}^{n \times p}, B \in \mathbb{R}^{p \times q}$ is the matrix $AB \in \mathbb{R}^{n \times q}$ with elements $(AB)_{ij} = \sum_{k=1}^{p}(A_{ik}B_{kj})$ for $i \in \{1, \ldots, n\}, j \in \{1, \ldots, q\}$. Observe that the number of columns of the first matrix must be equal to the number of rows of the second matrix. One can check readily that addition and multiplication for matrices have similarly properties as for real-valued numbers—except commutation: AB is not necessarily BA.

Table B.1 Properties of example matrices

A	$\begin{pmatrix}1&0\\0&1\end{pmatrix}$	$\begin{pmatrix}0&1\\-1&0\end{pmatrix}$	$\begin{pmatrix}-1&1\\0&1\end{pmatrix}$	$\begin{pmatrix}1&1\\1&1\end{pmatrix}$	$\begin{pmatrix}1&0\\0&1\\0&0\end{pmatrix}$
$A^\top$	$\begin{pmatrix}1&0\\0&1\end{pmatrix}$	$\begin{pmatrix}0&-1\\1&0\end{pmatrix}$	$\begin{pmatrix}-1&0\\1&1\end{pmatrix}$	$\begin{pmatrix}1&1\\1&1\end{pmatrix}$	$\begin{pmatrix}1&0&0\\0&1&0\end{pmatrix}$
A^{-1}	$\begin{pmatrix}1&0\\0&1\end{pmatrix}$	$\begin{pmatrix}0&-1\\1&0\end{pmatrix}$	$\begin{pmatrix}-1&1\\0&1\end{pmatrix}$	–	–
diagonal	yes	no	no	no	yes
symmetric	yes	no	no	yes	–
invertible	yes	yes	yes	no	–
orthogonal	yes	yes	no	no	–
pos. definite	yes	no	no	no	–
pos. semi-definite	yes	yes	no	yes	–
rank[A]	2	2	2	1	2
trace[A]	2	0	0	2	–
det[A]	1	1	-1	0	–
eigenvectors	$\begin{pmatrix}1\\0\end{pmatrix},\begin{pmatrix}0\\1\end{pmatrix}$	–	$\begin{pmatrix}1\\0\end{pmatrix},\begin{pmatrix}1\\2\end{pmatrix}$	$\begin{pmatrix}1\\-1\end{pmatrix},\begin{pmatrix}1\\1\end{pmatrix}$	–
eigenvalues	1, 1	–	$-1, 1$	0, 2	–
singular values	1, 1	1, 1	$\sqrt{3/2 \pm \sqrt{5/4}}$	0, 2	1, 1

The *multiplication of a matrix* $A \in \mathbb{R}^{n\times p}$ *with a scalar* $b \in \mathbb{R}$ is the matrix $bA \in \mathbb{R}^{n\times p}$ defined through $(bA)_{ij} := bA_{ij}$ for $i \in \{1, \ldots, n\}, j \in \{1, \ldots, p\}$. Three examples for addition and multiplication are

$$\begin{pmatrix} 1 & 1 \\ 1 & 2 \\ 1 & 3 \end{pmatrix} + \begin{pmatrix} 2 & -4 \\ 2 & -5 \\ 2 & -6 \end{pmatrix} + \begin{pmatrix} 3 & 7 \\ 3 & 8 \\ 3 & 9 \end{pmatrix} = \begin{pmatrix} 1+2+3 & 1-4+7 \\ 1+2+3 & 2-5+8 \\ 1+2+3 & 3-6+9 \end{pmatrix} = \begin{pmatrix} 6 & 4 \\ 6 & 5 \\ 6 & 6 \end{pmatrix},$$

$$\begin{pmatrix} 1 & 2 & 3 \\ 4 & 5 & 6 \end{pmatrix} \cdot \begin{pmatrix} 0.1 \\ 0.2 \\ 0.3 \end{pmatrix} = \begin{pmatrix} 1\cdot 0.1 + 2\cdot 0.2 + 3\cdot 0.3 \\ 4\cdot 0.1 + 5\cdot 0.2 + 6\cdot 0.3 \end{pmatrix} = \begin{pmatrix} 1.4 \\ 3.2 \end{pmatrix},$$

and

$$-2\begin{pmatrix} 1 & 2 \\ 3 & 4 \end{pmatrix} = \begin{pmatrix} (-2)\cdot 1 & (-2)\cdot 2 \\ (-2)\cdot 3 & (-2)\cdot 4 \end{pmatrix} = \begin{pmatrix} -2 & -4 \\ -6 & -8 \end{pmatrix}.$$

identity matrix

Finally, the matrix $\mathrm{I}_{p\times p} \in \mathbb{R}^{p\times p}$ defined through $(\mathrm{I}_{p\times p})_{ii} = 1$ for $i \in \{1, \ldots, p\}$ and $(\mathrm{I}_{p\times p})_{ij} = 0$ for $i, j \in \{1, \ldots, p\}$ with $i \neq j$ is called the *identity matrix*. One can check readily that $A\mathrm{I}_{p\times p} = A$ for $A \in \mathbb{R}^{n\times p}$ and $\mathrm{I}_{p\times p}A = A$ for $A \in \mathbb{R}^{p\times n}$, which generalizes the identities $a \cdot 1 = 1 \cdot a = a$ for $a \in \mathbb{R}$.

Transpose of Matrices and Symmetric Matrices

The transposition of a matrix interchanges the matrix's rows and columns. This operation plays an important role in manipulating inner products, for example.

matrix transposition

symmetric matrix

Definition B.2.1

Transposes of Matrices and Symmetric Matrices The *transpose* of a matrix $A \in \mathbb{R}^{n\times p}$ is the matrix $A^\top \in \mathbb{R}^{p\times n}$ defined through $(A^\top)_{ij} := A_{ji}$ for $i \in \{1, \ldots, p\}$, $j \in \{1, \ldots, n\}$. A square matrix $A \in \mathbb{R}^{p\times p}$ that satisfies $A = A^\top$ is called *symmetric*.

We use the convention $A_{ij}^\top := (A^\top)_{ij}$. The definition of transposes applies in particular to vectors: for example,

$$\begin{pmatrix}1\\2\end{pmatrix}^\top = \begin{pmatrix}1 & 2\end{pmatrix}.$$

This observation allows us to reformulate the standard inner product: for all $\boldsymbol{b}, \boldsymbol{c} \in \mathbb{R}^p$ (which means $\boldsymbol{b}, \boldsymbol{c} \in \mathbb{R}^{p\times 1}$ in the language of matrices),

$$\langle \boldsymbol{b}, \boldsymbol{c}\rangle = \sum_{j=1}^{p} b_j c_j = \sum_{j=1}^{p} (\boldsymbol{b}^\top)_{1j}(\boldsymbol{c})_{j1} = (\boldsymbol{b}^\top \boldsymbol{c})_{11} = \boldsymbol{b}^\top \boldsymbol{c},$$

where we have also used the definition of the standard inner product (Page X) and the definition of matrix–matrix multiplications including the fact that $\boldsymbol{a}^\top \boldsymbol{b} \in \mathbb{R}^{1\times 1} = \mathbb{R}$. And similarly, we find for all $A \in \mathbb{R}^{n\times p}$ and $\boldsymbol{b} \in \mathbb{R}^p$, $\boldsymbol{c} \in \mathbb{R}^n$ that

$$\langle A\boldsymbol{b}, \boldsymbol{c}\rangle = \sum_{i=1}^{n}\sum_{j=1}^{p} A_{ij} b_j c_i = \sum_{j=1}^{p}\sum_{i=1}^{n} b_j (A^\top)_{ji} c_i = \langle \boldsymbol{b}, A^\top \boldsymbol{c}\rangle. \tag{B.1}$$

Hence, the transposition allows us to swap matrices from one argument of the inner product to the other one.

A type of matrices that are naturally symmetric are diagonal square matrices.

Definition B.2.2

Diagonal Matrices A matrix $A \in \mathbb{R}^{n\times p}$ that satisfies $A_{ij} = 0$ for all $i \in \{1, \dots, n\}$ and $j \in \{1, \dots, p\}$ with $i \neq j$ is called *diagonal*.

diagonal matrix

Both square *and* non-square matrices can be diagonal—cf. ◘ Table B.1. But since $A^\top \in \mathbb{R}^{p\times n}$ for $A \in \mathbb{R}^{n\times p}$, only square diagonal matrices, where $n = p$, are symmetric.

We conclude with useful rules for working with transposes.

Lemma B.2.1

Properties of Transposition It holds that 1. $(A^\top)^\top = A$ for every $A \in \mathbb{R}^{n\times p}$ (involution), 2. $(A + cB)^\top = A^\top + cB^\top$ for every $A, B \in \mathbb{R}^{n\times p}$ and $c \in \mathbb{R}$ (linearity); and 3. $(AB)^\top = B^\top A^\top$ for every $A \in \mathbb{R}^{n\times p}, B \in \mathbb{R}^{p\times q}$ (reversion under multiplication).

Proof of Lemma B.2.1 The proof consists of simple calculations:

For 1., we find by applying Definition B.2.1 on transposes twice that

$$((A^\top)^\top)_{ij} = (A^\top)_{ji} = A_{ij}$$

for all $i \in \{1, \ldots, n\}$ and $j \in \{1, \ldots, p\}$, as desired.

For 2., we find by alternating use of Definition B.2.1 and the definitions of the basic matrix operations that

$$(A + cB)^\top_{ij} = (A + cB)_{ji} = A_{ji} + cB_{ji} = A^\top_{ij} + cB^\top_{ij}$$

for all $i \in \{1, \ldots, n\}, j \in \{1, \ldots, p\}$, as desired.

For 3., we find by alternating use of Definition B.2.1 and the definition of the matrix–matrix multiplication that

$$(AB)^\top_{ij} = (AB)_{ji} = \sum_{k=1}^{p} A_{jk}B_{ki} = \sum_{k=1}^{p} A^\top_{kj}B^\top_{ik}$$

$$= \sum_{k=1}^{p} B^\top_{ik}A^\top_{kj} = (B^\top A^\top)_{ij}$$

for all $i \in \{1, \ldots, q\}, j \in \{1, \ldots, n\}$, as desired. □

Positive (Semi-)Definite Matrices

In the definition of Gaussian graphical models of ► Sect. 3.2, we have required the covariance matrices to be positive definite. This has three advantages: the covariance matrix is invertible (1. in Lemma B.2.5 below), which ensures a well-defined precision matrix; the determinant of the covariance matrix is non-zero (3. in Lemma B.2.6 below), which ensures a well-defined density; and the diagonal matrices of the covariance matrix are again positive definite (Lemma B.2.2 below), which ensures that the properties of the Gauss distribution transfer to its marginals. Thus, positive definiteness greatly facilitates our derivations in ▶ Chap. 3 and, similarly, facilitates many other derivations in mathematics more generally.

Definition B.2.3

Positive (Semi-)Definite Matrices A square matrix $A \in \mathbb{R}^{p\times p}$ that satisfies $\boldsymbol{b}^\top A\boldsymbol{b} \geq 0$ for all $\boldsymbol{b} \in \mathbb{R}^p \setminus \{\boldsymbol{0}_p\}$ is called *positive semi-definite*. A square matrix $A \in \mathbb{R}^{p\times p}$ that satisfies $\boldsymbol{b}^\top A\boldsymbol{b} > 0$ for all $\boldsymbol{b} \in \mathbb{R}^p \setminus \{\boldsymbol{0}_p\}$ is called *positive definite*.

positive (semi-) definite matrix

It holds that $\boldsymbol{b}^\top A\boldsymbol{b} = \cos[\angle_{\boldsymbol{b},A\boldsymbol{b}}]\|\boldsymbol{b}\|_2\|A\boldsymbol{b}\|_2$, where $\angle_{\boldsymbol{b},A\boldsymbol{b}}$ is the angle between $\boldsymbol{b}$ and $A\boldsymbol{b}$. Hence, the angle between a $\boldsymbol{b} \in \mathbb{R}^p \setminus \{\boldsymbol{0}_p\}$ and $A\boldsymbol{b}$ must not be larger than 90° for positive semi-definite matrices and smaller than 90° for positive definite matrices:

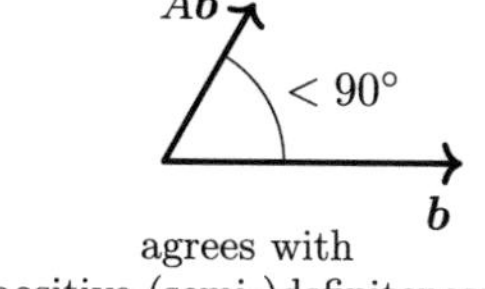

agrees with positive (semi-)definiteness: $\cos[\angle_{\boldsymbol{b},A\boldsymbol{b}}] > 0$

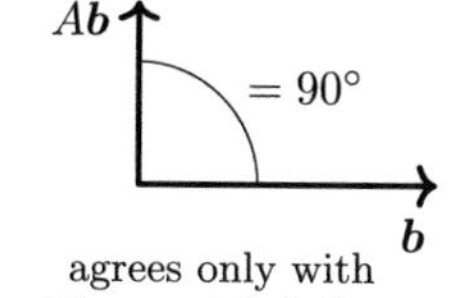

agrees only with positive semi-definiteness: $\cos[\angle_{\boldsymbol{b},A\boldsymbol{b}}] = 0$

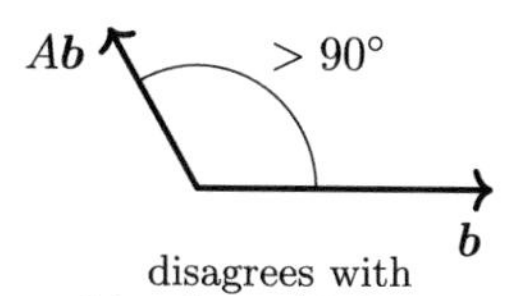

disagrees with positive (semi-)definiteness: $\cos[\angle_{\boldsymbol{b},A\boldsymbol{b}}] < 0$

So in other words, positive (semi-)definite matrices preserve the general direction of every vector.

Positive (semi-)definiteness is sometimes defined only for matrices that are symmetric, but we keep these two concepts disentangled.

In statistics, the most prominent example for a positive semi-definite matrix is the Gram matrix $X^\top X$—see Exercise 1.2. More generally, one can check that every matrix of the form $A^\top A$ for a $A \in \mathbb{R}^{n\times p}$ is positive semi-definite.

Important for working with marginals of Gauss distributions is that positive definiteness (as well as symmetry) extends to square submatrices on the diagonal.

Lemma B.2.2

Symmetry and Positive Definiteness of Square Submatrices If $M \in \mathbb{R}^{p\times p}$ is a symmetric, positive definite matrix of the form

$$M = \begin{pmatrix} A & B \\ B^\top & C \end{pmatrix},$$

then A and C are also symmetric and positive definite.

Verify that the stated form of M ensures that A and C are square matrices. We leave the proof of the lemma as an exercise.

Determinant of Matrices

The determinant function assigns to every square matrix a scalar. The determinant appears, for example, in the densities of Gauss distributions, which makes it essential to our treatment of Gaussian graphical models.

matrix determinant

Definition B.2.4

Determinant of Matrices The *determinant function* $\det : \mathbb{R}^{p\times p} \to \mathbb{R}$ is defined as

$$\det : A \mapsto \sum_{m\in\mathcal{M}^p} \left(\operatorname{sign}[m]\prod_{i=1}^{p} A_{im[i]}\right),$$

where $\mathcal{M}^p := \{m : \{1,\ldots,p\} \to \{1,\ldots,p\},\ m \text{ is bijective}\}$ is the set of *permutations* of $\{1,\ldots,p\}$, and $\operatorname{sign}[m] := 1$ if the permutation consists of an even number of successive interchanges of two indexes and $\operatorname{sign}[m] := -1$ otherwise. This formulation of the determinant is called the *Leibniz formula*.

A function $m : \{1,\ldots,p\} \to \{1,\ldots,p\}$ is called bijective if for each $j \in \{1,\ldots,p\}$, there is exactly one $i \in \{1,\ldots,p\}$ such that $j = m[i]$; for example, the function $m : \{1,2,3\} \to \{1,2,3\}$ with $m[1] = 1$, $m[2] = 3$, and $m[3] = 2$ is bijective and, therefore, a permutation, while the function $m : \{1,2,3\} \to \{1,2,3\}$ with $m[1] =$

1, $m[2] = 2$, and $m[3] = 2$ is not bijective and, therefore, not a permutation. Hence, a permutation reshuffles indexes and, therefore, can be seen as a sequence of operations that each interchanges two indexes; for example, $m : \{1, 2, 3\} \to \{1, 2, 3\}$ with $m[1] = 1$, $m[2] = 3$, and $m[3] = 2$ interchanges just indexes 2 and 3, which means that $\text{sign}[m] = -1$, while $m : \{1, 2, 3\} \to \{1, 2, 3\}$ with $m[1] = 2$, $m[2] = 3$, and $m[3] = 1$ first interchanges indexes 1 and 2 and then 2 and 3 (or equivalently, first interchanges indexes 2 and 3 and then 1 and 3), which means that $\text{sign}[m] = 1$.

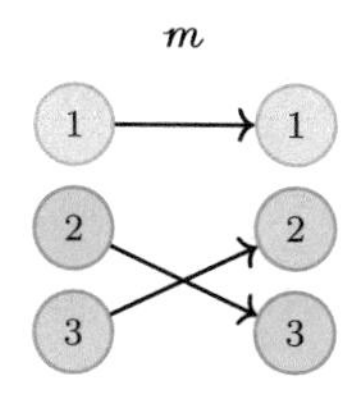

permutation with $\text{sign}[m] = -1$

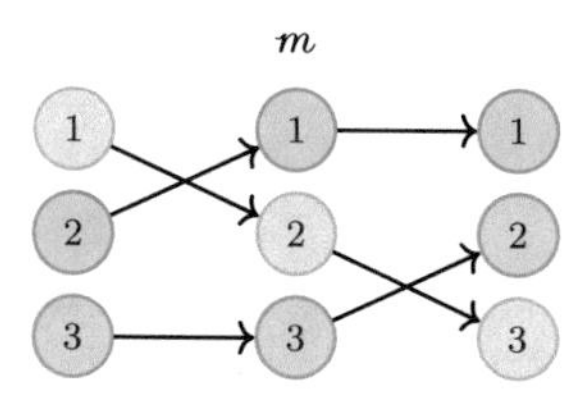

permutation with $\text{sign}[m] = 1$

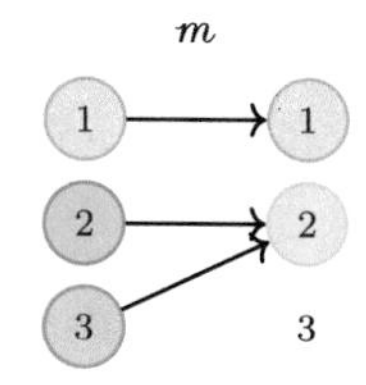

not a permutation because not bijective

Consequently, the determinant of a matrix $A \in \mathbb{R}^{1\times1}$ is $\det[A] = A_{11}$; the determinant of a matrix $A \in \mathbb{R}^{2\times2}$ is $\det[A] = A_{11}A_{22} - A_{12}A_{21}$, and so forth.

Geometrically speaking, the determinant in absolute value is the volume of the parallelepiped spanned by the matrix's columns. We can verify this readily for (2×2)-matrices $A = (\boldsymbol{a}, \boldsymbol{b}) \in \mathbb{R}^{2\times2}$. Basic geometry teaches us that the volume of the parallelepiped spanned by $\boldsymbol{a}$ and $\boldsymbol{b}$ is $\text{vol}_{\boldsymbol{a},\boldsymbol{b}} = \|\boldsymbol{a}\|_2\|\boldsymbol{b}\|_2 \sin[\angle_{\boldsymbol{a},\boldsymbol{b}}]$, where $\angle_{\boldsymbol{a},\boldsymbol{b}}$ is the angle between $\boldsymbol{a}$ and $\boldsymbol{b}$. But $\sin^2[\angle_{\boldsymbol{a},\boldsymbol{b}}] + \cos^2[\angle_{\boldsymbol{a},\boldsymbol{b}}] = 1$ and $\cos[\angle_{\boldsymbol{a},\boldsymbol{b}}] = \langle\boldsymbol{a}, \boldsymbol{b}\rangle/(\|\boldsymbol{a}\|_2\|\boldsymbol{b}\|_2)$, so that $\text{vol}_{\boldsymbol{a},\boldsymbol{b}} = \sqrt{\|\boldsymbol{a}\|_2^2\|\boldsymbol{b}\|_2^2 - \langle\boldsymbol{a}, \boldsymbol{b}\rangle^2}$. A quick computation then yields

$$
\begin{aligned}
\text{vol}_{\boldsymbol{a},\boldsymbol{b}} &= \sqrt{\|\boldsymbol{a}\|_2^2\|\boldsymbol{b}\|_2^2 - \langle\boldsymbol{a}, \boldsymbol{b}\rangle^2} && \text{above insights}\\
&= \sqrt{(a_1^2 + a_2^2)(b_1^2 + b_2^2) - (a_1b_1 + a_2b_2)^2} && \text{definition of Euclidean norms and standard inner products}\\
&= \sqrt{a_1^2b_1^2 + a_1^2b_2^2 + a_2^2b_1^2 + a_2^2b_2^2 - a_1^2b_1^2 - 2a_1b_1a_2b_2 - a_2^2b_2^2} && \text{expanding the squared terms}\\
&= \sqrt{a_1^2b_2^2 + b_1^2a_2^2 - 2a_1b_2b_1a_2} && \text{consolidating}\\
&= \sqrt{(a_1b_2 - b_1a_2)^2} && \text{summarizing the terms}
\end{aligned}
$$

$$
\begin{aligned}
&= |a_1 b_2 - b_1 a_2| && \text{simplifying} \\
&= |A_{11}A_{22} - A_{12}A_{21}| && A = (\boldsymbol{a}, \boldsymbol{b}) \\
&= |\det[A]|\,, && \text{above definition of the determinant}
\end{aligned}
$$

as desired. Some illustrations:

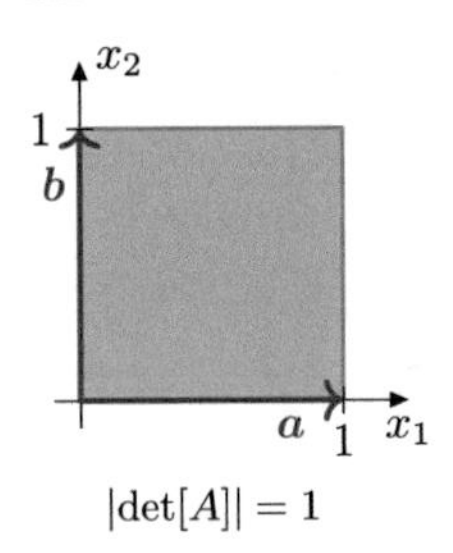

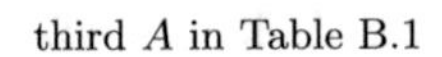

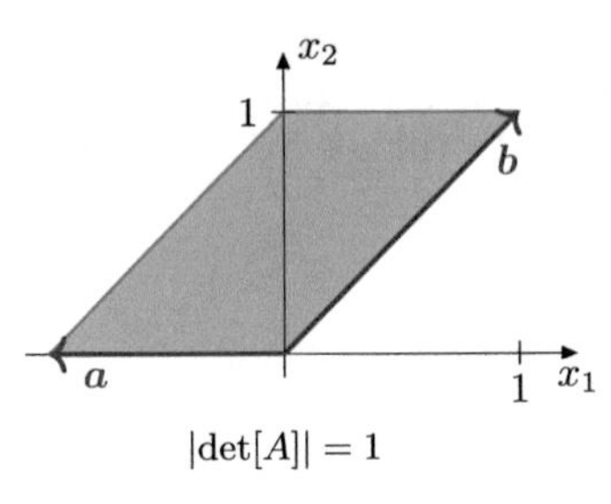

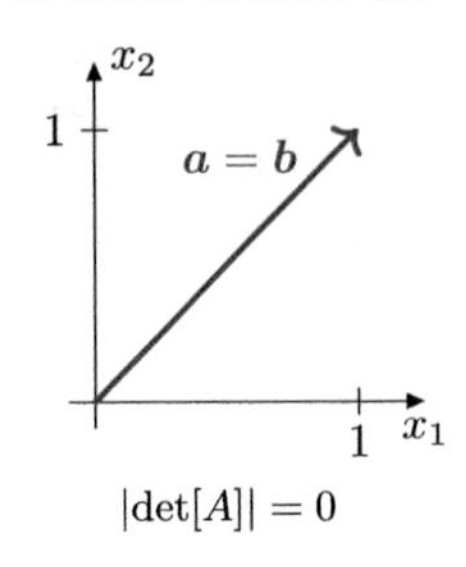

The following lemma contains the most important properties of determinants.

Lemma B.2.3

Basic Properties of Determinants Let $A, B \in \mathbb{R}^{p \times p}$ be two square matrices. Then, 1. $\det[AB] = \det[A]\det[B]$ (multiplicativity); 2. $\det[A^\top] = \det[A]$ (invariance under transposition); and 3. $\det[A] = \prod_{i=1}^{p} A_{ii}$ if A is diagonal; in particular $\det[\mathrm{I}_{p\times p}] = 1$ (diagonal case).

We leave the proof as an exercise.

We finally show that the determinants of positive definite matrices are positive.

Lemma B.2.4

Determinant of Positive Definite Matrices The determinant of a positive definite matrix is strictly positive.

Proof of Lemma B.2.4 We prove the claim via the intermediate value theorem.

Verify first that the determinant function is continuous. Hence, for every matrix $A \in \mathbb{R}^{p\times p}$, the function $f_A : w \mapsto \det[(1-w)\mathrm{I}_{p\times p} + wA]$ is continuous. Moreover, $f_A[0] = 1$ by 3. in Lemma B.2.3. Thus, by the intermediate value theorem, a necessary condition for $f_A[1] < 0$ is that $f_A[w] = 0$ for a $w \in [0, 1]$.

Verify now that for every positive definite $A \in \mathbb{R}^{p \times p}$, the matrix $(1-w)\mathrm{I}_{p \times p} + wA$ is also positive definite for every $w \in [0, 1]$. By 1. in Lemma B.2.5 and 3. in Lemma B.2.6, it then holds that $\ell_A[w] \neq 0$. Hence, in view of the above condition, $\ell_A[1] = \det[A] > 0$, as desired. □

Inverse of Matrices

Recall that it holds for every number $a \in \mathbb{R}$ that $a \neq 0$ if and only if there is another number, namely $1/a \in \mathbb{R} \setminus \{0\}$, that satisfies $a \cdot (1/a) = (1/a) \cdot a = 1$. We call $1/a$ the *reciprocal number* of a. For example, the reciprocal number of 2 is 1/2: indeed, $2 \cdot (1/2) = (1/2) \cdot 2 = 1$. Matrix inverses now generalize this notion of reciprocal numbers to matrices.

Definition B.2.5

Inverse of Matrices A square matrix $A \in \mathbb{R}^{p \times p}$ for which there is another matrix $A^{-1} \in \mathbb{R}^{p \times p}$ such that $AA^{-1} = A^{-1}A = \mathrm{I}_{p \times p}$ is called *invertible*. We then call A^{-1} the *matrix inverse* of A.

matrix inverse

In $\mathbb{R}^{1 \times 1}$, matrix inverses indeed become reciprocal numbers: a matrix $A = a \in \mathbb{R}^{1 \times 1}$ is invertible if and only if $a \neq 0$, and the inverse of A is then $A^{-1} = 1/a$.

The notion of matrix inverses harmonizes with positive definiteness:

Lemma B.2.5

Inverse of Positive Definite Matrices Let $A \in \mathbb{R}^{p \times p}$ be a positive definite matrix. Then, 1. A is invertible; 2. the inverse A^{-1} is also positive definite; and 3. the diagonal elements of A are positive: $A_{ii} > 0$ for all $i \in \{1, \ldots, p\}$.

On the other hand, let $A \in \mathbb{R}^{p \times p}$ be a symmetric and positive semi-definite matrix. Then, 4. A is invertible if and only if A is positive definite.

The second example in ◘ Table B.1 illustrates that invertible matrices do not need to be positive definite and the third example that the fourth claim is false for matrices that are not symmetric. We omit the proof of the lemma.

The basic properties of matrix inversion are:

Lemma B.2.6

Properties of Inversion Let $A \in \mathbb{R}^{p\times p}$ be an invertible matrix. Then, 1. A^{-1} is invertible with inverse $(A^{-1})^{-1} = A$ (involution); 2. $(A^\top)^{-1} = (A^{-1})^\top$ (transposition commutes with inversion); in particular, if A is symmetric, then also A^{-1} is symmetric; 3. $\det[A], \det[A^{-1}] \neq 0$ and $\det[A^{-1}] = 1/\det[A]$ (determinant of a matrix and of the inverse matrix are reciprocal).

Proof of Lemma B.2.6 The proof consists of elementary manipulations of the above definitions.

1. follows readily from the definition of invertible matrices in Definition B.2.5: just swap A and A^{-1}.

2. follows from a short calculation:

$$\begin{aligned}
A^{-1} &= A^{-1}\mathrm{I}_{p\times p} && \text{property of the identity matrix}\\
&= A^{-1}(\mathrm{I}_{p\times p})^\top && \text{identity matrix is square and symmetric}\\
&= A^{-1}(A^{-1}A)^\top \\
& && A \text{ invertible by assumption; Definition B.2.5}\\
&= A^{-1}A^\top(A^{-1})^\top \\
& && (A^{-1}A)^\top = A^\top(A^{-1})^\top \text{ according to 3. in Lemma B.2.1}\\
&= A^{-1}A(A^{-1})^\top \\
& && A \text{ symmetric by assumption; Definition B.2.1}\\
&= \mathrm{I}_{p\times p}(A^{-1})^\top && A \text{ invertible; Definition B.2.5}\\
&= (A^{-1})^\top\,, && \text{property of identity matrix}
\end{aligned}$$

as desired.

3. follows from 1. and 3. in Lemma B.2.3:

$$\det[A]\det[A^{-1}] = \det[AA^{-1}] = \det[\mathrm{I}_{p\times p}] = 1\,.$$

Indeed, this equality implies that neither factor on the right-hand side can be zero and the desired equality then follows by dividing through $\det[A] \neq 0$. □

Trace of Matrices

The trace function enables concise formulations of maximum (regularized) likelihood estimators for Gaussian graphical models in ▶ Sect. 3.3. In mathematics more broadly, the trace function is used, for example, in generalizing the standard inner product from vectors to matrices.

Definition B.2.6

Trace of Matrices The *trace function* trace : $\mathbb{R}^{p\times p} \to \mathbb{R}$ is defined as

$$\text{trace} \; : \; A \mapsto \sum_{i=1}^{p} A_{ii} \, .$$

matrix trace

Hence, the trace sums the elements of the diagonal of a matrix. The trace of the identity matrix $\mathrm{I}_{p\times p}$ is the ambient dimension: $\text{trace}[\mathrm{I}_{p\times p}] = p$. The trace of a scalar $A = a \in \mathbb{R}^{1\times 1}$ is the scalar itself: $\text{trace}[A] = a$. The latter implies in particular that $\langle \boldsymbol{a}, \, \boldsymbol{b}\rangle = \text{trace}[\boldsymbol{a}^\top \boldsymbol{b}]$ for $\boldsymbol{a}, \boldsymbol{b} \in \mathbb{R}^p$, which motivates generalizing the inner product from vectors to matrices through $\langle A, \, B\rangle := \text{trace}[A^\top B]$ for $A, B \in \mathbb{R}^{n\times p}$.

Important for us are the following properties of the trace:

Lemma B.2.7

Linearity and Symmetry of the Trace Function The trace function is linear in the following sense: for all $A, B \in \mathbb{R}^{p\times p}$ and $c \in \mathbb{R}$, it holds that

$$\text{trace}[cA] = c\,\text{trace}[A] \quad \text{and}$$

$$\text{trace}[A + B] = \text{trace}[A] + \text{trace}[B] \, .$$

The trace function is also symmetric in the following sense: for all $A \in \mathbb{R}^{n\times p}$ and $B \in \mathbb{R}^{p\times n}$, it holds that

$$\text{trace}[AB] = \text{trace}[BA] \, .$$

Proof The proof consists of three short calculations.
The linearity follows from

$$\begin{aligned}
\text{trace}[cA] &= \sum_{i=1}^{p} (cA)_{ii} && \text{Definition B.2.6 of the trace} \\
&= \sum_{i=1}^{p} cA_{ii} \\
& && \text{definition of scalar–matrix multiplication} \\
&= c \sum_{i=1}^{p} A_{ii} && \text{linearity of the sum} \\
&= c\,\text{trace}[A] && \text{Definition B.2.6 of the trace}
\end{aligned}$$

and

$$\begin{aligned}
\text{trace}[A+B] &= \sum_{i=1}^{p} (A+B)_{ii} \\
& && \text{Definition B.2.6 of the trace} \\
&= \sum_{i=1}^{p} (A_{ii} + B_{ii}) \\
& && \text{definition of matrix–matrix addition} \\
&= \sum_{i=1}^{p} A_{ii} + \sum_{i=1}^{p} B_{ii} && \text{linearity of the sum} \\
&= \text{trace}[A] + \text{trace}[B]\,. \\
& && \text{Definition B.2.6 of the trace}
\end{aligned}$$

The symmetry follows from

$$\begin{aligned}
\text{trace}[AB] &= \sum_{i=1}^{n} (AB)_{ii} && \text{Definition B.2.6 of the trace} \\
&= \sum_{i=1}^{n} \sum_{j=1}^{p} A_{ij} B_{ji} \\
& && \text{definition of matrix–matrix multiplication} \\
&= \sum_{j=1}^{p} \sum_{i=1}^{n} B_{ji} A_{ij} && \text{rewriting the sum}
\end{aligned}$$

$$= \sum_{j=1}^{p} (BA)_{jj}$$

definition of matrix–matrix multiplication

$$= \operatorname{trace}[BA]\,.$$ Definition B.2.6 of the trace

□

Eigenvectors and Eigenvalues of Matrices

The matrices we consider in graphical modeling are all symmetric and positive definite. It turns out that for every such matrix, there is an orthogonal basis of special vectors on which the matrix has the effect of a scalar multiplication. We call these vectors eigenvectors.

> **Definition B.2.7**
>
> **Eigenvectors and Eigenvalues of Matrices** A vector $\boldsymbol{q} \in \mathbb{R}^p \setminus \{\boldsymbol{0}_p\}$ with $A\boldsymbol{q} = m\boldsymbol{q}$ for a square matrix $A \in \mathbb{R}^{p \times p}$ and a number $m \in \mathbb{R}$ is called an *eigenvector* of A. The number m is then called the corresponding *eigenvalue* of A.

eigenvector/eigenvalue of a matrix

The eigenvectors are those vectors for which the matrix operation is a multiplication with a scalar. The eigenvalue determines if this scalar multiplication stretches ($|m| > 1$), shortens ($|m| < 1$), or keeps the vector's length ($|m| = 1$) and if it flips ($\text{sign}[m] = -1$) or retains ($\text{sign}[m] = 1$) the vector's direction.

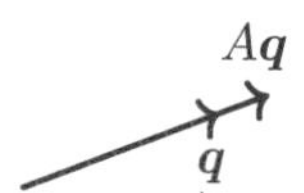

$\boldsymbol{q}$ is an eigenvector of A with eigenvalue $m > 1$

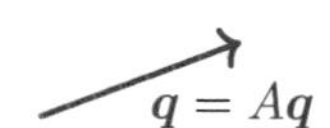

$\boldsymbol{q}$ is an eigenvector of A with eigenvalue $m = 1$

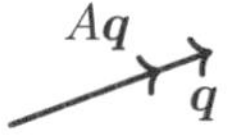

$\boldsymbol{q}$ is an eigenvector of A with eigenvalue $0 < m < 1$

Aq q

$\boldsymbol{q}$ is an eigenvector of A with eigenvalue $m = 0$

Aq q

$\boldsymbol{q}$ is an eigenvector of A with eigenvalue $m < 0$

Aq q

$\boldsymbol{q}$ is not an eigenvector of A

Eigenvectors and eigenvalues are also useful in physics, for example. Let $\boldsymbol{b}[t] \in \mathbb{R}^p$ characterize the state of a physical system at time t and $A \in \mathbb{R}^{p\times p}$ how the system evolves with time:

$$\frac{\partial}{\partial t}\boldsymbol{b}[t] = A\boldsymbol{b}[t] .$$

We speak of a *linear dynamical system.* If A has an eigenvector $\boldsymbol{q} \in \mathbb{R}^p$ with eigenvalue $m \in \mathbb{R}$, one can verify readily that a solution of the system is

$$\boldsymbol{b}[t] = e^{mt}\boldsymbol{q} .$$

This solution remains bounded if and only if $m \leq 1$; we then speak of a stable system. Thus, eigenvectors and eigenvalues can tell us something about a system's stability.

Important for us is that symmetric matrices admit an orthonormal basis of eigenvectors. To show this, we first define the concept of orthogonality.

orthogonal matrix

Definition B.2.8

Orthogonal Matrices An invertible matrix $A \in \mathbb{R}^{p\times p}$ that satisfies $A^{-1} = A^\top$ is called *orthogonal.*

Consider a matrix $A \in \mathbb{R}^{p\times p}$ with columns $\boldsymbol{a}_1, \ldots, \boldsymbol{a}_p \in \mathbb{R}^p$, that is, $A = (\boldsymbol{a}_1, \ldots, \boldsymbol{a}_p)$. As in ▶ Sect. 2.1, one can show readily that $(A^\top A)_{ij} = \langle \boldsymbol{a}_i, \boldsymbol{a}_j\rangle$. For orthogonal matrices, this becomes $(A^{-1}A)_{ij} = \langle \boldsymbol{a}_i, \boldsymbol{a}_j\rangle$, which means in view of Definition B.2.5 of matrix inverses that $\langle \boldsymbol{a}_i, \boldsymbol{a}_j\rangle = \|\boldsymbol{a}_i\|_2^2 = 1$ for $i = j$ and $\langle \boldsymbol{a}_i, \boldsymbol{a}_j\rangle = 0$ for $i \neq j$ and, therefore, that $\boldsymbol{a}_1, \ldots, \boldsymbol{a}_p$ is an orthonormal basis of $\mathbb{R}^p$. You can check that the reverse statement is also true: if $\boldsymbol{a}_1, \ldots, \boldsymbol{a}_p \in \mathbb{R}^p$ is an orthonormal basis of $\mathbb{R}^p$, then $A = (\boldsymbol{a}_1, \ldots, \boldsymbol{a}_p) \in \mathbb{R}^p$ is orthogonal. We conclude that orthogonal matrices are those matrices whose columns form an orthonormal basis of the ambient space.

The orthonormality of the columns ensures in particular that the parallelepiped spanned by these columns has volume one. In the language of determinants:

Lemma B.2.8

Determinant of Orthogonal Matrices The determinant of an orthogonal matrix $A \in \mathbb{R}^{p \times p}$ is either one or minus one: $|\det[A]| = 1$.

A proof follows readily from Lemma B.2.6 on determinants; we leave the details as an exercise. The reverse statement is not true: see again the illustrations on Page 320 for the determinant.

We can now state the main result.

Lemma B.2.9

spectral decomposition

Spectral Decomposition For each symmetric square matrix $A \in \mathbb{R}^{p \times p}$, there are eigenvectors $\boldsymbol{q}_1, \ldots, \boldsymbol{q}_p \in \mathbb{R}^p$ with eigenvalues $m_1, \ldots, m_p \in \mathbb{R}$ such that $\langle \boldsymbol{q}_i, \boldsymbol{q}_j \rangle = 0$ for all $i, j \in \{1, \ldots, p\}$, $i \neq j$, and $\|\boldsymbol{q}_i\|_2 = 1$ for all $i \in \{1, \ldots, p\}$, and we can write

$$A = QDQ^\top,$$

where $Q = (\boldsymbol{q}_1, \ldots, \boldsymbol{q}_p) \in \mathbb{R}^{p \times p}$ is orthogonal ($Q^\top = Q^{-1}$) and $D \in \mathbb{R}^{p \times p}$ is diagonal ($D_{ij} = 0$ for $i \neq j$) with diagonal entries $D_{ii} = m_i$ for $i \in \{1, \ldots, p\}$. We call this factorization of symmetric matrices *spectral decomposition* or *eigendecomposition*.

We omit the proof. The lemma says that each symmetric matrix has eigenvectors that form an orthonormal basis of the ambient space, and therefore, each symmetric matrix is a concatenation of a change of basis, a stretching along the new basis vectors, and a change back to the original basis.

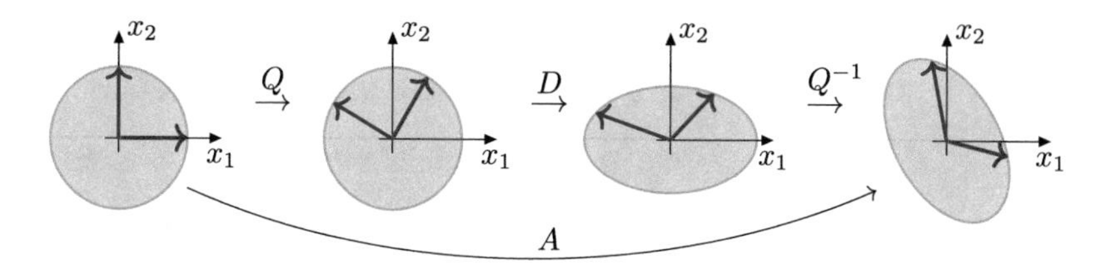

We also find the following lemma:

Lemma B.2.10

Eigenvalues of Positive (Semi-)Definite Matrices The eigenvalues of a positive semi-definite matrix are non-negative. The eigenvalues of a positive definite matrix are strictly positive.

Combined with the lemma above, we find that matrices that are symmetric and positive semi-definite have eigenvectors, each one with a non-negative eigenvalue, that form an orthonormal basis of the $\mathbb{R}^p$. This observation allows us in particular to define square-roots of symmetric, positive semi-definite matrices:

Corollary B.2.1

Square-Roots of Symmetric and Positive (Semi-)Definite Matrices Consider a symmetric and positive semi-definite matrix $A \in \mathbb{R}^{p\times p}$ with spectral decomposition $A = QDQ^\top$. Define $A^{\frac{1}{2}} \in \mathbb{R}^{p\times p}$ as $A^{\frac{1}{2}} := QD^{\frac{1}{2}}Q^\top$ with $(D^{\frac{1}{2}})_{ij} := \sqrt{D_{ij}}$. Then, $A^{\frac{1}{2}}$ is symmetric (use 3. in Lemma B.2.1 and the fact that $D^{\frac{1}{2}}$ is a square diagonal matrix) and $A = A^{\frac{1}{2}}A^{\frac{1}{2}}$ (use the fact that $Q^\top = Q^{-1}$). Further, if A is invertible, then also $A^{\frac{1}{2}}$ is invertible, and its inverse is $A^{-\frac{1}{2}} = QD^{-\frac{1}{2}}Q^\top$ with $(D^{-\frac{1}{2}})_{ij} := 1/\sqrt{D_{ij}}$ for $i = j$ and $(D^{-\frac{1}{2}})_{ij} := 0$ otherwise.

Proof of Lemma B.2.10 Let $A \in \mathbb{R}^{p\times p}$ be a positive semi-definite matrix and $\boldsymbol{q} \in \mathbb{R}^p \setminus \{\boldsymbol{0}_p\}, m \in \mathbb{R}$ an eigenvector/eigenvalue pair: $A\boldsymbol{q} = m\boldsymbol{q}$. On the one hand, because A is positive semi-definite, Lemma B.2.3 implies that $\boldsymbol{q}^\top A\boldsymbol{q} \geq 0$. On the other hand,

$$
\begin{aligned}
\boldsymbol{q}^\top A\boldsymbol{q} &= \boldsymbol{q}^\top(m\boldsymbol{q}) && \boldsymbol{q}, m \text{ is an eigenvector/eigenvalue pair to } A \\
&= m\boldsymbol{q}^\top\boldsymbol{q} && \text{linearity of matrix–matrix multiplication} \\
&= m\|\boldsymbol{q}\|_2^2\,. && \text{definition of the } \ell_2\text{-norm}
\end{aligned}
$$

Combining the two insights and noting that $\|\boldsymbol{q}\|_2^2 > 0$ for $\boldsymbol{q} \neq \boldsymbol{0}_p$ by the positive definiteness of norms, we find that $m \geq 0$.

The second statement can be proved in a very similar way. □

Singular Value Decomposition

We now review the singular value decomposition, which is used for computing the prediction errors in ▸ Sect. 1.2 and Exercise 1.2, for example. The singular value decomposition roughly says that every matrix can be factorized into three parts: a change of basis, a scaling of the axes in this coordinate system, and another change of basis. Hence, the singular value decomposition generalizes the spectral decomposition above.

The general idea is as now follows: Consider the absolute value of the diagonal matrix in Lemma B.2.9, that is, define a diagonal matrix $S \in \mathbb{R}^{p\times p}$ through $S_{ij} := |D_{ij}|$. Verify then that the matrix $U \in \mathbb{R}^{p\times p}$ defined through $U_{ij} := \text{sign}[D_{jj}]Q_{ij}$ is orthogonal (cf. the discussion after Definition B.2.8) and that $US = QD$. Verify similarly that the matrix $V := Q$ is also orthogonal, which implies that $V^\top = Q^{-1}$. We can then write the spectral decomposition for symmetric matrices in Lemma B.2.9 as

$$A = USV^\top .$$

The main difference from the earlier formulation is that the diagonal matrix S here contains the eigenvalues in absolute value. Or stated differently, the diagonal matrix here contains the non-negative square-roots of the eigenvalues of $A^\top A = AA$. The key observation is now that $A^\top A$ is always a square symmetric matrix—irrespective of what the base matrix A is—which makes it possible to generalize the decomposition to arbitrary matrices.

singular value decomposition

Lemma B.2.11

Singular Value Decomposition We can write every matrix $A \in \mathbb{R}^{n \times p}$ as

$$A = USV^\top$$

with $U \in \mathbb{R}^{n \times n}$ and $V \in \mathbb{R}^{p \times p}$ orthogonal (that is, $U^{-1} = U^\top$ and $V^{-1} = V^\top$) and $S \in \mathbb{R}^{n \times p}$ diagonal (that is, $S_{ij} = 0$ if $i \neq j$). We call such a factorization a *singular value decomposition* of A. The diagonal entries of S are the non-negative square-roots of the eigenvalues of $A^\top A$. We call these entries the *singular values* of A. The number of non-zero elements in the diagonal matrix, which equals the maximal number of linearly independent columns of A and also equals the maximal number of independent rows of A, is called the *rank* of A.

singular value

rank of a matrix

We omit the proof. The singular value decomposition generalizes the spectral decomposition as written above from symmetric to arbitrary matrices. The difference in the factorizations is that the two orthogonal matrices U, V here might be completely unrelated; in particular, they do not even need to have the same dimensions.

Specific Results for Gaussian Graphical Models

We finally use the above concepts to derive specific results needed in ▶ Sect. 3.4 on neighborhood selection.

We first give an alternative formulation of determinants. This version is used to differentiate the log-determinant function: see Exercise 3.3.

Definition B.2.9

Cofactor Matrices The *cofactor matrix* $C \equiv C[A] \in \mathbb{R}^{p\times p}$ for a matrix $A \in \mathbb{R}^{p\times p}$ is defined through $C_{ij} := (-1)^{i+j} m_{ij}$ for $i,j \in \{1,\ldots,p\}$, where $m_{ij} := \det[A_{\{i\}^\complement\{j\}^\complement}]$ is the determinant of the $((p-1)\times(p-1))$-matrix that results from deleting the ith row and the jth column of A.

cofactor matrix

Lemma B.2.12

Properties of Cofactor Matrices Let $A \in \mathbb{R}^{p\times p}$ be a square matrix and C its cofactor matrix according to Definition B.2.9. Then, (i) the values of $C_{1j},\ldots,C_{pj}$ do not depend on A_{ij}, and (ii) $A^{-1} = C^\top/\det[A]$.

Claim (i) follows readily from the definition of the cofactors; Claim (ii) should be contrasted with *Cramer's rule*—we omit the details.

Lemma B.2.13

Laplace Expansion of Determinants Let $A \in \mathbb{R}^{p\times p}$ be a square matrix and C its cofactor matrix according to Definition B.2.9. Then,

Laplace expansion

$$\det[A] = \sum_{k=1}^{p} C_{kj}A_{kj} = \sum_{k=1}^{p} C_{ik}A_{ik}\,,$$

for all $i,j \in \{1,\ldots,p\}$. This identity is called the *Laplace expansion* of the determinant.

These formulas expand the determinant along the rows/-columns of the matrix. We omit the proof.

Now, we relate special block matrices to their submatrices. We will need these results for proving that Gaussian graphical models are amenable to neighborhood selection: see ► Sect. 3.4.

Lemma B.2.14

Determinant of Special Block Matrices For every square matrix $A \in \mathbb{R}^{(p+q)\times(p+q)}$ of the form

$$A = \begin{pmatrix} \mathrm{I}_{p\times p} & B \\ \mathbf{0}_{q\times p} & C \end{pmatrix}$$

with $B \in \mathbb{R}^{p\times q}$ and $C \in \mathbb{R}^{q\times q}$, it holds that $\det[A] = \det[C]$.

Similarly, for every square matrix $A \in \mathbb{R}^{(q+p)\times(q+p)}$ of the form

$$A = \begin{pmatrix} C & B \\ \mathbf{0}_{q\times p} & \mathrm{I}_{q\times q} \end{pmatrix}$$

with $B \in \mathbb{R}^{p\times q}$ and $C \in \mathbb{R}^{p\times p}$, it holds that $\det[A] = \det[C]$.

Proof of Lemma B.2.14 We apply the Leibniz formula of Definition B.2.4 to matrices that have the described shape.

For our case of $((p+q)\times(p+q))$-matrices, the Leibniz formula is

$$\det[A] = \sum_{m\in\mathscr{M}^{p+q}} \left(\mathrm{sign}[m]\prod_{i=1}^{p+q} A_{im[i]}\right),$$

where $\mathscr{M}^{p+q}$ is the set of permutations of $\{1,\ldots,p+q\}$.

To prove the first claim, we first use the fact that $\det[A^\top] = \det[A]$ by 2. in Lemma B.2.3. Hence, we consider the matrix

$$A^\top = \begin{pmatrix} \mathrm{I}_{p\times p} & \mathbf{0}_{p\times q} \\ B^\top & C^\top \end{pmatrix}.$$

The upper part of matrix consists of an identity matrix and all zeros otherwise; therefore, it holds for all $i \in \{1,\ldots,p\}$ that $A^\top_{im[i]} = 1$ if $m[i] = i$ and $A^\top_{im[i]} = 0$ otherwise. Hence, the sum in the above equality can be restricted to permutations that keep the first p indexes unchanged, or stated differently, it is sufficient to consider permutations of the last q indexes:

$$\det[A^\top] = \sum_{m \in \mathscr{M}^q} \left(\operatorname{sign}[m] \prod_{j=1}^{p} A_{jj}^\top \prod_{i=1}^{q} A_{(p+i)(p+m[i])}^\top \right),$$

where $\mathscr{M}^q$ is the set of permutations of $\{1, \ldots, q\}$.

Recall now that $A_{jj}^\top = (\mathrm{I}_{p\times p})_{jj} = 1$ and $A_{(p+i)(p+m[i])}^\top = C_{im[i]}^\top$. Plugging this into the above equality gives

$$\det[A^\top] = \sum_{m \in \mathscr{M}^q} \left(\operatorname{sign}[m] \prod_{i=1}^{q} C_{im[i]}^\top \right).$$

In view of Definition B.2.4, the right-hand side of this identity is equal to $\det[C^\top]$, so that we can conclude that $\det[A] = \det[C]$ (using again 2. in Lemma B.2.3), as desired.

The second claim can be proved along the same lines. □

Lemma B.2.15

Submatrices of Inverse Matrices Consider a symmetric and positive matrix $M \in \mathbb{R}^{(p+q)\times(p+q)}$ of the form

$$M = \begin{pmatrix} A & B \\ B^\top & C \end{pmatrix}$$

with $A \in \mathbb{R}^{p\times p}, B \in \mathbb{R}^{p\times q}, C \in \mathbb{R}^{q\times q}$. We write its inverse M^{-1} (which exists and is also positive definite by 1. and 2. in Lemma B.2.5 and symmetric by 2. in Lemma B.2.6) in the form

$$M^{-1} = \begin{pmatrix} \widetilde{A} & \widetilde{B} \\ \widetilde{B}^\top & \widetilde{C} \end{pmatrix}$$

with $\widetilde{A} \in \mathbb{R}^{p\times p}, \widetilde{B} \in \mathbb{R}^{p\times q}, \widetilde{C} \in \mathbb{R}^{q\times q}$. It then holds that

$$\text{(i) } C^{-1} = \widetilde{C} - \widetilde{B}^\top \widetilde{A}^{-1} \widetilde{B} \quad \text{and} \quad \text{(ii) } \frac{\det[C]}{\det[M]} = \frac{1}{\det[\widetilde{A}^{-1}]}.$$

The theorem relates submatrices of a matrix with the submatrices of the inverse matrix. We use these relationships in Lemma 3.4.1 with $M = \Sigma$ to connect the coordinates of Gauss-distributed vectors through linear regressions. These linear regressions are the basis of neighborhood selection in ► Sect. 3.4.

Proof of Lemma B.2.15 We can base the proof on the above insights on matrix algebra.

For proving (i), we first calculate

$$MM^{-1} = \begin{pmatrix} A & B \\ B^\top & C \end{pmatrix} \begin{pmatrix} \widetilde{A} & \widetilde{B} \\ \widetilde{B}^\top & \widetilde{C} \end{pmatrix} = \begin{pmatrix} A\widetilde{A} + B\widetilde{B}^\top & A\widetilde{B} + B\widetilde{C} \\ B^\top\widetilde{A} + C\widetilde{B}^\top & B^\top\widetilde{B} + C\widetilde{C} \end{pmatrix}.$$

Since $MM^{-1} = \mathrm{I}_{(p+q)\times(p+q)}$ by Definition B.2.5 of matrix inverses, the matrix equality yields in particular

$$B^\top\widetilde{A} + C\widetilde{B}^\top = \mathbf{0}_{q\times p} \quad \text{and} \quad B^\top\widetilde{B} + C\widetilde{C} = \mathrm{I}_{q\times q}\,.$$

Since $\widetilde{A}$ and C are square submatrices on the diagonal of M^{-1} and M, respectively, they are also invertible according to Lemmas B.2.2 and B.2.5. We can, therefore, multiply the first equation by $\widetilde{A}^{-1}$ from the right and the second equation by C^{-1} from the left to find

$$\begin{aligned} B^\top\widetilde{A}\widetilde{A}^{-1} + C\widetilde{B}^\top\widetilde{A}^{-1} &= \mathbf{0}_{q\times p}\widetilde{A}^{-1} \quad \text{and} \\ C^{-1}B^\top\widetilde{B} + C^{-1}C\widetilde{C} &= C^{-1}\,\mathrm{I}_{q\times q}\,. \end{aligned}$$

Using the properties of matrix–matrix multiplications and the fact that $\widetilde{A}\widetilde{A}^{-1} = \mathrm{I}_{p\times p}$ and $C^{-1}C = \mathrm{I}_{q\times q}$ by Definition B.2.5 of matrix inverses, this becomes

$$B^\top + C\widetilde{B}^\top\widetilde{A}^{-1} = \mathbf{0}_{q\times p} \quad \text{and} \quad C^{-1}B^\top\widetilde{B} + \widetilde{C} = C^{-1}\,.$$

We can rearrange the equalities then as

$$B^\top = -\,C\widetilde{B}^\top\widetilde{A}^{-1} \quad \text{and} \quad C^{-1} = \widetilde{C} + C^{-1}B^\top\widetilde{B}\,.$$

The rest is then a simple calculation:

$$\begin{aligned} C^{-1} &= \widetilde{C} + C^{-1}B^\top\widetilde{B} \quad \text{right-hand side of the previous display} \\ &= \widetilde{C} + C^{-1}(-C\widetilde{B}^\top\widetilde{A}^{-1})\widetilde{B} \\ &\qquad \text{substituting } B^\top \text{ via the left-hand side of the previous display} \end{aligned}$$

$$= \widetilde{C} - \widetilde{B}^\top \widetilde{A}^{-1} \widetilde{B}\,,$$

$C^{-1}(-C) = -\mathrm{I}_{q\times q}$ by the linearity of matrix–matrix multiplications and Definition B.2.5

as desired.

For proving (ii), we first calculate

$$\begin{aligned}
\det[M^{-1}] &= \det\begin{pmatrix} \widetilde{A} & \widetilde{B} \\ \widetilde{B}^\top & \widetilde{C} \end{pmatrix} && \text{writing } M^{-1} \text{ as stated in the lemma}\\
&= \det\left[\begin{pmatrix} \widetilde{A} & \mathbf{0}_{p\times q} \\ \widetilde{B}^\top & \mathrm{I}_{q\times q} \end{pmatrix}\begin{pmatrix} \mathrm{I}_{p\times p} & \widetilde{A}^{-1}\widetilde{B} \\ \mathbf{0}_{q\times p} & \widetilde{C} - \widetilde{B}^\top \widetilde{A}^{-1} \widetilde{B} \end{pmatrix}\right]\\
&&& \text{separating the matrix into two factors}\\
&= \det\begin{pmatrix} \widetilde{A} & \mathbf{0}_{p\times q} \\ \widetilde{B}^\top & \mathrm{I}_{q\times q} \end{pmatrix}\det\begin{pmatrix} \mathrm{I}_{p\times p} & \widetilde{A}^{-1}\widetilde{B} \\ \mathbf{0}_{q\times p} & \widetilde{C} - \widetilde{B}^\top \widetilde{A}^{-1} \widetilde{B} \end{pmatrix}\\
&&& \text{using 1. in Lemma B.2.3}\\
&= \det\begin{pmatrix} \widetilde{A} & \widetilde{B} \\ \mathbf{0}_{p\times q} & \mathrm{I}_{q\times q} \end{pmatrix}\det\begin{pmatrix} \mathrm{I}_{p\times p} & \widetilde{A}^{-1}\widetilde{B} \\ \mathbf{0}_{q\times p} & \widetilde{C} - \widetilde{B}^\top \widetilde{A}^{-1} \widetilde{B} \end{pmatrix}\\
&&& \text{using 2. in Lemma B.2.3 for the first determinant}\\
&= \det[\widetilde{A}]\det[\widetilde{C} - \widetilde{B}^\top \widetilde{A}^{-1} \widetilde{B}]\\
&&& \text{using the second part of Lemma B.2.14 for the first term and the first part for the second terms}\\
&= \det[\widetilde{A}]\det[C^{-1}]\,. && \text{Claim (i)}
\end{aligned}$$

Hence, using again that $\widetilde{A}$ and C are invertible and then using the fact that the determinants of matrices and their inverses are reciprocal according to 3. in Lemma B.2.6, we find

$$\frac{1}{\det[M]} = \frac{1}{\det[\widetilde{A}^{-1}]\det[C]}\,,$$

which can be rearranged to

$$\frac{\det[C]}{\det[M]} = \frac{1}{\det[\widetilde{A}^{-1}]}\,,$$

as desired. □

We finally prove a statement in the main part of the book.

Lemma B.2.16

Parameters in Neighborhood Selection With the notation on Page 93, it holds that

$$\Theta_{ij} = -\frac{\Theta_{ii}(\underline{\boldsymbol{\beta}}^i)_j + \Theta_{jj}(\underline{\boldsymbol{\beta}}^j)_i}{2} \qquad \text{for all } i, j \in \{1, \ldots, d\}.$$

This equation expresses arbitrary elements of the precision matrix by diagonal elements and the regression vectors defined in Lemma 3.4.1. The equation is the motivation for the neighborhood selection estimator (3.6).

Proof of Lemma B.2.16 The proof is simple yet slightly tedious algebra.

Recall first that $\underline{\boldsymbol{\beta}}^j \in \mathbb{R}^d$ augments the $(d-1)$-dimensional regression vector $\boldsymbol{\beta}^j$ of Lemma 3.4.1 with a coordinate of value -1 that is inserted at the jth position (see Page 93). Recall also that the precision matrix $\Theta \in \mathbb{R}^{d \times d}$ is symmetric and positive definite (see Page 86) and, therefore, (i) has strictly positive diagonal elements (see 3. in Lemma B.2.5) and (ii) is symmetric (see 2. in Lemma B.2.6).

We now derive for all $i, j \in \{1, \ldots, d\}$

$$\boldsymbol{\beta}^j = -(\Theta_{j\{j\}^\complement})^\top / \Theta_{jj} \qquad \text{by definition in Lemma 3.4.1}$$

$$\Rightarrow \quad (\Theta_{j\{j\}^\complement})^\top = -\Theta_{jj}\boldsymbol{\beta}^j$$

rearranging; note that $\Theta_{jj} > 0$ by (i)

$$\Rightarrow \quad \begin{pmatrix} \Theta_{j1} \\ \vdots \\ \Theta_{j(j-1)} \\ \Theta_{j(j+1)} \\ \vdots \\ \Theta_{jd} \end{pmatrix} = -\Theta_{jj} \begin{pmatrix} (\boldsymbol{\beta}^j)_1 \\ \vdots \\ (\boldsymbol{\beta}^j)_{j-1} \\ (\boldsymbol{\beta}^j)_j \\ \vdots \\ (\boldsymbol{\beta}^j)_{d-1} \end{pmatrix}$$

writing the previous equation more explicitly

$$\Rightarrow \quad \begin{pmatrix} \Theta_{j1} \\ \vdots \\ \Theta_{j(j-1)} \\ \Theta_{j(j+1)} \\ \vdots \\ \Theta_{jd} \end{pmatrix} = -\Theta_{jj} \begin{pmatrix} (\underline{\boldsymbol{\beta}}^j)_1 \\ \vdots \\ (\underline{\boldsymbol{\beta}}^j)_{j-1} \\ (\underline{\boldsymbol{\beta}}^j)_{j+1} \\ \vdots \\ (\underline{\boldsymbol{\beta}}^j)_d \end{pmatrix}$$

definition of the augmented vector $\underline{\boldsymbol{\beta}}^j$

$$\Rightarrow \quad \begin{pmatrix} \Theta_{j1} \\ \vdots \\ \Theta_{j(j-1)} \\ \Theta_{jj} \\ \Theta_{j(j+1)} \\ \vdots \\ \Theta_{jd} \end{pmatrix} = -\Theta_{jj} \begin{pmatrix} (\underline{\boldsymbol{\beta}}^j)_1 \\ \vdots \\ (\underline{\boldsymbol{\beta}}^j)_{j-1} \\ (\underline{\boldsymbol{\beta}}^j)_j \\ (\underline{\boldsymbol{\beta}}^j)_{j+1} \\ \vdots \\ (\underline{\boldsymbol{\beta}}^j)_d \end{pmatrix}$$

$(\underline{\boldsymbol{\beta}}^j)_j = -1$ by definition

$$\Rightarrow \quad \Theta_{ji} = -\Theta_{jj}(\underline{\boldsymbol{\beta}}^j)_i \,.$$

taking the ith coordinate on either side

Similarly, $\Theta_{ij} = -\Theta_{ii}(\underline{\boldsymbol{\beta}}^i)_j$. Moreover, since Θ is symmetric by (ii), it holds that $\Theta_{ij} = \Theta_{ji}$. In summary,

$$\Theta_{ij} = -\frac{\Theta_{ii}(\underline{\boldsymbol{\beta}}^i)_j + \Theta_{jj}(\underline{\boldsymbol{\beta}}^j)_i}{2},$$

as desired. □

Bibliography

Aitchison, J. (1982). The statistical analysis of compositional data. *Journal of the Royal Statistical Society, Series B: Statistical Methodology, 44*(2), 139–160.

Albert, A. (1972). *Regression and the Moore–Penrose pseudoinverse*. Elsevier.

Almal, S., & Padh, H. (2012). Implications of gene copy-number variation in health and diseases. *Journal of Human Genetics, 57*(1), 6.

Anscombe, F. (1948). The transformation of Poisson, binomial and negative-binomial data. *Biometrika, 35*(3/4), 246–254.

Antoniadis, A. (2010). Comments on: ℓ_1-penalization for mixture regression models. *Test, 19*, 257–258.

Arlot, S., & Celisse, A. (2010). A survey of cross-validation procedures for model selection. *Statistics Surveys, 4*, 40–79.

Bakin, S. (1999). Adaptive regression and model selection in data mining problems, PhD thesis, The Australian National University, Canberra.

Banerjee, O., El Ghaoui, L., & d'Aspremont, A. (2008). Model selection through sparse maximum likelihood estimation for multivariate Gaussian or binary data. *Journal of Machine Learning Research, 9*, 485–516.

Bellec, P., & Tsybakov, A. (2017). Bounds on the prediction error of penalized least squares estimators with convex penalty. *Modern Problems of Stochastic Analysis and Statistics, 208*, 315–333.

Belloni, A., & Chernozhukov, V. (2013). Least squares after model selection in high-dimensional sparse models. *Bernoulli, 19*(2), 521–547.

Belloni, A., Chernozhukov, V., & Wang, L. (2011). Square-root lasso: Pivotal recovery of sparse signals via conic programming. *Biometrika, 98*(4), 791–806.

Besag, J. (1974). Spatial interaction and the statistical analysis of lattice systems. *Journal of the Royal Statistical Society, Series B: Statistical Methodology, 36*(2), 192–236.

Bickel, P., Klaassen, C., Ritov, Y., & Wellner, J. (1993). *Efficient and adaptive estimation for semiparametric models*. Johns Hopkins University Press.

Bickel, P., Ritov, Y., & Tsybakov, A. (2009). Simultaneous analysis of lasso and Dantzig selector. *The Annals of Statistics, 37*(4), 1705–1732.

Bien, J., Gaynanova, I., Lederer, J., & Müller, C. (2018a). Non-convex global minimization and false discovery rate control for the TREX. *Journal of Computational and Graphical Statistics, 27*(1), 23–33.

Bien, J., Gaynanova, I., Lederer, J., & Müller, C. (2018b). Prediction error bounds for linear regression with the TREX. *Test, 28*(2), 451–474.

Bien, J., & Wegkamp, M. (2013). Discussion of: Correlated variables in regression: Clustering and sparse estimation. *Journal of Statistical Planning and Inference, 143*(11), 1859–1862.

Borgelt, C., & Kruse, R. (2002). *Graphical models: Methods for data analysis and mining*. Wiley.

Boucheron, S., Lugosi, G., & Massart, P. (2013), *Concentration inequalities: A nonasymptotic theory of independence*. Oxford University Press.

Boyd, S., & Vandenberghe, L. (2004). *Convex optimization*. Cambridge University Press.

Bu, Y., & Lederer, J. (2017). Integrating additional knowledge into estimation of graphical models. arXiv:1704.02739.

Bunea, F., Lederer, J., & She, Y. (2014). The group square-root lasso: Theoretical properties and fast algorithms. *IEEE Transactions on Information Theory, 60*(2), 1313–1325.

Cai, T., Liu, W., & Luo, X. (2011). A constrained ℓ_1 minimization approach to sparse precision matrix estimation. *Journal of the American Statistical Association, 106*(494), 594–607.

Celisse, A. (2008), Model selection via cross-validation in density estimation, regression, and change-points detection, PhD thesis, Université Paris Sud-Paris XI.

Chatterjee, S., & Jafarov, J. (2015). Prediction error of cross-validated lasso. arXiv:1502.06291.

Chételat, D., Lederer, J., & Salmon, J. (2017). Optimal two-step prediction in regression. *Electronic Journal of Statistics, 11*(1), 2519–2546.

Chichignoud, M., Lederer, J., & Wainwright, M. (2016). A practical scheme and fast algorithm to tune the lasso with optimality guarantees. *Journal of Machine Learning Research, 17*(1), 1–20.

Dalalyan, A., Hebiri, M., & Lederer, J. (2017). On the prediction performance of the lasso. *Bernoulli, 23*(1), 552–581.

Dettling, M., & Bühlmann, P. (2004). Finding predictive gene groups from microarray data. *Journal of Multivariate Analysis, 90*(1), 106–131.

Diesner, J., & Carley, K. (2005). Exploration of communication networks from the Enron email corpus. In *SIAM International Conference on Data Mining* (pp. 3–14).

Dobra, A., Hans, C., Jones, B., Nevins, J., Yao, G., & West, M. (2004). Sparse graphical models for exploring gene expression data. *Journal of Multivariate Analysis, 90*(1), 196–212.

Dudley, R. (2002), *Real analysis and probability* (Vol. 74). Cambridge University Press.

Durrett, R. (2010), *Probability: Theory and examples* (4th ed.). Cambridge University Press.

Edwards, D. (2012), *Introduction to graphical modelling*. Springer.

Efron, B., Hastie, T., Johnstone, I., & Tibshirani, R. (2004). Least angle regression. *Annals of Statistics, 32*(2), 407–499.

Engl, H., Hanke, M., & Neubauer, A. (1996). *Regularization of inverse problems* (Vol. 375). Springer.

Fan, J., & Li, R. (2001). Variable selection via nonconcave penalized likelihood and its oracle properties. *Journal of the American Statistical Association, 96*(456), 1348–1360.

Frank, I., & Friedman, J. (1993). A statistical view of some chemometrics regression tools. *Technometrics, 35*(2), 109–135.

Friedman, J., Hastie, T., & Tibshirani, R. (2008). Sparse inverse covariance estimation with the graphical lasso. *Biostatistics, 9*(3), 432–441.

Fultz, N., Bonmassar, G., Setsompop, K., Stickgold, R., Rosen, B., Polimeni, J. , & Lewis, L. (2019). Coupled electrophysiological, hemodynamic, and cerebrospinal fluid oscillations in human sleep. *Science, 366*(6465), 628–631.

Gallavotti, G. (2013), *Statistical mechanics: A short treatise*. Springer.

Geisser, S. (1975). The predictive sample reuse method with applications. *Journal of the American Statistical Association, 70*(350), 320–328.

Gold, D., Lederer, J., & Tau, J. (2020). Inference for high-dimensional nested regression. *Journal of Econometrics, 217*(1), 79–111.

Golub, G., Heath, M., & Wahba, G. (1979). Generalized cross-validation as a method for choosing a good ridge parameter. *Technometrics, 21*(2), 215–223.

Greenshtein, E., & Ritov, Y. (2004). Persistence in high-dimensional linear predictor selection and the virtue of overparametrization. *Bernoulli, 10*(6), 971–988.

Grimmett, G. (1973). A theorem about random fields. *Bulletin of the London Mathematical Society, 5*(1), 81–84.

Hastie, T., Tibshirani, R., & Wainwright, M. (2015), *Statistical learning with sparsity: The lasso and generalizations*. Chapman and Hall.

Hebiri, M., & Lederer, J. (2013). How correlations influence lasso prediction. *IEEE Transactions on Information Theory, 59*(3), 1846–1854.

Hiriart-Urruty, J.-B., & Lemaréchal, C. (2004). *Convex analysis and minimization algorithms*. Springer.

Hoerl, A., & Kennard, R. (1970). Ridge regression: Biased estimation for nonorthogonal problems. *Technometrics, 12*(1), 55–67.

Homrighausen, D., & McDonald, D. (2013a). The lasso, persistence, and cross-validation. In *Proceedings of machine learning research* (Vol. 28, pp. 1031–1039).

Homrighausen, D., & McDonald, D. (2013b). Risk-consistency of cross-validation with lasso-type procedures. *Statistica Sinica, 27*(3), 1017–1036.

Homrighausen, D., & McDonald, D. (2014). Leave-one-out cross-validation is risk consistent for lasso. *Machine Learning, 97*(1–2), 65–78.

Huang, S.-T., Düren, Y., Hellton, K., & Lederer, J. (2019). Tuning parameter calibration for prediction in personalized medicine. arXiv:1909.10635.

Javanmard, A., & Montanari, A. (2014). Confidence intervals and hypothesis testing for high-dimensional regression. *Journal of Machine Learning Research, 15*(1), 2869–2909.

Judson, R., Salisbury, B., Schneider, J., Windemuth, A., & Stephens, J. (2002). How many SNPs does a genome-wide haplotype map require? *Pharmacogenomics, 3*(3), 379–391.

Karush, W. (1939), Minima of functions of several variables with inequalities as side constraints, aster's thesis, University of Chicago.

Kidd, J. et al. (2008). Mapping and sequencing of structural variation from eight human genomes. *Nature, 453*(7191), 56–64.

Kim, Y., Choi, H., & Oh, H.-S. (2008). Smoothly clipped absolute deviation on high dimensions. *Journal of the American Statistical Association, 103*(484), 1665–1673.

Knight, K., & Fu, W. (2000). Asymptotics for lasso-type estimators. *Annals of Statistics, 28*(5), 1356–1378.

Kuhn, H., & Tucker, A. (1951). Nonlinear programming. In *Proceedings of Second Berkeley Symposium* (pp. 481–492). University of California Press.

Kurtz, Z., Müller, C., Miraldi, E., Littman, D., Blaser, M., & Bonneau, R. (2015). Sparse and compositionally robust inference of microbial ecological networks. *PLoS Computational Biology, 11*(5), e1004226.

Laszkiewicz, M., Fischer, A., & Lederer, J. (2020). Thresholded adaptive validation: Tuning the graphical lasso for graph recovery. arXiv:2005.00466.

Lauritzen, S. (1996). *Graphical models*. Oxford University Press.

Lederer, J. (2013). Trust, but verify: Benefits and pitfalls of least-squares refitting in high dimensions. arXiv:1306.0113.

Lederer, J., & Müller, C. (2015). Don't fall for tuning parameters: Tuning-free variable selection in high dimensions with the TREX. In *AAAI Conference on Artificial Intelligence*.

Lederer, J., Yu, L., & Gaynanova, I. (2019). Oracle inequalities for high-dimensional prediction. *Bernoulli, 25*(2), 1225–1255.

Lepski, O., Mammen, E., & Spokoiny, V. (1997). Optimal spatial adaptation to inhomogeneous smoothness: An approach based on kernel estimates with variable bandwidth selectors. *Annals of Statistics, 25*(3), 929–947.

Lepskii, O. (1991). On a problem of adaptive estimation in Gaussian white noise. *Theory of Probability and its Applications, 35*(3), 454–466.

Li, W., & Lederer, J. (2019). Tuning parameter calibration for ℓ_1-regularized logistic regression. *Journal of Statistical Planning and Inference, 202*, 80–98.

Mazumder, R., & Hastie, T. (2012). The graphical lasso: New insights and alternatives. *Electronic Journal of Statistics, 6*, 2125–2149.

Meinshausen, N. (2007). Relaxed lasso. *Computational Statistics and Data Analysis, 52*(1), 374–393.

Meinshausen, N. (2013). Sign-constrained least squares estimation for high-dimensional regression. *Electronic Journal of Statistics, 7*, 1607–1631.

Meinshausen, N., & Bühlmann, P. (2006). High-dimensional graphs and variable selection with the lasso. *Annals of Statistics, 34*(1), 1436–1462.

Merriam-Webster.com (2019). Oracle. Retrieved November 11, 2019 from https://www.merriam-webster.com

Mills, R., Luttig, C., Larkins, C., Beauchamp, A., Tsui, C., Pittard, W., & Devine, S. (2006). An initial map of insertion and deletion (INDEL) variation in the human genome. *Genome Research, 16*(9), 1182–1190.

Negahban, S., Yu, B., Wainwright, M., & Ravikumar, P. (2012). A unified framework for high-dimensional analysis of M-estimators with decomposable regularizers. *Statistical Science, 27*(4), 538–557.

Obozinski, G., Jacob, L., & Vert, J.-P. (2011). Group lasso with overlaps: The latent group lasso approach. arXiv:1110.0413.

Osborne, M., Presnell, B., & Turlach, B. (2000). On the lasso and its dual. *Journal of Computational and Graphical Statistics, 9*(2), 319–337.

Oztoprak, F., Nocedal, J., Rennie, S., & Olsen, P. (2012), Newton-like methods for sparse inverse covariance estimation. In *Advances in neural information processing systems* (pp. 755–763).

Park, T., & Casella, G. (2008). The Bayesian lasso. *Journal of the American Statistical Association, 103*(482), 681–686.

Penrose, R. (1955). A generalized inverse for matrices. *Mathematical Proceedings of the Cambridge Philosophical Society, 51*(3), 406–413.

Perrone, V., Jenatton, R., Seeger, M., & Archambeau, C. (2018). Scalable hyperparameter transfer learning. In *Advances in neural information processing systems* (pp. 6845–6855).

Preston, C. (1973). Generalized Gibbs states and Markov random fields. *Advances in Applied Probability, 5*(2), 242–261.

Schneider, U., & Ewald, K. (2017). On the distribution, model selection properties and uniqueness of the lasso estimator in low and high dimensions. arXiv:1708.09608.

Sherman, S. (1973). Markov random fields and Gibbs random fields. *Israel Journal of Mathematics, 14*(1), 92–103.

Simon, N., Friedman, J., Hastie, T., & Tibshirani, R. (2013). A sparse-group lasso. *Journal of Computational and Graphical Statistics, 22*(2), 231–245.

Spirtes, P., Glymour, C., Scheines, R., Heckerman, D., Meek, C., Cooper, G. , & Richardson, T. (2000). *Causation, prediction, and search.* MIT Press.

Städler, N., Bühlmann, P., & van de Geer, S. (2010). ℓ_1-penalization for mixture regression models. *Test, 19*, 209–285.

Stock, J., & Trebbi, F. (2003). Retrospectives: Who invented instrumental variable regression? *Journal of Economic Perspectives, 17*(3), 177–194.

Stone, M. (1974). Cross-validatory choice and assessment of statistical predictions. *Journal of the Royal Statistical Society, Series B: Statistical Methodology, 36*(2), 111–133.

Sun, T., & Zhang, C.-H. (2010). Comments on: ℓ_1-penalization for mixture regression models. *Test, 19*, 270–275

Sun, T., & Zhang, C.-H. (2012). Scaled sparse linear regression. *Biometrika, 99*(4), 879–898.

Taheri, M., Lim, N., & Lederer, J. (2020). Efficient feature selection with large and high-dimensional data. arXiv:1609.07195.

Tibshirani, R. (1996). Regression shrinkage and selection via the lasso. *Journal of the Royal Statistical Society, Series B: Statistical Methodology, 58*(1), 267–288.

Tibshirani, R. (2013). The lasso problem and uniqueness. *Electronic Journal of Statistics, 7*, 1456–1490.

Tikhonov, A. (1943). On the stability of inverse problems. *Doklady Akademii Nauk SSSR, 39*(5), 195–198.

van de Geer, S. (2007), The deterministic lasso. In *JSM Proceedings*.

van de Geer, S., & Bühlmann, P. (2009). On the conditions used to prove oracle results for the lasso. *Electronic Journal of Statistics, 3*, 1360–1392.

van de Geer, S., & Bühlmann, P. (2011). *Statistics for high-dimensional data: Methods, theory and applications*. Springer.

van de Geer, S., Bühlmann, P., Ritov, Y., & Dezeure, R. (2014). On asymptotically optimal confidence regions and tests for high-dimensional models. *Annals of Statistics, 42*(3), 1166–1202.

van de Geer, S., & Lederer, J. (2013). The lasso, correlated design, and improved oracle inequalities. In *From probability to statistics and back: High-dimensional models and processes–a festschrift in honor of Jon A. Wellner', IMS* (pp. 303–316).

van der Vaart, A. (2000). *Asymptotic statistics* (Vol. 3). Cambridge University Press.

Wainwright, M. (2009). Sharp thresholds for high-dimensional and noisy sparsity recovery using ℓ_1-constrained quadratic programming (lasso). *IEEE Transactions on Information Theory, 55*(5), 2183–2202.

Wainwright, M. (2014). Structured regularizers for high-dimensional problems: Statistical and computational issues. *Annual Review of Statistics and Its Application, 1*, 233–253.

Yuan, M., & Lin, Y. (2006). Model selection and estimation in regression with grouped variables. *Journal of the Royal Statistical Society, Series B: Statistical Methodology, 68*(1), 49–67.

Yuan, M., & Lin, Y. (2007). Model selection and estimation in the Gaussian graphical model. *Biometrika, 94*(1), 19–35.

Zhang, C.-H. (2010). Nearly unbiased variable selection under minimax concave penalty. *The Annals of Statistics, 38*(2), 894–942.

Zhang, C.-H., & Zhang, T. (2012). A general theory of concave regularization for high-dimensional sparse estimation problems. *Statistical Science, 27*(4), 576–593.

Zhao, P., & Yu, B. (2006). On model selection consistency of lasso. *Journal of Machine Learning Research, 7*, 2541–2563.

Zou, H., & Hastie, T. (2005). Regularization and variable selection via the elastic net. *Journal of the Royal Statistical Society, Series B: Statistical Methodology, 67*(2), 301–320.

Zuber, J.-B., & Itzykson, C. (1977). Quantum field theory and the two-dimensional Ising model. *Physical Review D, 15*(10), 2875.

Index

D

E

F

I

J

K

L

M

R

S

T

U

V

W

Z

Printed in the United States
by Baker & Taylor Publisher Services